Preventive Aspects of Coronary Heart Disease

Books Available in Cardiovascular Clinics Series

Preventive Aspects of Coronary Heart Disease

Edward D. Frohlich, M.D. / Editor

Alton Ochsner Distinguished Scientist
Vice President for Academic Affairs
Alton Ochsner Medical Foundation
New Orleans, Louisiana

CARDIOVASCULAR CLINICS
Albert N. Brest, M.D. / Editor-in-Chief

James C. Wilson Professor of Medicine
Director, Division of Cardiology
Jefferson Medical College
Philadelphia, Pennsylvania

 F. A. DAVIS COMPANY ● Philadelphia

Printed in the United States of America

Last digit indicates print number: 10 9 8 7 6 5 4 3 2 1

Printed on acid-free paper effective with Volume 17, Number 1.

NOTE: As new scientific information becomes available through basic and clinical research, recommended treatments and drug therapies undergo changes. The author(s) and publisher have done everything possible to make this book accurate, up-to-date, and in accord with accepted standards at the time of publication. However, the reader is advised always to check product information (package inserts) for changes and new information regarding dose and contraindications before administering any drug. Caution is especially urged when using new or infrequently ordered drugs.

Library of Congress Cataloging in Publication Data

Cardiovascular clinics. 20/3

    Philadelphia, F. A. Davis, 1969–
      v. ill. 27 cm.
    Editor: v. 1– A. N. Brest
    Key title: Cardiovascular clinics, ISSN 0069-0384.
    1. Cardiovascular system—Diseases—Collected works. I. Brest, Albert N., ed.
    [DNLM: W1 CA77N]
RC681.A1C27   616.1   70-6558
ISBN 0-8036-3869-8   MARC-S

Preface

Identification of *factors of risk*, as originally termed by Kannel and his colleagues in the Framingham Study[1] has taught us much about the pathogenesis and natural history of coronary artery disease and the means to reverse the major cause of disability and death in this country—the morbidity and mortality associated with the cardiovascular diseases. Indeed, since that publication, epidemiologists and clinical investigators concerned with other areas of disease have employed the concept of *risk factors* for other diseases, syndromes, and for the goals of mass public health treatment programs.

In this regard, we have learned of cardiovascular risk factors, coronary heart disease risk factors, hypertension risk factors, renal disease risk factors, risk factors predisposing the individual to neoplastic diseases, and so forth. But the one area with the most thorough and reproducible studies that has resulted in a precise elucidation of specific factors that confer increased risk of enhanced morbidity and mortality, has related to *coronary heart disease.* Other diseases have received less precise delineation of risk factors.

This book details the risk factors underlying coronary heart disease. Some of these factors were identified early on by the Framingham team, others were identified later; but each factor that is discussed here confers significant and independent risk to the morbidity and mortality that result from the atherosclerotic disease process that culminates in coronary heart disease.

Over the past four decades we have witnessed the emergence of amazingly sophisticated means for cardiovascular diagnosis and therapy. As a result of profound advances we have seen a dramatic reduction in cardiovascular morbidity and mortality. For the first time, cardiovascular deaths have been reduced to the extent that they no longer exceed the sum of deaths from all other causes in the United States.

The vast impact of this on the public health is comparable to that of the introduction of antibiotics and their effects on previously lethal diseases. With the advent of penicillin we have seen the amazing near-disappearance of rheumatic fever and its sequelae, rheumatic carditis and valvular heart disease, of luetic heart disease and aneurysms, and of the various forms of endocarditis, myocarditis, and pericarditis.

During this same span of years we have witnessed the remarkable development of an array of technological achievements that include the means for invasive diagnostic procedures such as cardiac catheterization, and noninvasive methods of echocardiography, Doppler studies, and magnetic, radioisotopic, and positron imagery that provides detailed diagnostic and even prognostic information. These innovations, along with extracorporeal means for perfusion, blood banking, and synthetic grafts also have permitted surgical interventions that would not have been conceived at the outset of this cardiovascular odyssey.

Another major advance has been the appearance of new pharmacological modalities: the diuretics, the beta-adrenergic receptor and angiotensin converting enzyme inhibitors, the calcium antagonists and other antihypertensive agents, a spectrum of antiarrhythmic compounds, anticoagulants and fibrinolytic therapy, and the promise of still more innovative and novel modes of therapy that will appear via genetic engineering and other wizardry of the pharmaceutical chemists and molecular biologists.

During these years of highly productive clinical investigation, there has been a parallel series of contributions from our colleagues in the area of cardiovascular epidemiology. These advances have included the demonstration of validity and efficacy of various therapeutic programs by the unique development of complex multicenter trials.

Underlying these areas of clinical achievements have been important long-term population-based studies. The crowning epidemiological achievement has been the Framingham Heart Study and its ability to identify the specific *factors of risk;* by the power of biostatistical analysis, specific risk factors that impart independent risk of premature cardiovascular morbidity and mortality were identified. Some of these factors clearly are not modifiable—advancing years, male gender, and black race. Others are at least partially modifiable—predisposition to diabetes mellitus, increasing body mass, and hyperuricemia. By virtue of the important aforementioned multicenter intervention trials, we have unimpeachable evidence that cigarette consumption, rising systolic and diastolic arterial pressures, hyperlipidemia, diabetes mellitus, and possibly even left ventricular hypertrophy are modifiable, and their correction should reduce morbidity and mortality associated with cardiovascular illnesses.

This is the message of the relatively new era of preventive cardiology—and of this monograph. However, rather than to repeat all of the exciting breakthroughs that have occurred over recent decades, we have chosen areas in which new concepts are being introduced. To be sure, some of these messages concern many of the established risk factors, but their lessons are abundantly clear: correction of each of these factors will improve cardiovascular and overall health. These are the concerns of preventive cardiology as it carries its discipline into the 1990s. Its teachings must certainly be transferred to the everyday practice of cardiovascular medicine for the public health to be improved. This is the challenge to today's cardiovascular physician.

Edward D. Frohlich, M.D.

1. Kannel, WB, Dawber, TR, Kagan, A, et al: Factors of risk in the development of coronary heart disease: Six years' follow-up experience. Ann Intern Med 55:33, 1961.

Editor's Commentary

No aspect of cardiology is more important than prevention. Of particular importance is prevention of atherosclerotic coronary disease, which is the leading cause of mortality in the Western world. Attention to contributory factors can curb the development of coronary disease, and, in addition, can benefit general health. This volume of CARDIOVASCULAR CLINICS not only explores the classic risk factors such as lipids, hypertension, and smoking, but also examines numerous other topics of special interest such as the reversibility of atherosclerosis, preventive cardiology in the young, prevention of sudden cardiac death, isolated systolic hypertension in the elderly, psychosocial factors in coronary disease, and the risk of left ventricular hypertrophy. Thus, this book should amply serve the interests of a broad audience. I am very grateful to Edward Frohlich for his guidance in the development of this material, and we are both deeply indebted to the contributing authors for their superb contributions.

Albert N. Brest, M.D.
Editor-in-Chief

Contributors

Roger T. Anderson, B.A.
Behavioral Medicine Branch
Division of Epidemiology and Clinical Applications
National Heart, Lung, and Blood Institute
Bethesda, Maryland

Mark L. Armstrong, M.D.
Professor of Medicine
Division of Cardiovascular Diseases
University of Iowa College of Medicine
Iowa City, Iowa

Gerald S. Berenson, M.D.
Professor of Medicine
Department of Medicine
Chief, Division of Cardiology
Louisiana State University
New Orleans, Louisiana

Ann E. Bowler, M.S.
Epidemiologic Consultant
National High Blood Pressure Education Program
National Heart, Lung, and Blood Institute
Bethesda, Maryland

W. Virgil Brown, M.D.
President and CEO
Medlantic Research Foundation
Washington, DC

Jerome D. Cohen, M.D.
Professor of Medicine
Director of Preventive Cardiology Programs

ix

St. Louis University School of Medicine
St. Louis, Missouri

Susan M. Czajkowski, Ph.D.
Behavioral Medicine Branch
Division of Epidemiology and Clinical Applications
National Heart, Lung, and Blood Institute
Bethesda, Maryland

Francis G. Dunn, M.B., Ch.B., F.R.C.P.
Consultant Cardiologist
Department of Cardiology
Stobhill General Hospital
Honorary Lecturer in Cardiology
University of Glasgow
Glasgow, Scotland

Edward D. Frohlich, M.D.
Alton Ochsner Distinguished Scientist
Vice President for Academic Affairs
Alton Ochsner Medical Foundation
New Orleans, Louisiana

Curt D. Furberg, M.D., Ph.D.
Professor of Medicine and Chairman
Department of Public Health Sciences
Bowman Gray School of Medicine
Winston-Salem, North Carolina

Edward Genton, M.D.
Ochsner Clinic
New Orleans, Louisiana

David G. Harrison, M.D., Ph.D.
Associate Professor of Medicine
University of Iowa College of Medicine
Iowa City, Iowa

David Heber, M.D., Ph.D.
Associate Clinical Professor of Medicine
Chief, Division of Clinical Nutrition
Department of Medicine
University of California Los Angeles
Los Angeles, California

Donald D. Heistad, M.D.
Professor of Internal Medicine and Pharmacology
University of Iowa College of Medicine
Iowa City, Iowa

Wm. James Howard, M.D.
Director of Clinical Research
Medlantic Research Foundation
Washington, D.C.

Leonard G. Hudzinski, Ph.D.
Director, Ochsner Center for the Elimination of Smoking
Ochsner Medical Institutions
New Orleans, Louisiana

Carolyn C. Johnson, M.S., N.C.C.
Instructor, Department of Medicine
Louisiana State University Medical Center
New Orleans, Louisiana

J. Antonio G. Lopez, M.D.
Fellow Associate
Division of Cardiovascular Diseases
University of Iowa College of Medicine
Iowa City, Iowa

Morton H. Maxwell, M.D.
Clinical Professor of Medicine and Co-Director of Division of Clinical Nutrition
University of California Los Angeles School of Medicine
Los Angeles, California

Marjorie B. Megan
Research Associate
Division of Cardiovascular Diseases
University of Iowa College of Medicine
Iowa City, Iowa

Theresa S. Nicklas, L.D.N., Dr.P.H.
Assistant Professor of Medicine
Department of Medicine
Louisiana State University Medical Center
New Orleans, Louisiana

Margaret C. Oalmann, Dr.P.H.
Professor, Department of Pathology
Louisiana State University School of Medicine
New Orleans, Louisiana

Jeffrey L. Probstfield, M.D.
Scientific Project Officer
Division of Epidemiology and Clinical Applications
National Heart, Lung, and Blood Institute
Clinical Trials Branch
Bethesda, Maryland

Edward J. Roccella, Ph.D., M.P.H.
Coordinator, National High Blood Pressure Education Program
Office of Prevention, Education and Control
National Heart, Lung, and Blood Institute
Bethesda, Maryland

Henry B. Sadlo, M.D.
Department of Medicine (Cardiology)
Emory University School of Medicine
Atlanta, Georgia

Sally A. Shumaker, Ph.D.
Behavioral Medicine Branch
Division of Epidemiology and Clinical Applications
National Heart, Lung, and Blood Institute
Bethesda, Maryland

Joseph Stokes III, M.D. (*deceased*)
Boston University School of Medicine
Boston, Massachusetts

Jack P. Strong, M.D.
Boyd Professor and Head
Department of Pathology
Louisiana State University School of Medicine
New Orleans, Louisiana

Sathanur R. Srinivasan, Ph.D.
Professor, Department of Medicine and Biochemistry
Louisiana State University Medical Center
New Orleans, Louisiana

Stephen M. Weiss, Ph.D.
Chief, Behavioral Medicine
Division of Epidemiology and Clinical Applications
National Heart, Lung, and Blood Institute
Bethesda, Maryland

Nanette K. Wenger, M.D.
Professor of Medicine (Cardiology)
Emory University School of Medicine
Director, Cardiac Clinics
Grady Memorial Hospital
Atlanta, Georgia

Mark D. Wittry, M.D.
St. Louis University School of Medicine
St. Louis, Missouri

Contents

PART 1

Cardiovascular Risks:
Lessons from the Community

CHAPTER 1

Cardiovascular Risk Factors

Joseph Stokes III, M.D.

The purpose of this chapter is to summarize the current knowledge regarding the risk factors for coronary heart disease (CHD) and other important clinical manifestations of atherosclerosis, including untimely death. It is an extraordinarily complex subject. For example, a review by Hopkins and Williams[1] classified 246 factors that had been identified by one or more studies over the last 40 years as being associated with CHD alone. The prime objective of most of these studies was to identify those causes of atherosclerosis that can be modified in order either to prevent or to delay the development of this ubiquitous disease. Unfortunately, few of the factors catalogued by these authors would even meet a rigorous definition of a *risk factor* and of those that could, only serum lipids, blood pressure, and cigarette smoking have been clearly identified as causative.

DEFINITIONS

The Framingham Study introduced the term *risk factor* in its seminal publication by Kannel and colleagues in 1961.[2] It was invented to fill the logical void between the concepts of *association* and *causation* and is best defined as *a factor associated with either a disease or a condition and suspected of being causative.* Unfortunately, this last qualifying phrase is often forgotten by many investigators.

CHARACTERISTICS OF RISK

The concept of risk is essential to both epidemiology and preventive cardiology. The term begs at least three questions: of what, to whom, and by when? The *what* for this chapter is CHD and other manifestations of atherosclerosis. The *whom* refers generally either to the healthy patients undergoing a health maintenance examination or to others undergoing cardiovascular risk assessment. However, on occasion the risks to communities can be assessed, such as the situation in the current community intervention trials being supported by the National Heart, Lung and Blood Institute. The question *by when?* varies—from time to time it covers a lifetime, but most cardiovascular risk assessment estimates are from between

3

6 and 10 years. The Health Risk Appraisal program of the Carter Center at Emory University estimates the risk of death from various causes over the subsequent 10 years.[3] Risk is usually expressed in three ways: absolute, relative, and attributable, each of which has important implications regarding both causal inference and prevention. For instance, the relative risk of dyslipidemia decreases for men with increasing age. However, the attributable risk of this factor is little changed by advancing years owing to the fact that age (or, more precisely, *time*) has such a powerful effect on increasing the absolute risk.

CRITERIA FOR CAUSATION

In order to derive causal inference from factors associated with the development of cardiovascular disease (CVD), epidemiology applies a sequence of logical steps that include its timing (that is, a cause must invariably precede an effect), its strength and consistency, and whether or not it is supported by biological rationale. Even though CVD meets all four criteria, the most conclusive evidence for those risk factors that are modifiable is gained by intervention trials because if one modifies a cause, one should invariably observe an effect. Unfortunately, intervention trials can be performed efficiently only on high-risk cohorts. For example, the Lipid Research Clinics Primary Prevention Trial was performed only on men with an average serum total cholesterol of 295 mg per dl.[4] Such trials are also expensive and require at least 5 to 7 years to conduct, as will be reviewed in later chapters of this book.

CONCEPTUAL MODEL

The most useful conceptual model by which to classify the plethora of risk factors for CVD was first suggested by McKeown[5] as a means of classifying all causes of health and disease. McKeown points out that pathogenesis begins with conception, with those biological characteristics determined by our *genetic* inheritance. Even before birth, the fetus is exposed to various *environmental* supports and hazards and, after birth, must cope with a variety of factors in its physical, biological, and social environment, some of which may be powerful and over which the individual has little or no control. Therefore, epidemiologists tend to classify both genetic factors and factors in the macroenvironment as either fixed or nonmodifiable. Nevertheless, most of the great victories of public health have been won by such environmental interventions as the chlorination of common water sources and the elimination of smallpox virus from the microbiologic environment. Indeed, there is substantial evidence that the great epidemic of CHD that has afflicted all developed societies during the first half of the 20th century may be largely explained by maladaptation to the agricultural and industrial revolutions, the first of which substantially increased the dietary intake of saturated fat, whereas the latter markedly reduced requisite energy expenditure.

We cope with these powerful pathogenic factors by means of certain behaviors, the most important of which McKeown refers to as *health behaviors,* such as diet, physical activity, and cigarette smoking. Such behaviors are important to clinical health maintenance and preventive medicine because they are the best means available to physicians and other health professionals for modifying pathogenic traits, such as serum lipids and blood pressure, thereby either to prevent or to delay the development of diseases, such as atherosclerosis and its various clinical manifestations.

THE IMPORTANT RISK FACTORS FOR CARDIOVASCULAR DISEASE

GENETIC FACTORS

Astute clinicians have long recognized that coronary disease clusters in families, which we now know is explained not only by the fact that these individuals share the same genes but also that they often eat from a common kitchen and share many of the same health habits. The genetic factors that explain part of this familial aggregation are listed in Table 1–1. Age remains a powerful predictor of CVD—a fact that annoys those who struggle to remain at low risk yet still face CHD as the most likely cause of death merely because of the passage of time. Although there is no evidence that the susceptibility to atherosclerosis changes with age, there are good reasons for assuming that the disease develops owing to a time-dose product. This is certainly borne out by the fact that children with homozygous familial hypercholesterolemia can die from CHD as early as the fifth or sixth year of life.

The sex differences in CHD are also profound. Pathologists have been able to identify differences in male and female coronary arteries in newborns. During the childbearing years, women exhibit only about one quarter the risk of developing CHD compared with men of comparable age. Although this difference diminishes after menopause, women continue to be significantly less likely than men to develop CHD even after the age of 65.[6,7]

The reasons for this relative protection are not fully understood. Much of it is probably due to the influence that a woman's endocrine environment between menarche and menopause has on serum lipids and blood pressure. Estrogens elevate serum high-density lipoprotein cholesterol (HDL-C), which decreases the total cholesterol: high-density lipoprotein cholesterol (TC:HDL–C) ratio—the best serum lipid summary estimate of dyslipidemia.[8]

Genetic factors, as yet poorly understood, contribute to the four atherogenic traits listed in Table 1–1, although the specificity of gene action is better understood for dyslipidemia and diabetes than it is for either hypertension or obesity. Indeed, it was only recently that it was generally accepted that humans exhibit the same genetic determinant of obesity that had been identified earlier in other animal models.[9]

Epidemiologists have also questioned whether or not a strong family history is

Table 1–1. Genetic Determinants of Coronary Heart Disease

Age
Sex
Menopause
Genetic contribution to:
  Hypertension
  Dyslipidemia
  Diabetes
  Obesity

---

an independent predictor of CHD when the other genetic factors listed in Table 1–1 are included in the analytic model. Myers and associates[10] have completed an analysis of family history of CHD reported by the 5209 subjects of the original Framingham study cohort. Reported parental CHD death proved to be an independent predictor for CHD for men but not for women in an analytic model that included age, sex, systolic blood pressure, serum total cholesterol, glucose intolerance, and Metropolitan Relative Weight along with several other risk factors. The failure of family history to make a statistically significant contribution to CHD risk for women is better explained by the lower incidence of CHD in that sex than it is by any inherent biological differences between men and women.

ENVIRONMENTAL FACTORS

As mentioned earlier, many consider atherosclerosis to be a disease of maladaptation. In addition, the fascinating possibility of environmental sanitation as a means of controlling the disease has encouraged the search for environmental factors, such as water quality. The search has been further stimulated by geopathologic studies that reveal marked differences in CHD mortality among various countries. As illustrated in Figure 1–1, death rates per 100,000 for CHD in 1977 among men 35 to 74 years old varies from almost 900 in Finland to less than 100 in Japan. Because other studies of Japanese migrants[11] indicate that this difference is not genetic, attention focused on cultural and physical environmental factors. The cur-

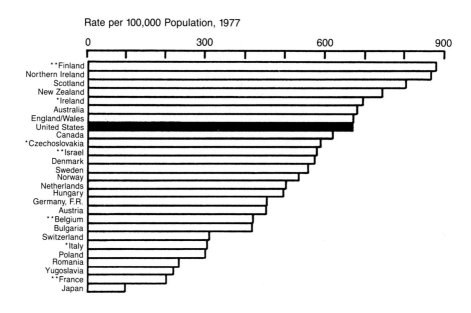

Rate per 100,000 Population, 1977

*1975 data
**1976 data
Source: Prepared by NHLBI; data from the World Health Organization

Figure 1–1. Death rates for coronary heart disease by country: men 35–74 years of age.
SOURCE: Report of the Intersociety Commission for Heart Disease Resources: Optimal resources for primary prevention of atherosclerotic diseases. Circulation. 70:1A–205A, 1984.

rent assumption is that cultural dietary practices explain the low rate for Japan. However, Schroeder's[12] suggestion that water quality might be involved stimulated a spate of studies testing the hypothesis that either soft water or trace metal deficiency is a risk factor for CHD. Sharret and Feinlieb[13] reviewed this evidence in 1983 and concluded that proof was lacking and that many of the studies were methodologically flawed.

However, interest has persisted regarding the relationship of socioeconomic status to the risk of CVD. A curious pattern exists by which CHD is more prevalent among the affluent in developing countries, whereas the inverse gradient is seen in developed countries, such as the United States and Great Britain.[14] There is also evidence that cigarette smoking, obesity, and nonhygienic dietary practices are more common among the poor. This evidence, combined with the fact that disease and disability rates also exhibit an inverse socioeconomic gradient, led the Black Commission in Great Britain to suggest that the health of the British might be better served by income supports for the poor than by allocating more resources to the British National Health Service.

BEHAVIORAL FACTORS

Diet

The concept that diet might play a role in the pathogenesis of atherosclerosis can be traced back to Anitschkow,[15] who concluded that dietary cholesterol was the source of the cholesterol in atheromas. This idea was broadened to include dietary fat and was supported by the observation in Norway that deaths from CHD fell dramatically in 1944 and 1945, when the Nazis diverted almost all dairy and other dietary fat to the production of munitions.[16] Keys and associates[17] then began a 40-year search to define the role of diet in the pathogenesis of atherosclerosis. Table 1–2 lists those dietary factors that have been shown to affect the concentration of serum low-density lipoprotein cholesterol (LDL-C), which is generally considered to be the prime serum lipid variable causing atherosclerosis. Both weight gain and steady-state obesity, particularly that of central distribution, have been shown to be associated with elevated LDL-C. There is now general agreement that dietary saturated fatty acids represent the most important factor in elevating LDL-C. However, a recent Framingham study indicates that the percentage of calories derived from fat may be an even more important factor.[18] Monounsaturates have long been

Table 1–2. Dietary Factors Affecting Serum Low-Density Lipoprotein Cholesterol Concentration

Caloric imbalance (weight gain)
Percentage calories derived from fat
Saturated fatty acids
Monounsaturated fatty acids
  Polyunsaturated fatty acids
  Omega 6
  Omega 3
  Cholesterol
  Fiber

considered neutral in their effect on serum lipids and cholesterol. However, a study by Bonanome and Grundy[19] suggests that monounsaturates may be beneficial. Although controversy still prevails regarding the mechanism of their action, poly-unsaturated fatty acids consistently lower LDL-C, and omega 3 fatty acids, found primarily in fish oils, also have a beneficial effect on lowering triglycerides.[20]

Earlier studies in the rat indicated that dietary cholesterol was not an important determinant of serum total cholesterol because in that species exogenous cholesterol merely reduced the rate of endogenous synthesis. Later studies indicated that the rate of endogenous cholesterol synthesis was far lower in humans than it was in rats, and, therefore, dietary intake greater than 250 to 300 mg per day had a hypercholesterolemic effect. In addition, at least one study in the United States found dietary cholesterol to be related to the development of CHD.[21] Finally, pectin and other soluble fiber can lower LDL-C somewhat,[22,23] although the dose required is larger than most individuals can easily tolerate. Studies suggest that oat bran also can be beneficial. Therefore, the current prudent dietary recommendations of the American Heart Association are that the percentage of calories from fat be kept less than 30 percent, with no more than 10 percent being derived from saturated fat. The American Heart Association also suggests that dietary cholesterol should be restricted to less than 300 mg per day. Chapters 10 and 11 provide further detail on dietary and pharmacologic treatment of dyslipidemia.

Physical Activity

Physical activity has been gaining recognition as an important health behavior.[24,25] It serves not only as a means of maintaining caloric balance but also as a means of preventing CHD. The Framingham Study has reported an inverse relationship between physical activity and the risk of CVD mortality (Fig. 1–2); it appears that physical activity may be particularly beneficial in older age groups. Several means have been suggested as to how exercise exerts its effect. Vigorous exercise elevates serum HDL-C, particularly the light HDL-C fraction. Herbert and colleagues[26] suggest that this is due to decreased catabolism of the particle rather than increased production. However, most attention has been directed at the effect of exercise on obesity and caloric balance. Not only does physical activity generate direct caloric expenditure and appetite inhibition, but it also exerts a conditioning effect that may be most important by increasing caloric expenditure during usual daily activities.

However, it is also evident that vigorous exercise can precipitate primary cardiac arrest. Siscovick and co-workers[27] studied this phenomenon and concluded that although the risk of cardiac arrest is transiently increased during vigorous exercise, habitual exercise is associated with an overall decrease in risk. The fact that those who are poorly conditioned are at greatest risk should advise physicians to counsel caution in initiating an exercise program for sedentary patients. Chapters 12 and 13 provide additional information on the effects of exercise and guidance for its safe implementation.

Cigarette Smoking

Cigarette smoking, dealt with in Chapters 14 and 15, is one of the three major risk factors for CVD and one about which the evidence is strong enough to define a causative role. The Framingham Study has found that cigarette smoking not only is associated with all manifestations of CHD[28] but also with both cardiovascular and total mortality (Fig. 1–3). Although smokers exhibit a relative risk for squa-

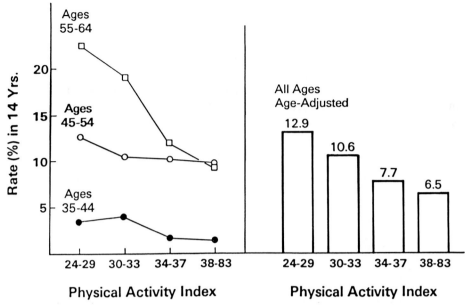

Figure 1–2. Risk of cardiovascular mortality according to physical activity status: men 35 to 64 years of age.
SOURCE: The Framingham Study.

mous cell carcinoma of the lung that is greater than their risk for CHD, the population-attributable risk for smokers is greater for coronary disease owing to the fact that the incidence of CHD is far greater than it is for lung cancer. Fortunately, those who quit smoking lose their increased risk of CHD within 24 months of quitting.[28] Unfortunately, switching to filter cigarettes does not appear to represent a safe alternative (Fig. 1–4).

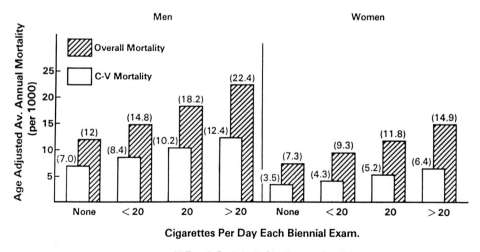

Figure 1–3. Risk of death according to cigarette habit: 20–year follow-up: subjects 45–74 years of age.
SOURCE: The Framingham Study.

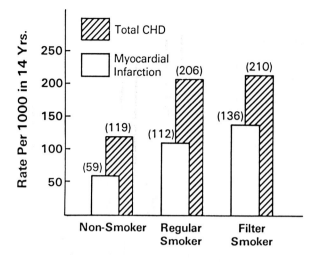

Figure 1–4. Risk of coronary heart disease according to cigarette smoking: filter vs. nonfilter: men under 55 years of age.
SOURCE: The Framingham Study.

Alcohol Use

Many studies have demonstrated either an inverse (Fig. 1–5) or a U-shaped relationship between alcohol use and CVD.[29] These observations are tempered by the clear relationship between heavy alcohol use and elevated blood pressure and the fact that noncardiovascular mortality begins to increase as alcohol consumption rises above 2 drinks per day. Therefore, for those who are capable of temperate alcohol use, it is probably prudent to advise continued consumption at or below 1 to 2 drinks per day. However, in view of the tremendous social and medical costs of alcohol use, it is unwise to recommend alcohol to those who do not regularly imbibe, and it is particularly important not to recommend its use for any individual with a strong family history of alcohol abuse.

Stress and Type A/B Behavior

It would be easy for a review such as this to become deeply mired in the sticky issues related to stress and coronary-prone behavior as risk factors for CHD. The

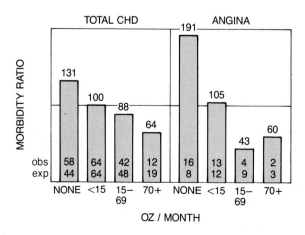

Figure 1–5. Risk of CHD and angina according to alcohol intake: men 50–62 years of age: 18-year follow-up.
SOURCE: The Framingham Study.

issues are not easily dealt with on a rational level because many individuals and a few investigators hold deeply felt beliefs that stress is an important cause of CVD. These beliefs are frequently reflected in actions taken by retirement boards and those assessing disability claims. The mere assessment of stress is a complex subject, and at least three methods have been suggested to measure type A/B behavior.

The summative evaluation of type A behavior as a risk factor for CHD suggests that it makes little or no contribution for men, but that it may represent a significant factor for women, particularly those working women who achieve higher educational levels than their spouses.[30] In addition, several investigators, including a fascinating report from the Rancho Bernardo study in California, suggest that men married to such wives are also at increased risk of CHD.[31] Nevertheless, the evidence certainly does not warrant modification of type A behavior as either an effective or efficient means of reducing the risk of CHD. Chapter 9 includes additional information related to this controversy.

Other Relevant Behaviors

The effectiveness of thrombolytic therapy of acute coronary thrombosis adds urgency to encouraging patients with symptoms of this syndrome not to delay seeking coronary care. In addition, physicians should also be aware that patient compliance with their prescribed regimens is far less than perfect. This compliance issue is relevant because both primary and secondary prevention of CHD often requires adherence to drug regimens that not only entail significant out-of-pocket costs but also have significant adverse side effects.

In addition, birth control pills have been demonstrated to increase the risk of stroke,[32] particularly in older women who smoke and who experience withdrawal headaches. Fortunately, a study by Stampfer and associates[33] from the Nurses Health study indicates that the use of the pill does not increase the risk of CHD after discontinuing its use. It also appears that postmenopausal estrogen use by women may be beneficial not only in preventing osteoporosis but also in reducing the risk of CHD, although full agreement on this issue has not yet been reached.[34]

ATHEROGENIC TRAITS

Atherogenic traits are those anatomic, physiologic, or biochemical traits that, if combined with age, sex, and cigarette smoking, can best predict both the occurrence and prognosis of CHD and other clinical manifestations of atherosclerosis. Two of these traits, dyslipidemia and hypertension, have been shown to play causative roles, inasmuch as intervention trials have demonstrated that correcting these traits reduces the incidence of cardiovascular events. Experimental and epidemiologic evidence also indicates that dyslipidemia (that is, elevated LDL-C, depressed HDL-C, elevated TG, and an elevated TC:HDL-C ratio) is a *necessary* cause, inasmuch as it is virtually impossible to produce atherosclerosis without modifying in some way the normal pattern of serum lipids. This implies that the optimum level of serum total cholesterol for the adult male may be as low as 140 mg per dl.

Dyslipidemia

With the exception of age, dyslipidemia is the most powerful predictor of CHD.[35] These conclusions stem from studies both between and within populations. The relationship has been established as being both strong and independent and is entirely congruent with a spectrum of studies, ranging from laboratory to clinical observations. Hypercholesterolemia alone predicts all major clinical manifestations of atherosclerotic disease, with the possible exception of cerebrovascular disease.

The World Health Organization has begun to monitor cardiovascular mortality systematically in those developed countries with reliable application of international classification of disease. An initial report by Simons[36] from 19 of these countries indicated that 45 percent of the interpopulation variance can be explained by serum total cholesterol, and that this could be increased to 55 percent by the use of the TC:HDL-C ratio. However, rates in Japan, France, and Italy were lower than could be explained by lipid values alone. Holman and co-workers[37] have reported that both dietary fat and serum total cholesterol are correlated with the extent of atherosclerosis, based on approximately 3100 postmortem examinations carried out in the international atherosclerosis project. A report by the Inter-Society Commission for Heart Disease Resources on the optimum resources for primary prevention of atherosclerotic diseases[38] and the chapter by Gotto and Farmer[39] provide excellent summaries of these data.

The landmark publication in 1961 from the Framingham Study by Kannel and colleagues[2] identified serum cholesterol and blood pressure as the most important risk factors for CHD except for age and sex. Subsequently, the Framingham Study has published almost 40 reports extending its analysis of the role not only of serum total cholesterol but also of various cholesterol lipoprotein subfractions and triglyceride.[35] The Framingham Study has also emphasized that the ratio of either TC:HDL-C or LDL-C:HDL-C is the best summary estimate of risk.[8] This factor is important because some individuals with serum total cholesterol values of less than 200 mg per dl may still be at high risk by virtue of a very low HDL-C. Conversely, other individuals, particularly women, with serum total cholesterol values above 240 mg per dl may *not* be at high risk by virtue of high HDL-C value. Serum total cholesterol has proved a highly statistically significant predictor of all clinical manifestations of CHD, intermittent claudication, and total cardiovascular disease.[40] However, serum total cholesterol is not predictive of stroke and transient ischemic attacks (TIA), and its predictive power weakens in individuals over the age of 50.

The pathogenesis of atherosclerosis is complex. Although dyslipidemia may be unique as representing the only *necessary* risk factor for atherosclerotic diseases, hypertension, cigarette smoking, glucose intolerance, obesity, physical inactivity, certain clotting factors (detailed in Chapter 8), and left ventricular hypertrophy measured either by electrocardiogram or by echocardiogram (see Chapter 5) also contribute to risk. Reduced vital capacity and tachycardia also serve as proxy measures of risk and may play a pathogenic role.

This complexity is illustrated in Figure 1–6, which reports the 8-year incidence of CVD in four sets of 35-year-old men in the original Framingham cohort. The lowest-risk men have low-normal blood pressures, do not smoke, and do not exhibit any evidence of glucose intolerance or left ventricular hypertrophy on electrocardiogram. The highest-risk cohort exhibits all these risk factors. However, for each cohort, there is a curvilinear relationship between the level of serum total cholesterol and risk.

The data regarding serum triglycerides are far less consistent. Adding triglycerides to LDL-C and HDL-C in a risk-estimation model usually does not improve the predictive value. However, a study by Anderson and others[41] reports the relationship of nonfasting very low-density lipoprotein (VLDL) levels as measured at the initial Framingham examination in relation to cardiovascular mortality. These

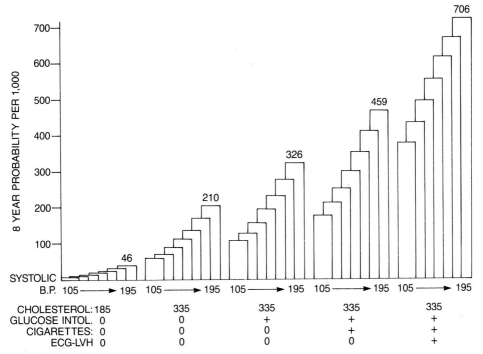

Figure 1–6. Risk of cardiovascular disease according to serum cholesterol at specified levels of other risk factors. (ECG–LVH = electrocardiographic evidence of left ventricular hypertrophy. SPB = systolic blood pressure.)
Source: Stokes, J III: Dyslipidemia as a risk factor for cardiovascular disease and untimely death: The Framingham Study. (From Gotto, AM, et al, (eds): Atherosclerosis Review, proceedings of Paris symposium, 18:49, Raven Press, New York, 1988.)

observations indicated VLDL is strongly related to both overall mortality and cardiovascular mortality in men and women. This relationship is stronger for VLDL than it is for total cholesterol and remains significant with both overall and cardiovascular mortality in a multivariate Cox regression analysis with both total cholesterol and LDL-C in the model.

Hypertension

Hypertension is the most important consistent *contributing* cause of atherosclerosis and the atherogenic trait that has been most successfully modified to prevent stroke and, to a lesser extent, CHD. On the one hand, the presumption is that hypertension creates conditions in the arterial endothelium that encourages the development of atheromas, such as those described by Ross.[42] On the other hand, hypertension is difficult to define as a precise, qualitative risk factor because the relationship between the blood pressure and the risk of CVD is log-linear and does not exhibit any threshold. This relationship can be observed for blood pressures such as those between 120 and 140 mmHg systolic, which are generally considered to be normal. It is this fact that encourages the aphorism that the lower the blood pressure the better so long as one does not faint every time one stands up. Epidemiologists tend to prefer systolic to diastolic pressure because the former can be measured more reliably, and elevated systolic pressure alone confers an increased

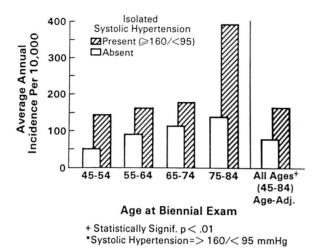

Figure 1-7. Risk of myocardial infarction with isolated systolic hypertension: 24-year follow-up: men 45–84 years of age. SOURCE: The Framingham Study.

risk even when the diastolic pressure is normal (Fig. 1–7). In addition, the two are so co-linear that it is difficult to use both in analytic models such as the multiple logistic.

Hypertension is a particularly powerful predictor of TIA and stroke, and intervention studies have demonstrated that the drug treatment of hypertension is far more successful in cerebrovascular disease than it is in CHD. Indeed, the Hypertension Detection and Follow-Up Program is one of the few intervention trials that showed that antihypertensive therapy could significantly reduce the risk of CHD. The inverse holds for the treatment of dyslipidemia, which has been far more successful in preventing CHD than other atherosclerotic manifestations. Hypertension is discussed in detail in Chapters 3 and 4.

Glucose Intolerance

Diabetes makes an important independent contribution to the risk of CVD, particularly for women.[44] Indeed, epidemiologic studies over the last 40 years have largely confirmed the clinical aphorism that it is rare to encounter symptomatic coronary disease in any premenopausal woman unless she has diabetes, hypertension, or both. Although it is also associated with dyslipidemia, diabetes makes its additional contribution to risk in analytic models that include lipid variables.

Obesity

Obesity is probably the most neglected of the atherogenic traits. This neglect stems from the fact that of the original prospective studies of CHD in the United States, only Framingham and Albany could demonstrate any consistent relationship. The Framingham Study originally observed that obesity was predictive of the development of CHD and was also closely related to levels of serum total cholesterol, blood pressure, blood glucose, and uric acid. However, if obesity was contained in an analytic model that included these other variables, it did not make an independent contribution to risk. However, after 26 years of follow-up of the original Framingham cohort, Hubert and colleagues[45] reported that obesity *did* make an independent contribution to the risk of cardiovascular disease, particularly among younger subjects studied. They also observed that it did not exert its effect exclusively through its association with serum lipids, blood pressure, and blood glucose.

The distribution of obesity is also important in determining its association with serum lipids, morbidity, and mortality. Following the initial observation of Vague,[46] Larsson, Bjorntorp and others[47] have made major contributions to this important concept. The Framingham Study has shown that the subscapular skin-fold as a measure of central obesity makes a stronger and independent contribution to the risk of developing CVD over a 22-year period of follow-up.[48]

The most powerful effect of obesity on both cardiovascular morbidity and mortality is due to its impact on cardiovascular risk factors. Not only does obesity increase blood pressure, blood glucose, and risk of type II diabetes, but it also is associated with an increase in the LDL-C, a decrease in the HDL-C, an increase in the fasting triglycerides, and an increase in the TC:HDL-C ratio.[49] Obesity is also associated with physical inactivity, which may explain why it makes an independent contribution to risk other than its association with blood pressure, serum lipids, and diabetes. There is a highly consistent correlation between body mass index and serum total cholesterol. Once serum total cholesterol levels have been established, change of body weight is the most important determinant of change in serum lipid levels. The effects of weight loss are discussed further in Chapter 10.

In essence, the prevention of obesity in childhood and adolescence (as outlined in the next chapter) may be the most important means of preventing dyslipidemia. Weight reduction is one of the most efficient means of correcting dyslipidemia once it has developed.

Hematologic/Rheologic Factors

The rediscovery of coronary thrombosis has renewed interest in hematocrit, clotting factors, and decreased fibrinolysis as risk factors for CVD. Hematocrit makes its strongest contribution to the risk of stroke.[40] A recent Framingham study indicates that fibrinogen may be a risk factor and may represent one mechanism whereby cigarette smoking contributes to risk.[50] However, studies have led to inconsistent findings, and the strength of the association is not such that it has strong implication for prevention. Chapter 8 outlines possible methods of controlling thrombogenic factors.

Other Traits

Electrocardiographic abnormalities, and most particularly left ventricular hypertrophy (LVH), as determined both by electrocardiogram and echocardiogram, are independent risk factors for CHD. The assumption that LVH is a summative measure of the severity of hypertension is borne out by the fact that LVH is a more powerful risk factor for TIA and stroke than it is for CHD.[40] (See Chapter 5.)

Other factors, such as diminished vital capacity and tachycardia, have been reported as excellent proxy measures of CVD risk, particularly for sudden cardiac death.[51] However, the pathogenic rationale suggests that they mark risk rather than play any pathogenic roles. Nevertheless, these other factors are useful in risk estimation and as simple clinical indices of risk.

RISK PROFILES OF ATHEROGENIC DISEASE

Each atherogenic disease has its own unique profile of risk factors, and variations are also observed between the various manifestations of CHD itself (that is,
angina, myocardial infarction, and sudden death). The 30-year follow-up data from
the original Framingham cohort indicate that dyslipidemia, hypertension, cigarette
smoking, glucose intolerance, and LVH per electrocardiogram are the major contributors to CHD incidence, although for men both dyslipidemia and cigarette
smoking become less predictive after the age of 55.[40] With the exception of age,
hypertension and LVH are the major contributors for TIA and stroke, with hematocrit and cigarette smoking making an additional contribution for men and glucose
intolerance for women. Dyslipidemia makes little or no contribution to stroke. Cigarette smoking is the dominant risk factor for peripheral vascular disease. Lipids,
blood pressure, and glucose intolerance are also important, as is hematocrit for
men.

SECULAR TRENDS

The United States has enjoyed a marked reduction of CVD mortality, as
reflected in Figure 1–8. Coronary heart disease mortality began to fall in 1968, and
many studies (Table 1–3) have attempted to identify its causes.[52] Goldman and
Cook[52] have estimated that 50 percent of the reduction could be ascribed to cessation of cigarette smoking and dietary changes reflected in improvement in dyslipidemia. They estimated only 14 percent of the fall as being due to the treatment of
hypertension, and that most of the remainder is due to improved coronary care
following the development of clinical manifestations of the disease.

Framingham studies regarding secular trends of CHD are perplexing. The
decline in cardiovascular mortality in the United States has been well documented
and is reflected in the Framingham Study. For instance, unpublished analysis by
D'Agostino and associates reveals a reduction in cardiovascular mortality among
men 55 to 64 years old of almost 20 percent between 1953 and 1973. The comparable decline among women in the same age group was greater than 30 percent.
In contrast, prevalence rates have *increased* over the past 20 years, and incidence
rates have remained constant. These data suggest that the decline in mortality for
CVD in the United States may be primarily due to better survival after the onset
of CHD rather than due to a decrease in incidence. In essence, it would appear that
secondary prevention may have been more effective than have methods of primary
prevention of CVD.

CLINICAL METHODS OF RISK ASSESSMENT

Clinicians now have available to them a variety of efficient means of estimating
the risk of various cardiovascular events.[53] It is now possible to construct risk assessment models, based on the Framingham Study data, which can predict that about
half of the new coronary events will occur in the top quintile of multivariate risk
using the seven risk factors of age, sex, serum total cholesterol, systolic blood pressure (see Chapters 3 and 4), presence or absence of cigarette smoking (see Chapter
14), glucose intolerance, and LVH per electrocardiogram (see Chapter 5). If available, the HDL-C can also be added to the model. By adding other electrocardio-

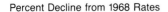

Percent Decline from 1968 Rates

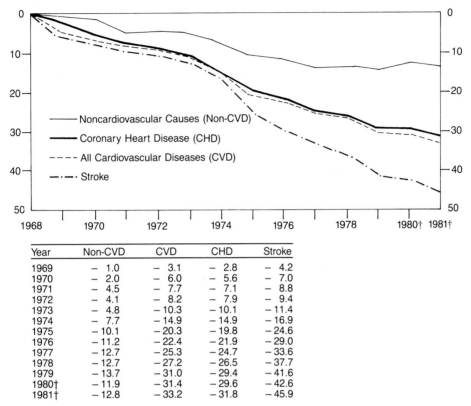

Year	Non-CVD	CVD	CHD	Stroke
1969	− 1.0	− 3.1	− 2.8	− 4.2
1970	− 2.0	− 6.0	− 5.6	− 7.0
1971	− 4.5	− 7.7	− 7.1	− 8.8
1972	− 4.1	− 8.2	− 7.9	− 9.4
1973	− 4.8	− 10.3	− 10.1	− 11.4
1974	− 7.7	− 14.9	− 14.9	− 16.9
1975	− 10.1	− 20.3	− 19.8	− 24.6
1976	− 11.2	− 22.4	− 21.9	− 29.0
1977	− 12.7	− 25.3	− 24.7	− 33.6
1978	− 12.7	− 27.2	− 26.5	− 37.7
1979	− 13.7	− 31.0	− 29.4	− 41.6
1980†	− 11.9	− 31.4	− 29.6	− 42.6
1981†	− 12.8	− 33.2	− 31.8	− 45.9

Figure 1–8. Trends in mortality for cardiovascular disease and noncardiovascular causes of death: decline by age-adjusted death rates US 1968–81.
SOURCE: Report of the Intersociety Commission for Heart Disease Resources: Optimal resources for primary prevention of atherosclerotic diseases. Circulation, 70:1A, 1984.

Table 1–3. Estimated Causes of the 26% Decline in Deaths Due to Coronary Heart Disease (CHD) (USA 1968–1976)*

Cause	Estimated Number of Lives Saved	Contribution to Decline (%)
Reduction in cigarette smoking	176,000	28
Correction of dyslipidemia	168,000	27
Coronary care of acute myocardial infarction and coronary insufficiency	85,000	14
Treatment of hypertension	72,000	12
Other medical management of clinical manifestations of CHD	61,000	10
Emergency medical services (i.e., precoronary care)	25,000	4
Coronary artery bypass surgery	21,000	3
Unexplained	22,000	3
Total	630,000	101

*Adapted from Goldman and Cook.[52]

gram abnormalities, Metropolitan Relative Weight, heart rate, and diminished vital capacity, one can do somewhat better in estimating sudden cardiac death (see Chapter 6), about half of which such deaths will occur in the top decile of risk. Nevertheless, there are still serious limitations. Theoretical calculations indicate that inherent unreliability of measurement will limit risk estimations to about 78 percent of the total variance, and the current prospective studies of CVD within populations, such as the Framingham Study, have yet to explain more than 22 percent of the variance.

Risk estimation can be done from hard copy, by various hand-held computers offered by pharmaceutical companies, or by means of more sophisticated programs that can be run on personal computers. More general programs are also available, such as the Health Risk Appraisal system offered by the Carter Center of Emory University, which includes cardiovascular risk estimates as part of a comprehensive estimate of the risk of death from all causes over the subsequent 10 years.[3] Such methods are particularly useful in motivating patients to stop smoking and to reduce their risk otherwise by making changes in one or more health behaviors in order to modify one or more pathogenic traits.

SUMMARY

Atherosclerosis and its various clinical manifestations are now highly predictable and preventable diseases. Dyslipidemia appears to be a necessary cause, and hypertension and cigarette smoking are both powerful and modifiable contributing causes. Health professionals should incorporate cardiovascular risk assessment and risk factor modification within the context of their delivery of personal health services. Such services probably already have contributed to the decline of cardiovascular mortality, and the current levels of risk factors in the United States population indicate that substantial further reduction should be possible by creating a smoke-free environment by the year 2000 and by implementing the recommendations of the National Cholesterol and High Blood Pressure Education Programs.

ACKNOWLEDGMENT

The author appreciates the help of Ms. Ellen Yadon in the preparation of this manuscript.

REFERENCES

1. Hopkins, PN and Williams RR: A survey of 246 coronary risk factors. Atherosclerosis 40:1, 1981.
2. Kannel, WB, et al: Factors of risk in the development of coronary heart disease—six-year follow-up experience: The Framingham Study. Ann Intern Med 55:33, 1961.
3. Hall, JH and Zwemer, JD: Prospective Medicine: Health Hazard Appraisal. Methodist Hospital, Indiana, 1949.
4. The lipid research clinics coronary primary prevention trial results. 1. Reduction in incidence of coronary heart diesase. JAMA 251:351, 1984.
5. McKeown, T: Medicine in a Modern Society. Hafner Publishing, New York, 1966.
6. Kannel, WB, et al: Menopause and risk of cardiovascular disease: The Framingham Study. Ann Intern Med 85:447, 1976.
7. Colditz, GA, et al: Menopause and the risk of coronary heart disease in women. N Engl J Med 316:1105, 1987.

8. Castelli, WP, Abbott, RD, and McNamara, PM: Summary estimates of cholesterol used to predict coronary heart disease. Circulation 67:730, 1983.
9. Stunkard, AJ, et al: An adoption study of human obesity. N Engl J Med 314:193, 1986.
10. Myers, RH, et al: Family history as an independent risk factor for coronary heart disease: The Framingham Study. Submitted for publication.
11. Marmot, MG, et al: Epidemiologic studies of CHD and stroke in Japanese men living in Japan, Hawaii and California. Prevalence of coronary and hypertensive heart disease and associated risk factors. Am J Epidem 102:514, 1975.
12. Schroeder, HA: Relation between mortality from cardiovascular disease and treated water supplies: Variations in states and 163 large municipalities of the United States. JAMA 172:993, 1960.
13. Sharret, AR, and Feinlieb, M: Water constituents and trace elements in relation to cardiovascular disease. Prevent Med 4:20, 1975.
14. Marmot, MG: Epidemiology and the art of the soluable. Lancet 1:897, 1986.
15. Anitschkow, N: Experimental arteriosclerosis in animals. In Cowdry, EV (ed): Arteriosclerosis. McMillan Publishing Company, New York, 1950.
16. Malmros, H: The relation of nutrition to health. Acta Med Scand 246(Suppl):137, 1950.
17. Keys, A, et al: Lessons from serum cholesterol studies in Japan, Hawaii, and Los Angeles. Ann Intern Med 48:83, 1958.
18. Posner, BM, et al: Nutritional predictors of CHD over 20 years: The Framingham Study. Presentation at the 61st Scientific Session of the American Heart Association, 1988.
19. Bonanome, A and Grundy, SM: Effect of dietary stearic acid on plasma cholesterol and lipoprotein levels. N Engl J Med 318:1244, 1988.
20. Harris, WS, Connor, WE, and McMurry, MP: The comparative reductions of plasma lipids and lipoproteins by dietary polyunsaturated fats: Salmon oil vs. vegetable oil. Metabolism 32:179, 1983.
21. Shekelle, RB, et al: Diet, serum cholesterol and death from coronary heart disease: The Western Electric Study. N Engl J Med 304:65, 1981.
22. Keys, A, Grande, F, and Anderson, JT: Fiber and pectin in diet and serum cholesterol concentration in man. Proc Soc Exp Biol Med 106:555, 1961.
23. Khaw, K and Barrett-Connor, E: Dietary fiber and reduced ischemic heart disease mortality rates in men and women: A 12-year prospective study. Am J Epidem 126:1093, 1987.
24. Paffenbarger, RS Jr, et al: Physical activity, all-cause mortality, and longevity in college alumni. N Engl J Med 314:605, 1986.
25. Leon, AS, et al: Leisure-time physical activity levels and the risk of coronary heart disease and death. JAMA 258:2388, 1987.
26. Herbert, PN, et al: High-density lipoprotein metabolism in runners and sedentary men. JAMA 252:1034, 1984.
27. Siscovick, DS, et al: The incidence of primary cardiac arrest during vigorous exercise. N Engl J Med 311:874, 1984.
28. Stokes, J III and Rigotti, NA: Health consequences of cigarette smoking and the internist's role in smoking cessation. Adv Intern Med 33:431, 1988.
29. Marmot, MG: Alcohol and coronary heart disease. Interna J Epidem 13:160, 1984.
30. Haynes, SG and Feinlieb, M: Women, work and coronary heart disease: Prospective findings from the Framingham Study. Am J Pub Health 70:133, 1980.
31. Suarez, L and Barrett-Connor, E: Is an educated wife hazardous to your health? Am J Epidem 119:244, 1984.
32. Royal College of General Practitioners' Oral Contraception Study: Further analyses of mortality in oral contraceptive users. Lancet 1:541, 1981.
33. Stampfer, MJ, et al: A prospective study of post-menopausal estrogen therapy and coronary heart disease. N Engl J Med 313:1044, 1985.
34. Wilson, PWF, Garrison, RJ, and Castelli, WP: Postmenopausal estrogen use, cigarette smoking, and cardiovascular morbidity in women over 50. N Engl J Med 313:1038, 1985.
35. Stokes, J III: Dyslipidemia as a risk factor for cardiovascular disease and untimely death: The Framingham Study. In Stokes, J III and Mancini, M (eds): Atherosclerosis Reviews. Raven Press Limited, New York, 1988.
36. Simons, LA: Interrelations of lipids and lipoproteins with coronary artery disease mortality in 19 countries. Am J Cardiol 57:58, 1986.
37. Holman, RL, et al: The national history of atherosclerosis. Am J Path 34:209, 1958.
38. Report of the Inter-Society Commission for Heart Disease Resources: Optimal resources for primary prevention of atherosclerotic diseases. Circulation 70:1A, 1984.

39. Gotto, AM Jr and Farmer, JA: Risk factors for coronary artery disease. In Braunwald, E (ed): Heart Disease: A Textbook of Cardiovascular Medicine. WB Saunders, Philadelphia, 1988.
40. Stokes, J III, et al: The relative importance of selected risk factors for various manifestations of cardiovascular disease among men and women from 35 to 64 years old: 30 years of follow-up in the Framingham Study. Circulation 75(Suppl V):V65, 1987.
41. Anderson, KM, et al: Non-fasting VLDL and long-term cardiovascular disease mortality: The Framingham Study. Submitted for publication.
42. Ross, R: The pathogenesis of atherosclerosis: An update. N Engl J Med 314:488, 1986.
43. Hypertension Detection and Follow-Up Program Cooperative Group: Five-year findings of the Hypertension Detection and Follow-Up Program. I. Reduction in mortality of persons with high blood pressure, including mild hypertension. JAMA 242:2562, 1979.
44. Kannel, WB and McGee, DL: Diabetes and cardiovascular disease: The Framingham Study. JAMA 241:2035, 1979.
45. Hubert, HB, et al: Obesity as an independent risk factor for cardiovascular disease: 26-year follow-up of participants in the Framingham Study. Circulation 67:968, 1983.
46. Vague, J: The degree of masculine differentiation of obesities: A factor determining predisposition to diabetes, atherosclerosis, gout and uric calculus disease, Am J Clin Nutr 4:20, 1956.
47. Larsson, B, et al: Abdominal adipose tissue distribution, obesity and the risk of caridiovascular disease and death: 13-year follow-up of participants in the study of men born in 1913. Br Med J 388:1401, 1984.
48. Stokes, J III, Garrison, RJ, and Kannel, WB: The independent contributions of various indices of obesity to the 22-year incidence of coronary heart disease: The Framingham Study. In Vague, J (ed): Metabolic Complication of Human Obesities. Elsevier Science Publishers, New York, 1985.
49. Baumgarter RN, et al: Fatness and fat patterns: Associations with plasma lipids and blood pressures in adults, 18–57 years of age. Am J Epidem 126:614, 1987.
50. Kannel, WB, et al: Fibrinogen and the risk of cardiovascular disease. JAMA 258:1183, 1987.
51. Kannel, WB, Hubert, HB and Lew, EA: Vital capacity as a predictor of cardiovascular disease: The Framingham Study. Am Heart J 105:311, 1983.
52. Goldman, L and Cook, EF: The decline in ischemic heart disease mortality rates: An analysis of the comparative effects of medical interventions and changes in life style. Ann Intern Med 101:825, 1984.
53. Stokes, J III: The methods of clinical prevention. In Vanderschmidt, H, et al (ed): Handbook of Clinical Prevention. Williams and Wilkins, Baltimore, 1987.

CHAPTER 2

Prevention of Adult Heart Disease Beginning in the Pediatric Age*†

Gerald S. Berenson, M.D.
Sathanur R. Srinivasan, Ph.D.
Theresa A. Nicklas, LDN, Dr.P.H.
Carolyn C. Johnson, M.S., N.C.C.

The development of the concept of cardiovascular risk factors in children has advanced our understanding of the early natural history of coronary artery disease and essential hypertension.[1-3] Although clinical manifestations of cardiovascular disease (CVD) appear only later in life, it is now recognized that atherosclerosis and essential hypertension begin in childhood.[4] The precise initiating factors of these diseases remain unknown, but a number of determinants of their early onset have been clarified. Understanding these determinants will aid in beginning prevention in the pediatric age.

Studies in adults have shown the importance of cardiovascular risk factors in predicting future morbidity and mortality in presumably healthy and asymptomatic individuals. Efforts to extend such predictive models to children have taken place over the past 15 years. Detailed observations on free-living children have defined methods to obtain cardiovascular risk factor information, just as on adults. However, inasmuch as the development of CVD is a lifelong process, the early development of risk factors and how they change over time are of particular importance to the study of children and young adults.

Longitudinal observations show that levels of risk factor variables tend to remain within a given rank relative to peers.[5,6] This "tracking" of risk factor variables implies cardiovascular risk may be predictable from observations made in

*This research was supported by funds from the National Heart, Lung, and Blood Institute of the United States Public Health Service (USPHS) (HL-38844).

†This study would not have been possible without the generous support and participation of the young adults and their parents in Bogalusa, Louisiana, and in the Jefferson Parish (county) school system.

early life. Levels of serum total cholesterol and low-density lipoprotein cholesterol (LDL-C) track rather well, whereas blood pressure rankings persist somewhat less well. The fact that tracking does occur, however, suggests a potential for defining future cardiovascular risk in children. The identification of a child at high risk for the likelihood of future CVD, especially one with a positive family history of heart disease, is the first step toward beginning prevention.

The interrelationships of risk factors in children are similar to those observed in adults.[7,8] Excess body weight and fatness relate adversely to other risk factor variables, just as in adults. Interestingly, in childhood these relationships are greater in white children than they are in black children. A clustering of risk factors occurs slightly in young children but increases in older schoolchildren. Although not considered a major risk factor as such, obesity in childhood not only reflects a relationship to higher blood pressure levels and adverse serum lipid and lipoprotein changes but also to aberration of carbohydrate metabolism, reflected as higher insulin levels.

VALIDATION OF CARDIOVASCULAR RISK FACTORS IN CHILDREN

Inasmuch as the morbid events of CVD do not occur in the child and young adult age period, it is difficult to establish the significance of clinical and laboratory cardiovascular risk factor observations in children. Yet certain approaches have helped in this regard. Without elaborating in too great detail, echocardiographic studies have shown evidence of cardiac enlargement associated with higher blood pressure levels in children.[9,10] These blood pressure levels are much lower than usually accepted as abnormal in adults, but in those children with blood pressure persisting at the 90th percentile, the posterior wall and septal thickness are increased; wall stress is increased, along with certain hemodynamic changes, such as increased cardiac output and peripheral resistance.[11] Furthermore, studies with ultrasonic techniques have also demonstrated decreased elasticity of carotid arteries, especially in white boys with a parental history of myocardial infarction.[12]

Perhaps most significant are studies of actual anatomic changes that occur in the cardiovascular system seen at autopsy (Fig. 2–1). In the Bogalusa Heart Study, a pediatric pathology study has been conducted over the past 10 years.[4,13] Studies of the aorta and the coronary arteries in individuals who died mostly by accidental means were compared with antemortem risk factors. The observations regarding the evolution of lesions are in concert with those found earlier by autopsies conducted on soldiers in the Korean and Vietnam wars[12,14,15] and in the Community Pathology Study in the New Orleans area.[16,17] That is, fatty streaks begin to appear, especially in the aorta, in very young children, but fatty streaks and raised fibrous plaque lesions develop in the coronary vessels in the second and third decades of life. In the aorta, there is a remarkably close relationship between fatty streaks and serum cholesterol as well as LDL-C.[4] There is also a greater surface involvement with such lesions occurring in black young adults.[13] In contrast, the more significant fatty streaks and fibrous plaque lesions in the coronary vessels occur primarily in young male adults, especially in white men.[17] Here, the relationship is weak with serum total cholesterol and LDL-C but significant with serum triglycerides, systolic blood pressure, and high-density lipoprotein cholesterol (HDL-C, a negative association). The variations occurring in the different vascular sites may relate to some-

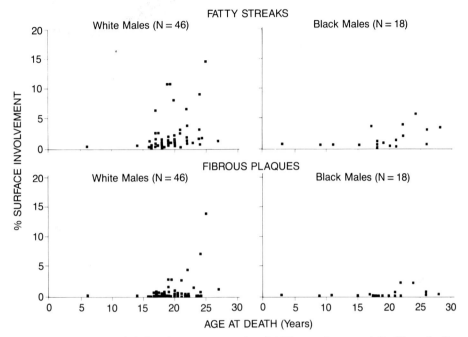

Figure 2–1. Atherosclerotic lesions in coronary arteries of children and young adults. (From the Bogalusa Heart Study.)

what different mechanisms in the pathogenesis of the disease. In the coronary vessels, a relationship to multiple cardiovascular risk factors exists and it is very likely that lesions relate to other mechanisms, for example, endothelium-platelet interactions. The relationship of antemortem studies of cardiovascular risk factors in children clearly has significance as indicated by the strong association of these factors with the development of atherosclerotic disease.

There have been many reviews on the management of high blood pressure levels in children, and recommendations have been made by an extensive task force report from the National Institutes of Health.[18] We also have conducted a clinical trial to control high blood pressure levels in children tracking at or above the 90th percentile.[19,20] Primary intervention was combined with very low-dose medication to modulate the blood pressure levels. Because there has been recent attention given to cholesterol levels among the general population, the following material focuses primarily on serum lipids and lipoproteins in children and on approaches to control hyperlipidemia through dietary and behavioral modifications.

LIPOPROTEINS IN CHILDREN AND ADOLESCENTS

The occurrence of lipoprotein abnormalities primarily related to inborn errors of metabolism (monogenic) is uncommon. For example, only about 10 percent of children with serum cholesterol levels above the 95th percentile can be categorized as having the genetically inherited condition of familial hypercholesterolemia. The

majority of individuals with high cholesterol levels have polygenic hypercholesterolemia, a condition more prevalent in populations in which diets are habitually rich
in saturated fat and cholesterol.[21]

Interindividual variability in serum cholesterol levels within a given population is determined by the interactions of environmental factors with an individual's
genotype. On an individual basis, although an individual's genotype sets a range
within which the serum cholesterol level (phenotype) will fall, environmental factors determine the phenotype's distribution within that range. Therefore, it is
important to understand the factors that alter serum cholesterol levels in childhood.
First, serum cholesterol levels vary at different age periods into adulthood, as shown
in Table 2–1. Furthermore, because serum cholesterol represents both atherogenic

Table 2–1. Serum Lipids and Lipoprotein Levels for
Infants, Children, and Young Adults (Bogalusa Heart
Study)

Age (Years)	Total Cholesterol		Triglycerides (mg/dl)	
	Median	*(90th P)*	*Median*	*(90th P)*
Birth	68	94	34	67
6 months	132	173	81	141
1–2	147	179	64	120
3–4	157	191	56	95
5–6	158	194	51	88
7–8	163	196	53	92
9–10	165	203	57	106
11–12	161	200	61	115
13–14	155	192	61	109
15–16	151	189	61	109
17–18	155	200	63	106
19–20	160	210	76	136
21–22	165	215	78	156
23–24	170	219	81	164
25–26	177	221	85	186

Age (Years)	Cholesterol Fractions (mg/dl)					
	HDL-C		LDL-C		VLDL-C	
	(10th P)	*Median*	*Median*	*(90th P)*	*Median*	*(90th P)*
Birth	18	35	29	43	2	9
6 mo	27	51	73	99	9	22
1–2	33	55	85	113	6	16
3–4	36	59	92	122	4	13
5–6	43	67	86	117	4	13
7–8	43	66	91	123	4	14
9–10	40	67	91	127	5	17
11–12	38	62	90	123	7	19
13–14	37	61	84	117	7	19
15–16	35	58	82	118	8	19
17–18	35	57	89	128	8	19
19–20	24	51	101	143	9	22
21–22	23	50	102	155	10	27
23–24	23	52	106	155	10	29
25–26	23	52	116	156	12	34

(LDL and very low-density lipoproteins [VLDL]) and antiatherogenic HDL particles, it is imperative that these alterations are studied in terms of individual lipoprotein fractions, especially the cholesterol and apolipoprotein (apo) components.
Although cholesterol screening is widely advocated, ultimately serum lipoproteins
should be defined for a guide to treatment[22] and perhaps even apolipoproteins to
detect subsets of individuals in families at high risk. [23]

LEVELS AT BIRTH AND CHANGES THROUGH ADOLESCENCE

It is evident that differences in serum cholesterol levels between divergent cul-
tures begin early in childhood.[24] Levels of children in populations having high rates
of coronary heart disease (CHD) are shifted toward higher values in comparison
with children from low-risk populations, although the levels at birth are around 70
mg per dl in all populations.

The serum lipoprotein profiles undergo considerable changes during two
important developmental phases, from birth through the first 2 years of life and
during sexual maturation. Percentile grids for age, race, and sex have been published.[3] Low levels of apo B–containing lipoproteins in neonates may be due to the
absence of exogenous fat in the lipid transport system. In infants, however, exogenous fat may play an important role in determining the mode of lipoprotein-lipid
transport, both qualitatively and quantitatively.[25] The mean levels of serum cholesterol essentially approach the young adult levels by 2 years of age.[26] Dynamic
changes occur in levels of serum lipoproteins (lipids, apo B and apo A-I) during
adolescence and sexual maturation that are determined by sex and race.[27–29] Serum
HDL cholesterol (HDL-C) declines in white adolescent males, whereas in females
and black males the decrease is mainly in LDL-C. On the one hand, serum LDL-
C begins to increase in the four race-sex groups at maturation, whereas HDL-C
continues to decrease in white males. On the other hand, VLDL cholesterol
(VLDL-C) increases in all children during puberty; unlike females, males continue
to show elevated levels after sexual maturation. Thus, lipoprotein transitions occur
during sexual maturation, establishing adult patterns of increased levels of both
VLDL-C and LDL-C and decreased levels of HDL-C in males versus females.

The most striking change during sexual maturation is the progressive increase
of the ratio of LDL-C to HDL-C in white males[27] (Fig. 2–2). In addition, the ratio
of HDL-C/apo A-I decreases markedly during this period, reflecting a disproportionate decrease of cholesterol, in relation to apo A-I, in HDL particles.[29] The fact
that this change is not seen in the other three race-sex groups has important clinical
implications for future development of CHD in white men.

Marked variation in the composition of lipoprotein particles occurs among
children.[29–34] For example, although the ratio of cholesterol to apo B in LDL varied
from 1.03 (10th percentile) to 1.37 (90th percentile), the ratio of cholesterol to apo
A-I in HDL varied from 0.27 (10th percentile) to 0.57 (90th percentile). It is obvious, therefore, that measuring lipoprotein cholesterol alone does not accurately
reflect lipoprotein concentration (particle number). Moreover, the lipoprotein
compositional differences noted in childhood may have a bearing on the predictions of CHD later in life. It is likely that a subgroup of children with disproportionate increase in apo B relative to cholesterol in LDL may be at an increased risk
because of the heritability and atherogenic potential of such LDL particles.[33,34] In
general, white children have relatively apo B-enriched LDL particles when compared with black children.[32] This may confer additional CHD risk on white males

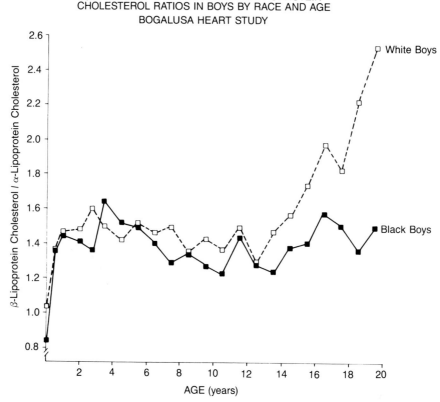

Figure 2–2. β-lipoprotein cholesterol/α-lipoprotein cholesterol ratios in boys by race and age. (From the Bogalusa Heart Study.)

who have already low levels of antiatherogenic HDL compared with the other race-sex groups.

BODY HABITUS

Both cross-sectional and longitudinal observations in children show a positive relation of various indices of obesity with VLDL-C and LDL-C and a negative association with HDL-C.[35–37] The finding that controlling for serum triglycerides (VLDL) eliminated the association between obesity and HDL-C suggests a direct relation of obesity to VLDL rather than HDL metabolism.[38] Obesity in childhood seems to have a threshold effect on lipoproteins, with increasing associations apparent at or above the 70th percentile of skinfold thickness.[39] In general, the associations are strongest in white males and weakest in black females, although black females tend to show higher indices of obesity.[37] The disturbances in carbohydrate metabolism are more strongly related to central body fat than to peripheral body fat even in childhood.[40] The significance of such associations is that a clustering of measures of central body fat, hyperinsulinemia, and adverse lipoprotein profile occurs early in life, especially in white males (Fig. 2–3). The relationship of even mild obesity (less than 15 percent above ideal body weight) to observations in car-

Mean HDL-C Levels Related to Sexual Maturation, Obesity,
and Insulin Levels in Nonsmoking, Nondrinking White Males (n = 767)
Bogalusa Heart Study

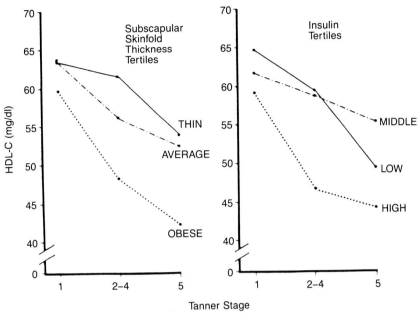

Figure 2–3. Mean HDL-C levels related to sexual maturation, obesity, and insulin levels in nonsmoking, nondrinking white males (n = 767). (From the Bogalusa Heart Study.)

bohydrate and lipid metabolism, especially in white males, has important implications for intervention early in life.

FAMILIAL AGGREGATION

The levels of serum lipids and lipoproteins aggregate in families.[41–45] Both heritability and common environment contribute in varying degrees to the phenomenon of familial aggregation.[44,46,47] It is of interest that heritability is predominant for LDL-C in whites, and for triglycerides in blacks, whereas environment is very significant for LDL-C in blacks and for HDL-C in whites.[44]

The familial aggregation of adverse levels of lipoproteins appears to account in part for the aggregation of CHD in families. Elevated levels of serum cholesterol in children are predictors of CHD mortality in their grandfathers.[42,48] However, the associations between paternal CHD and serum lipid/lipoprotein cholesterol levels in their offspring have been found by some workers,[49–52] although not by others.[53,54] The discrepancy may be due to the fact that some parents are too young to have reached the typical age for clinical onset of disease. Additionally, the measurement of the cholesterol moiety of the lipoproteins may not be sensitive enough to detect subtle differences in lipoprotein concentration and characteristics. Recently, child-parent associations have been examined in a community-based study of school-age children.[23] It appears that children whose fathers had a myocardial infarction are

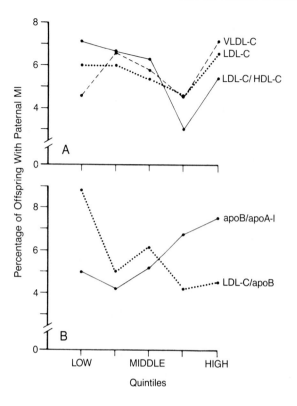

Figure 2–4. Percentage of offspring with paternal myocardial infarction.

more likely to be white, to be older, to smoke cigarettes, and to be more obese than are children whose fathers did not report a myocardial infarction.

Children whose fathers reported having had an infarction show significantly low mean levels of apo A-I and low LDL-C/apo B ratios, along with high apo B/apo A-I ratios. Furthermore, gradients in the relation of paternal myocardial infarction are evident across the ranges in values of both apo B/apo A-I ratio (a positive association) and the LDL-C/apo B ratio (a negative association) (Fig. 2–4). In contrast, cholesterol content of individual lipoprotein fractions in children is not related to paternal myocardial infarction. It appears that adverse apo A-I and apo B profiles may be evident in early life, long before the clinical symptoms begin. This finding has implication for preventive cardiology. Additional studies are necessary to evaluate the utility and practicality of measuring these apolipoproteins routinely.

LIFE-STYLE AND BEHAVIOR

As one would expect from adult studies, life-style patterns, such as cigarette smoking, alcohol consumption, and oral contraceptive use, have independent effects on lipoproteins of adolescents. In repeated cross-sectional studies, higher VLDL-C and lower HDL-C are encountered in cigarette smokers, especially for white females.[55,56] The findings of a longitudinal follow-up study indicate that continued cigarette smoking, even at moderate levels, during adolescence and early adulthood contributes to an adverse lipoprotein profile, especially in white males.[57]

Similar to cigarette smoking, oral contraceptive use produces adverse lipoprotein changes.[56,58] In general, oral contraceptive use appears to accentuate the adverse effects of smoking on lipoproteins. It is of interest that, with respect to HDL constituents, both cholesterol and apo A-I are related negatively to smoking and positively to alcohol consumption, independent of age and adiposity, especially in females, whereas oral contraceptive use is associated with apo A-I positively and HDL-C negatively, especially in black females.[38] Black-white differences in the effects of oral contraceptive use appear to be related to a greater use of high-estrogen formulations by blacks. Estrogen-progestin contents and their ratio in oral contraceptives are known to affect HDL-C differently.[59]

The relation of Type A behavior to elevated serum lipids and proneness to coronary atherosclerosis has been known for some time.[60] Children who are in the upper quintile for Type A–like behavior, such as hard-driving, fast eating, and loud talking, have a relative elevation of VLDL-C and LDL-C.[61]

DIETARY INFLUENCE

Dietary nutrients are the important environmental variables affecting serum lipoproteins, despite continuing controversy. Infants who consume commercial formulas that contain low or no cholesterol and high polyunsaturated fatty acids have lower serum lipid and lipoprotein levels than infants who consume cow's milk or human milk.[62,63] An impressive association between dietary components and serum lipoproteins is found during the early childhood period. For example, at 12 months, LDL-C is significantly related to animal fat, cholesterol, and energy intake.[62] Furthermore, changes in dietary cholesterol intake from 6 months to 4 years of age are associated positively with changes in LDL-C levels during this period, independent of energy intake or body weight[64] (Fig. 2–5). However, older,

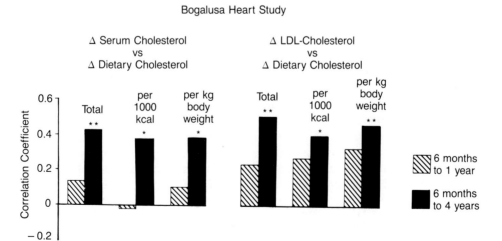

Figure 2–5. Spearman correlation coefficients of change in dietary cholesterol with change in serum total cholesterol and LDL-cholesterol. (From the Bogalusa Heart Study.)

school-aged children, like adults, show a weak (and sometimes no) association between nutrient intake and lipoprotein levels.[65-67] Categorical comparisons indicate that, in general, children with high serum cholesterol values show higher fat intakes (and lower carbohydrate intakes) than those with low serum cholesterol values.[65] It is of interest that longer eating spans result in significantly greater serum cholesterol values, reflecting greater intakes of calories, fat, and cholesterol.[65]

The findings that modifiable factors, such as diet, obesity, life-style, and behavioral patterns, influence lipoprotein levels in children underscore the potential for management of hyperlipoproteinemia and beginning primary prevention of CHD.

EATING PATTERNS OF AMERICAN CHILDREN

A look at what American children are now eating, as determined by the Bogalusa Heart Study and applicable to the dietary health of children in the United States in general, provides some background data before dietary recommendations can be made. The quantification and characterization of the dietary intake of children are of major importance. In the Bogalusa Heart Study, dietary data have been collected on infants, preschoolers, school-aged children, and adolescents[68] in an effort to evaluate environmental factors that affect cardiovascular risk beginning in early life.

INFANTS

Dietary data were obtained on a newborn infant cohort representing all live births in the community during an 18-month period. At the time of the study, 1974 to 1975, more than 78 percent of the infants received commercial formula at 1 month of age. Only 8 percent of the infants were breast-fed, and 4 percent consumed whole or evaporated cow's milk. Considerable variation occurs in infant diets, that is, the type of milk or formula and the introduction of foods. As might be expected, the use of whole or evaporated milk increases with age, whereas consumption of commercial formula decreases with age. The number of mothers breast-feeding in the United States has apparently increased, with newborns receiving breast milk plus formula more than doubling from the 1970s to 1980s. The exclusive use of cow's milk, evaporated milk, and prepared formula has decreased during this time.[69]

The early introduction of commercial baby foods into the infants' eating pattern was common, although current recommendations are to delay this habit. In the study of this infant cohort, by 1 month of age, over 10 percent of the infants were fed eggs, meat, desserts, and vegetables; 55 percent were fed strained fruit; and over 80 percent were fed cereal. By 4 to 6 months of age, the percentage of infants consuming commercial baby foods began to decline as more table foods were consumed. By 4 months of age, 50 percent of the infants were eating table foods, and by 1 year, virtually all infants were eating adult foods.

PRESCHOOLERS (AGED 6 MONTHS TO 4 YEARS)

There is a fourfold increase in sodium intake from age 6 months (0.88 g) to 4 years (3.21 g). When intake is expressed per kg of body weight, the nutrient density for preschoolers exceeds that of adolescents by 30 to 50 percent. Dietary total sodium intake of 4-year-olds approaches levels ingested by adolescents.[70]

The percentages of energy from selected dietary components presented in Table 2–2 for children 6 months to 17 years of age exceed the Recommended Daily Allowances at all ages. Carbohydrates provide approximately 49 to 55 percent of energy. The percentage of carbohydrate contributed by sucrose is double the 10 percent recommendation at 6 months and increases to 41 percent by 4 years. Mean percent of energy from protein (approximately 13 percent) approaches the recommended level at all ages studied, but the mean percent of energy from fat exceeds the 30 percent recommendation from 6 months (35 percent) to 17 years of age (40 percent) The low P/S ratio (less than 1.0) at all ages reflects a high saturated fat (14 to 16 percent) and low polyunsaturated fat (5 to 7 percent) diet.[71]

Mean dietary cholesterol intake per 1000 kcal was 106 mg at 6 months. The level increases to 193 mg at 2 years and then decreases slightly to 172 mg at 4 years of age. On a per kg body weight basis, dietary cholesterol averages 24 mg per kg body weight for preschoolers compared with 10 mg per kg body weight for 10-year-old children in Bogalusa. More than 65 percent of the 2- to 4-year-olds exceed the cholesterol recommendation of 100 mg per 1000 kcal.[71]

Of particular interest is the observation that tracking of dietary components begins as early as age 2 years. Sixty-nine percent of 2-year-old children in the upper tertile for dietary cholesterol intake remain in the upper tertile at age 4. This number is twice as many as would be expected by chance. Sixty-three percent of the children in the upper tertile for saturated fat intake at age 2 remain in the upper tertile at age 4. Similar results are noted for energy intake and several other dietary components.[72]

SCHOOL-AGED CHILDREN

School-aged children eat the typical American adult diet, characterized by high intakes of sodium, refined carbohydrates, and animal protein and fat and low intakes of potassium, complex carbohydrates, and vegetable protein and fat[73] (see Table 2).

Mean energy intake ranges from 2144 calories (age 10) to 2438 calories (age 17) (see Table 2–2). Boys consume more calories than girls. The mean protein density of the diet was consistent over time and varies from 13 to 14 percent of calories. Protein is mainly from animal sources, whereas half of the total energy intake comes from carbohydrate. Carbohydrate intake shows a sucrose to starch proportion of greater than one, which reflects a large sucrose intake. On the average, the percentage of calories from sucrose approaches 18 percent or greater. Mean fat intake contributes 39 to 41 percent of the total calories from ages 10 to 17 years. Saturated fat intake is high and produces a P/S ratio of less than 0.4. Dietary cholesterol intake increases from age 10 (302 mg) to age 17 (378 mg). On a per 1000 kcal basis, dietary cholesterol is approximately 125 to 150 mg per 1000 kcal and exceeds the 100 mg recommended in the Step 1 diet of the American Heart Association. There is no significant increase in sodium intake, ranging from 3 to 3.5 g in children 10 to 17 years of age.[68,70,73]

In general, the composition of children's diets is not vastly different from the diets of the majority of individuals in the United States.[74–77] No significant seasonal variations were observed in the food intakes.[65] Although food substitutions occur with seasons, and menus may vary from diets of Bogalusa children, the macronutrient composition of the diets is similar. Food market surveys have reported shifts in fat sources and availability,[78–80] and a change was documented in Bogalusa with

Table 2-2. Composition of Diets of Young Children and Adolescents by Age Compared with Current Dietary Recommendations (Bogalusa Heart Study)

Dietary Component	Age (Yr)									Current Dietary Recommendations (after age 2)*
	0.5 (n = 125)	1 (n = 99)	2 (n = 135)	3 (n = 106)	4 (n = 219)	10 (n = 871)	13 (n = 148)	15 (n = 108)	17 (n = 159)	
Energy (kcal)	949	1356	1922	2162	2258	2144	2361	2334	2438	
Protein (% kcal)	13	14	13	12	13	13	13	14	14	15%
Carbohydrate (% kcal)	55	49	48	51	49	49	47	50	46	55%
Sucrose (% kcal)	14	14	19	22	21	18	18	18	19	10%
Su/St Ratio†	1.10	0.93	1.36	1.44	1.34	1.07	1.08	0.95	1.19	<1
Fat (% kcal)	35	39	41	38	39	39	41	38	40	30%
Saturated Fat (% kcal)	16	17	16	14	14	15	15	13	14	10%
P/S ratio†	0.36	0.33	0.44	0.49	0.51	0.43	0.43	0.53	0.51	>1
Cholesterol (mg)	110	247	376	347	390	302	306	336	378	100 mg/1000 kcal
mg/1000 kcal	106	183	193	164	172	138	129	146	151	(not to exceed 300 mg/day)
Sodium (g)	0.88	1.85	2.67	2.97	3.21	3.51	3.39	3.59	3.67	1 g/1000 kcal
g/1000 kcal	0.90	1.35	1.39	1.37	1.43	1.67	1.47	1.57	1.59	(not to exceed 3 g/day)
g/kg body weight	0.12	0.19	0.22	0.21	0.20	0.10	0.07	0.06	0.06	

*American Heart Association; Surgeon General's 1990 Objectives for the Nation; The US Senate Select Committee on Nutrition and Human Needs; National Heart, Lung, and Blood Institute; American Society for Clinical Nutrition; American Medical Association; Food and Nutrition Board.

†Su/St ratio = sucrose/starch ratio. P/S ratio = polyunsaturated fatty acids/saturated fatty acids ratio.

a shift toward higher values in the P/S ratio (0.29 to 0.44) from 1973 to 1982. This shift could be explained by changes in the food industry and consumer habits;[78,81] however, the P/S ratio is still below 1.0. These observations indicate a continued need for improvement in the fatty acid composition of the American diet as well as for other components.

FOOD SOURCES OF DIETARY COMPONENTS

Dietary data collected in the Bogalusa Heart Study on children 6 months to 17 years of age provide quantitative information regarding the contribution of selected foods to the dietary intake. As expected, the majority of the nutrients come from milk or formula at 6 months of age, with a notable change in eating patterns at age 1 to include a larger variety of foods. The percent of total energy intake from meats increases from 6.2 percent (6 months) to 17 percent (4 years). Dairy products contribute 51 percent of the total energy intake at 6 months and 12 percent at 17 years. Vegetables contribute 5 to 8 percent at all ages. Fruits contribute 12 percent of energy intake at 6 months of age but only 4 percent in 17-year-olds. The major sources of total fat and saturated fat in rank order for preschool children are beef, milk, pork, and desserts. There is a decrease in percent of total fat coming from poultry and an increase in fat coming from pork from age 2 to age 17. The percent of cholesterol intake at ages two and 17 from milk (18 percent versus 11 percent), eggs (45 percent versus 24 percent), and beef (7 percent versus 19 percent) shows a decrease in egg consumption and an increase in beef consumption as children get older. The major food sources of sodium are processed breads, grains, cereals, veg-

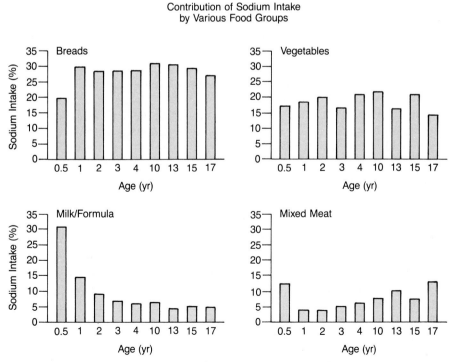

Figure 2–6. Contribution of sodium intake by various food groups.

etables, and mixed meats. The bread group contributes approximately one third of the total sodium intake in school-aged children. Vegetables contribute, on the average, 19 percent of the total sodium intake. Inasmuch as fresh vegetables are not high in sodium, the sodium is being added as a preservative to canned vegetables or during food preparation with salty meats and added salt. The combined contribution of sodium from mixed meats, pork, and beef increases with age (Fig. 2–6).

The percent of total sucrose intake from fruits decreases from 6 months of age (47 percent) to age 17 (11 percent). Percent of sucrose intake at 6 months and 17 years of age from milk (12 percent versus <1 percent), beverages (7 percent versus 21 percent), candy (11 percent versus 31 percent), and dessert (14 percent versus 20 percent) shows an increase in sugary foods and drinks and a decrease in milk consumption.

DIETARY GUIDELINES

The scope of measures for promotion of healthy eating habits are outlined. Necessary though these measures are, it must be recognized that change in eating behavior requires years for its full implementation. This time course will facilitate adoption of the criteria for optimal nutrition by the food-producing and food-distribution industries.

RECOMMENDATIONS BEFORE AGE TWO

Consistent tracking of dietary components, cardiovascular risk factors, and their interrelationships, beginning as early as age two, supports the recommendation that intervention should begin in early childhood. Although little change is advocated before age two, a "modified cardiovascular-eating approach" should be instituted during early childhood. If the following changes are made in infant feeding practices, this would approach the prudent recommendations of the American Heart Association and American Academy of Pediatrics. Keys to early prevention are breast-feeding from birth and delaying introduction of solid foods until four to six months of age. The adoption of healthy eating habits should focus on moderation rather than on elimination of certain foods during the first two years of life. A variety of nutritionally balanced foods should be gradually introduced. Energy intake should be based on growth requirements so as to maintain desirable body weight. The use of salt, sugar, and condiments in infant milk and in food preparation should be avoided.

RECOMMENDATIONS AFTER AGE TWO

The dietary goals for children from age two years would be to consume sufficient calories for adequate growth, containing no more than 30 percent from fat, with most of the energy difference coming from vegetable proteins and complex carbohydrates. Saturated, polyunsaturated, and monounsaturated fatty acids should provide 10 percent each of total calories. Cholesterol intake should be limited to less than 300 mg per day. These recommendations are similar to the Step 1 diet of the American Heart Association.

Salt intake should be no more than 5.0 g per day, and the fiber intake, particularly soluble fibers, should be increased. Many of the dietary suggestions made here have been made by others, notably the National Institutes of Health Consensus Conference[18] and the American Heart Association.[82] These suggestions have not been made, however, with a specific time and goal orientation. These dietary guidelines, recommended for the adult population, primarily should be ideal for optimal growth and are not, as has been shown, injurious for health when caloric intake is adequate.

PRACTICAL APPLICATION OF DIETARY RECOMMENDATIONS

Using the "food-group approach" to identify the major contributors of selected nutrients can be instrumental in developing realistic recommendations for dietary change. Substantial changes can be made in one's eating pattern through more selective food purchasing and food preparation techniques. For example, Figure 2–7 lists the major foods contributing to saturated fat in the diets of children. Mixed

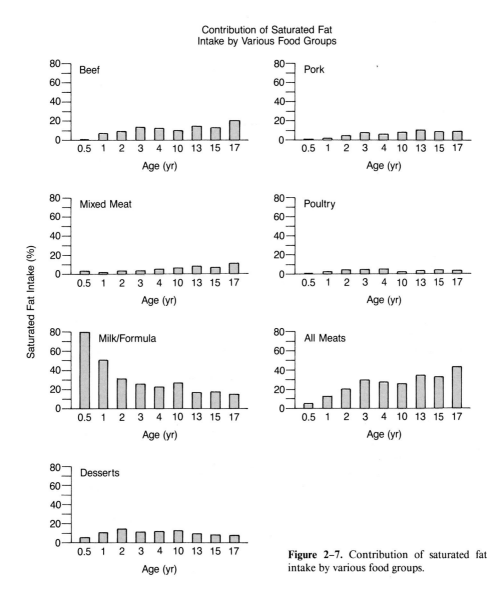

Figure 2–7. Contribution of saturated fat intake by various food groups.

meats, pork, beef, milk, desserts, and snacks are major contributors of saturated fat in children's diets. These food groups should become our major targets for lowering saturated fat intake. Prepackaged luncheon meats and hot dogs may contain 30 percent fat. A simple change from whole to low-fat or skim milk after age two would have a significant impact on the intake of saturated fat in children. The fatty, sugary desserts contributing 12 percent of the fat intake and 20 percent of the sucrose intake at age one year should be targeted for eating pattern intervention. Desserts yield twice the percentage of energy as either fruits or vegetables at age two years.

At all ages, the major source of sodium is the bread and cereal group. A switch to lower-salt varieties and less reliance on prepared and packaged mixes would have significant impact on sodium intake. How vegetables are purchased and prepared constitutes the second major food source of sodium to total daily intake. By purchasing fresh vegetables instead of canned vegetables and adding spices instead of salt during cooking and at the table, the amount of dietary sodium ingested would be decreased significantly.

Promotion of the current dietary goals at various ages can be accomplished more effectively by targeting major food sources for eating behavior change.

The following guidelines will assist individuals in adoping a healthier eating pattern:

Food Purchasing

1. Increase the proportion of lean beef (that is, tenderloin, round rump, sirloin tip), poultry, turkey, fish, shellfish, and low-fat dairy products in the diet. Ground meat can be made from lean cuts to achieve 5 to 8 percent fat instead of 25 percent. (Cooking techniques listed below can aid in reducing the fat content).
2. Increase the use of fruits and vegetables served in their natural state or with minimal preparation. Use whole-grain products.
3. Commercially prepared foods can be a major source of hidden fat. Rely on naturally sweet foods, such as fresh fruits and juices, for dessert items, using sugar only in moderation. Baked goods, in particular, often have highly saturated palm oil and coconut oil as ingredients to extend shelf life.
4. Choose commercially prepared foods more selectively. Use skim milk or low-fat milk (1 or 2 percent) instead of whole milk. Use cheeses made from skim or low-fat milk. Read labels for fat content. Some cheeses made from skim milk have fat contents as high as 8 or 9 percent. Use ice milk, sherbets, or sorbet rather than ice cream.

Food Preparation

1. Bake, broil, roast, or stew meats instead of frying.
2. Trim all visible fat from meats.
3. Drain all fat off cooked meat, such as ground meat.
4. Bake or roast meat on a meat rack so that fat drips off and can be discarded.
5. Remove the skin from chicken.
6. Use a nonstick spray made from vegetable oil or a nonstick pan to sautee foods that do not need a lot of oil, such as eggs, French toast, pancakes, and so forth.

Table 2–3. High-Fiber Foods

	Serving	Grams of Fiber
Breads and Cereals		
All-Bran, Extra Fiber	½ cup	13.0
Fiber-One	½ cup	12.0
All-Bran, Fruit & Almonds	⅔ cup	10.0
100% Bran	½ cup	8.4
All-Bran	½ cup	8.5
Bran Buds	⅓ cup	7.9
Oat Bran	⅓ cup	4.9
Legumes, Cooked		
Kidney beans	½ cup	7.3
Lima Beans	½ cup	4.5
Navy beans	½ cup	6.0
Vegetables, Cooked		
Brussel sprouts	½ cup	2.3
Carrots	½ cup	2.3
Corn	½ cup	2.9
Green peas	½ cup	3.6
Parsnip	½ cup	2.7
Potato, with skin	1 medium	2.5
Fruits		
Apple	1 medium	3.5
Banana	1 medium	2.4
Dried prunes	3	3.0
Orange	1 medium	2.6
Raisins	¼ cup	3.1
Strawberries	1 cup	3.0

7. Lightly steam fresh vegetables rather than boil them.
8. Increase the use of spices and herbs that contain no sodium, both in cooking and at the table.

Introduction of foods with high fiber, especially soluble fiber as in oat bran, can aid in lowering serum total cholesterol and LDL-C.[83] Table 2–3 lists high-fiber foods.

Because hyperlipidemia is so prevalent among children, we need to set forth a national policy to reduce the intake of saturated fat and cholesterol in our national diet—a goal that can be accomplished by both consumer education and modification of the food supply.

ROLE OF THE FOOD INDUSTRY

The food industry can contribute considerably through the use of more detailed labels and modification of prepared foods. Basically, industry needs to lower the saturated fat, cholesterol, and sodium content of its products. Such a policy should apply not only to food manufacturers but also to food distributors, from fast food chains to high-end restaurants to supermarkets. The food industry has the means as well as the capacity to influence the nutritional thinking of the public. The food industry has a great potential to offer foods that fit within guidelines of recommended food intake and healthy nutrition.

BEHAVIORAL APPROACHES TO BEGINNING PREVENTION

Traditional dietary recommendations by medical and dietary professionals generally have been unsuccessful. Various reasons underlie the development of behavioral strategies in dietary intervention with children. Behavioral approaches combined with medical and nutrition expertise offer viable means to aid primary prevention of cardiovascular risk factors. A behavioral approach, for example, is important in control of obesity, which has been a difficult area to attack in childhood. In the Bogalusa Heart Study, obesity shows a major interaction with serum lipids and lipoproteins, blood pressure, and even blood glucose and insulin levels. Indications are that, since the initial observations in 1973, children are becoming heavier and fatter.

Coupled with medical intervention, behavioral strategies serve to reinforce adoption of healthy life-styles. Two valuable techniques for behavioral health programs are counseling and contingency contracting. Individual, group, or family counseling has been successful in a wide range of behavioral health areas, including cholesterol-lowering dietary intervention. Singleton and associates,[84] using counseling with contingency contracting in an adult cholesterol reduction program, were successful in reaching goals by 60 percent of contract signers. A strong relationship was found between diet changes and lower serum cholesterol levels, as might be expected.

A positive family history of heart disease provides the impetus to recommend dietary counseling within a family context. An optimum setting for family counseling can be achieved by a behavior counselor, a nutrition counselor, or both. To effect change in children's dietary habits in an isolated context has not been successful (for example, attempts to treat childhood obesity). The growing child is an integral part of the family, subject to parental influence and development of life-styles of the family. Even though children make some meal and snack decisions, they basically eat what and how the family eats. By developing rapport within the family system, professionals can assess positive family functioning, such as intra-familial support and cooperation, or negative processes, such as competitiveness and sabotage. Once assessments have been made, counselors can begin the enhancement of social support within the family. This important psychosocial variable has been shown to be an essential determinant of adherence to medical protocols and a strong predictor of success.

Counseling provides the opportunity for development of social support between family members by (1) information transfer concerning benefits of supportive relationships, (2) specific problem-solving strategies, and (3) modeling strategies. These can best be illustrated by an example. The family is informed that working together to achieve specific goals will be a family project and that each family member will have a role in this project. Giving each other support leads to success and an opportunity for people who care about each other (information transfer). Mom acknowledges this but states that Dad, who is underweight and has no cholesterol problem, enjoys ice cream very much and brings a quart home every evening, which the family eats for dessert. The dilemma is how can she not allow the child to eat the ice cream, but, on the other hand, how can she ask her husband to give up something he enjoys? Counselors work with the family through a problem-solving process in which each family member takes an active part, and compromises are worked out (problem solving). Possible solutions are modeled within the counseling session, and the family makes an active decision together about which solution to try (modeling, decision making).

The contingency contract is a useful tool within the counseling paradigm. Culture in the United States places a great deal of value on a signed, written contract, and that value is put to good use in health programs. A contract consists of three major components: (1) a specific behavior to be performed or goal to be reached, (2) a specific time period, and (3) a specific reward for achievement. Once the problem solving and modeling are accomplished, the family is ready to set goals, which are then incorporated into the contract. It is the professional's responsibility to guide the family in the goal-setting process. Major goals are best accomplished by reduction to small, realistic, and achievable steps. This shaping process results in successive approximations to a desired objective and sidesteps failures that can hinder progress. Rewards that act as reinforcements are essential and can be given by the counselors or can be agreed on between family members.

The use of self-monitoring, a necessary tool in dietary management, is beneficial to clients as well as to professionals. The information provided by self-monitoring is required by professionals to understand eating behavior, not only kind and quantity of food intake and preparation but also total eating patterns. For this reason, counselors should make every effort to be creative when developing self-monitoring techniques, and careful training with clients should take place in the counseling session. It is unfortunately true that most adults tend to underestimate intake in monitoring, and children may simply forget. In addition, self-monitoring is judged by subjects to be unpleasant. Creativity, training, and ample reinforcement for accurate recording, along with an active support network within the family, will help to eliminate some of the aforementioned problems. Helping family members to use self-monitoring to observe their own behavior and to acquire an appreciation for dietary stimulus control will make recording challenging and productive.

STRATEGIES FOR PREVENTIVE CARDIOLOGY IN PEDIATRICS—HEART SMART PROGRAM

There are two intervention strategies for the control of CVD beginning in childhood. These are the *population strategy* and the *high-risk strategy*. The population strategy, or public health approach, involves intervention on the total population, including those with projected risk for CVD along with those who would not be considered at risk. In the public health approach, an attempt is made to shift the distribution of risk factors affecting the total population to achieve a lower risk (for example, shifting the total population of serum total cholesterol of 160 mg/dl average for children to that of 140 mg/dl). In approaching the pediatric population, the effort would be to encourage the adoption of healthy life-styles rather than to encourage behavior modification, as needed in older individuals.

POPULATION STRATEGY—PROGRAM FOR SCHOOLCHILDREN

A number of programs have been developed for schoolchildren (K–6) as an ideal target population to begin prevention of heart disease. One such model, the Heart Smart program, has been developed for elementary schoolchildren and encompasses the total school environment.[85,86] This program includes development of an extensive cardiovascular health curriculum,[87] modification of school lunch and snack foods,[88] development of an exercise program aimed at achievable and lifelong exercise habits,[89] and adoption of good behavioral skills, especially coping skills and decision making.[90] Of importance in this program is the development of a sense of self-image, self-identity, and responsibility for one's health in an effort to motivate young children to have an interest in their own health. An inoculation for good cardiovascular health behavior in young children should also apply to cigarette smoking, drug abuse, and even dropout in the later grades of school. This is an exciting program being developed for the total elementary school population of students, staff, and parents. Importantly, the school program focuses on the total school environment to affect a change and includes involving a supporting role for parents.[90]

HIGH-RISK STRATEGY—FAMILY HEALTH PROMOTION

Another component, which is described subsequently, is the Heart Smart Family Health Promotion program developed for a school setting. This is more akin to the high-risk approach as generally applied by a physician in practice. The high-risk strategy intervenes on individuals noted to have abnormal cardiovascular risk factors. In one sense, it is the approach of the physician who applies both primary and secondary treatment to patients. In the high-risk individual, when there is a strong genetic component, primary intervention may not be adequate, and intervention or treatment requires the use of medication to control the risk factors (for example, familial hypercholesterolemia).

Important to the application of medical, primary, and drug management of individuals is the use of behavioral concepts for the implementation of prevention. Recently, in a Jefferson Parish (county), Louisiana, elementary school, a family-based cardiovascular risk reduction program was developed to be implemented in a school setting.[91,92] A school cardiovascular screening identified children who had elevated blood pressure, weight, and blood lipids, based on percentile norms developed in the Bogalusa Heart Study.[2,3] These children and their parents were recruited to participate in a 12-week program aimed at dietary management; increased levels of physical activity and aerobic conditioning; and enhanced psychosocial aspects, such as social support, self-efficacy, and health knowledge and involvement. To accomplish this goal, counseling and contingency contracting as well as information transfer were used. A multidisciplinary team, including a behaviorist, a nutritionist, and an exercise physiologist, met with parents and children. Actual hands-on activities were emphasized. Brief lectures were given, mild and gradually increasing exercise activities were performed, and a series of dietary demonstrations were provided. These demonstrations taught food preparation, shopping, label reading, dining out, and snacking strategies.[93] Intrafamily and interfamily social support were fostered throughout the program via information transfer, staff modeling, problem solving, and reinforcement.

With regard to cardiovascular risk factors, beginning the program with children is a *reverse* screening to detect adults at high risk. Children at high risk were first identified in the schools and then parents were selected to be examined. As expected, the parents also demonstrated a high prevalence of risk factors, such as obesity, hypertension, and inactivity.[94] The risk factors were targeted and a behavioral, nutrition, and exercise program was begun. Self-monitoring was instituted at least 2 days per week by each family member; problem areas were pinpointed; and problem solving, modeling, and decision making were the protocols used in each session. Each family member voluntarily signed a contract targeting individualized programs within the family context, and predetermined rewards were offered for contract performance.

In this program, children and parents demonstrated positive changes in eating habits, physical activity, health knowledge, and blood pressure. Significant changes in eating behavior were noted for total energy intake and percentage of energy from sugar for intervention children and total energy for intervention fathers. Nonsignificant decreases in total fat, percent total fat, and percent total sugar occurred for intervention mothers and children over a short period of time. Both parents and children, however, increased exercise behaviors and improved aerobic fitness. Alcohol and beer consumption was decreased, and parent blood pressure levels significantly decreased. Blood pressure decreases in children were clinically but not statistically significant.

The *Heart Smart Family Health Promotion* demonstrated that positive dietary changes can occur within a model of counseling and contracting, when social support, self-monitoring, and positive reinforcement are active components of that model.

Complications to the aforementioned approach, which uses the family to help with cardiovascular risk reduction in children, obviously can occur when the family structure is weak or not existent. Furthermore, it is apparent that such an approach may be applicable to a clinic setting but may be difficult for a school or a physician in practice to achieve. Time constraints, background training, and lack of personnel with special expertise are problems with this approach unless it is organized to use a multidisciplinary team.

SUMMARY

Many advances have now been made in understanding the early natural history of coronary artery disease and essential hypertension, an understanding that these diseases begin in childhood and that CVD relates to clinical cardiovascular risk factors. Methods have now been established to determine risk factors in the pediatric age and, with a family history, to begin to identify children at potential risk for premature heart disease.

Advances have also been made in developing models for intervention and beginning prevention through both high-risk and population strategies directed at schoolchildren. Obviously, both approaches are needed and complement each other. An impressive future is ahead for effective preventive cardiology beginning with children by incorporation of cardiovascular health education and health promotion in elementary schools. Applying behavioral concepts to intervention programs can strengthen their chances of success. The overall good of having children adopt healthy life-styles with an understanding of their necessity is now attainable. It will be the responsibility of physicians to guide the direction of programs being promoted for children.

REFERENCES

1. Lauer, RM and Shekelle, RB: Childhood Prevention of Atherosclerosis and Hypertension. Raven Press, New York, 1980.
2. Berenson, GS, et al: Cardiovascular Risk Factors in Children: The Early Natural History of Atherosclerosis and Essential Hypertension. Oxford University Press, New York, 1980.

3. Berenson, GS (ed): Causation of Cardiovascular Risk Factors in Children: Perspectives on Cardio-vascular Risk Factors in Early Life. Raven Press, New York, 1986.

4. Newman, WP, et al: Relation of serum lipoprotein levels and systolic blood pressure to early atherosclerosis: The Bogalusa Heart Study. N Engl J Med 314:138, 1986.

5. Clarke, W, et al: Tracking of blood pressure, serum lipids and obesity in children: The Muscatine Study. Circulation 54(Suppl 2):23, 1976.

6. Webber, LS, et al: Tracking of cardiovascular disease risk factor variables in school-age children. J Chron Dis 36:647, 1983.

7. Webber, LS, et al: Occurrence in children of multiple risk factors for coronary artery disease: The Bogalusa Heart Study. Prev Med 8:407, 1979.

8. Shear, CL, et al: Body fat patterning and blood pressure in children and young adults: The Bogalusa Heart Study. Hypertension 9:236, 1987.

9. Schieken, RM, Clarke, WR, and Lauer, RM: Left ventricular hypertrophy in children with blood pressure in the upper quintile of the distribution: The Muscatine Study. Hypertension 3:669, 1981.

10. Burke, GL, et al: Blood pressure and echocardiographic measures in children: The Bogalusa Heart Study. Circulation 75:106, 1987.

11. Soto, LF, et al: Echocardiographic functions and blood pressure levels in children and young adults from a biracial population: The Bogalusa Heart Study. AJMS 297:271, 1989.

12. Riley WA, et al: Decreased arterial elasticity associated with cardiovascular disease risk factors in the young: The Bogalusa Heart Study. Arteriosclerosis 6:378, 1986.

13. Freedman, DS, et al: Black/white differences in aortic fatty streaks in adolescence and early adulthood: The Bogalusa Heart Study. Circulation 77:856, 1988.

14. Enos, WF, Holmes, RH, and Beyer, J: Coronary disease among United States soldiers killed in action in Korea: Preliminary report. JAMA 152:1090, 1953.

15. McNamara, JJ, Molot, MA, and Stremple, JF: Coronary artery disease in combat casualties in Vietnam. JAMA 216:1185, 1971.

16. Holman, RL, et al: The natural history of atherosclerosis: The early aortic lesions as seen in New Orleans in the middle of the 20th century. Am J Pathol 34:209, 1958.

17. Berenson, GS: A. O. Beckman Conference: Cardiovascular risk factors in children and early prevention of heart disease. Clin Chem 34:B115, 1988.

18. NIH Consensus Development Conference Statement: Lowering blood cholesterol to prevent heart disease. JAMA 253:2080, 1985.

19. Frank, GC, et al: An approach to primary preventive treatment of children with high blood pressure. J Am Coll Nutr 1:357, 1982.

20. Berenson, GS, et al: A model of intervention for prevention of early essential hypertension in the 1980s. Hypertension 5:41, 1983.

21. Brown, MS and Goldstein, JL: How LDL receptors influence cholesterol and atherosclerosis. Sci Am 251:58, 1984.

22. Cresanta, JL, et al: Prevention of atherosclerosis in childhood. Pediatr Clin N Am 33:835, 1986.

23. Freedman, DS, et al: The relation of apolipoproteins A-I and B in children to parental myocardial infarction. N Engl J Med 315:721, 1986.

24. Berenson, GS and Epstein, FH (Chairmen): Conference on blood lipids in children: Optimal levels for early prevention of coronary artery disease. Workshop Report: Epidemiologic Section, American Health Foundation. Prev Med 12:741, 1983.

25. Hahn, P: Development of lipid metabolism. Annu Rev Nutr 2:91, 1982.

26. Berenson, GS, et al: Cardiovascular disease risk factor variables during the first year of life. Am J Dis Child 133:1049, 1979.

27. Berenson, GS, et al: Dynamic changes of serum lipoproteins in children during adolescence and sexual maturation. Am J Epidemiol 113:157, 1981.

28. Morrison, JA, et al: Lipids, lipoproteins and sexual maturation during adolescence: The Princeton Maturation Study. Metabolism 28:641, 1979.

29. Srinivasan, SR, et al: Serum apolipoproteins A-I and B in 2854 children from a biracial community: The Bogalusa Heart Study. Pediatrics 78:189, 1986.

30. Srinivasan, SR, Webber, LS, and Berenson, GS: Lipid composition and interrelationships of major serum lipoproteins: Observations in children with different lipoprotein profiles: The Bogalusa Heart Study. Arteriosclerosis 2:335, 1982.

31. Freedman, DS, et al: Divergent levels of high density lipoprotein cholesterol and apolipoprotein A-I in children: The Bogalusa Heart Study. Arteriosclerosis 7:347, 1987.

32. Srinivasan, SR, et al: Relation of cholesterol to apolipoprotein B in low-density lipoproteins of children: The Bogalusa Heart Study. Arteriosclerosis 9:493, 1989.

33. Sniderman, A, et al: Association of coronary atherosclerosis with hyperapobetalipoproteinemia (increased protein but normal cholesterol levels in human plasma low density [β] lipiproteins). Proc Natl Acad Sci USA 77:606, 1980.

34. Sniderman, A, et al: Familial aggregation and early expression of hyperapobetalipoproteinemia. Am J Cardiol 55:291, 1985.

35. Morrison, JA and Glueck, CJ: Pediatric risk factors for adult coronary heart disease: Primary atherosclerosis prevention. Cardiovasc Rev Rep 2:1269, 1981.

36. Frerichs, RR, et al: Relation of serum lipids and lipoproteins to obesity and sexual maturity in white and black children. Am J Epidemiol 108:486, 1978.

37. Freedman, DS, et al: Relationship of changes in obesity to serum lipid and lipoprotein changes in childhood and adolescence. JAMA 254:515, 1985.

38. Freedman, DS, et al: Correlates of HDL cholesterol and apolipoprotein A-I levels in children: The Bogalusa Heart Study. Arteriosclerosis 7:354, 1987.

39. Aristimuno, GG, et al: Influence of persistent obesity in children on cardiovascular risk factors: The Bogalusa Heart Study. Circulation 69:895, 1984.

40. Freedman, DS, et al: Relation of body fat distribution to hyperinsulinemia in children and adolescents: The Bogalusa Heart Study. Am J Clin Nutr 46:403, 1987.

41. Shear, CL, et al: Childhood siblings aggregation of coronary artery disease risk factor variables in a biracial community. Am J Epidemiol 107:522, 1978.

42. Schrott, HG, et al: Increased coronary mortality in relations of hypercholesterolemic school children: The Muscatine Study. Circulation 59:320, 1979.

43. Morrison, JA, et al: Parent-offspring and sibling lipid and lipoprotein associations during and after sharing household environments: The Princeton School District Family Study. Metabolism 31:158, 1982.

44. Weinberg, R, Webber, LS, and Berenson, GS: Hereditary and environmental influence on cardiovascular risk factors for children. Am J Epidemiol 116:385, 1982.

45. Van Natta, P, et al: The East Baltimore Study: II Familial aggregation of plasma lipids in juveniles in a black inner city population. Am J Epidemiol 114:385, 1981.

46. Sing, CF and Orr, JD: Analysis of genetic and environmental sources of variation in serum cholesterol in Tecumseh, Michigan. IV. Separation of polygene from common environment effects. Am J Hum Genet 30:491, 1978.

47. Rao, DC, et al: The Cincinnati Lipid Research Clinic Family Study: Cultural and biological determinations of lipids and lipoprotein concentrations. Am J Human Genet 34:888, 1982.

48. Moll, PO, et al: Total cholesterol and lipoproteins in school children: Prediction of coronary heart disease in adult relatives. Circulation 67:127, 1983.

49. Rissanen, AM and Nikkilä, EA: Coronary artery disease and its risk factors in families of young men with angina pectoris and in controls. Br Heart J 39:875, 1977.

50. Ibsen, KK, Louis P, and Anderson, GE: Coronary heart risk factors in 177 children and young adults whose fathers died from ischemic heart disease before age 45. Acta Paediatr Scand 71:609, 1982.

51. Blonde, CV, et al: Parental history and cardiovascular disease risk factor variables in children. Prev Med 10:25, 1981.

52. Lee, J, Lauer, RM, and Clark, WR: Lipoproteins in the progeny of young men with coronary artery disease: Children with increased risk. Pediatrics 78:330, 1986.

53. Ten Kate, LP, et al: Familial aggregation of coronary heart disease and its relation to known genetic risk factors. Am J Cardiol 50:945, 1982.

54. Laskarzewski, P, et al: The relationship of paternal history of myocardial infarction, hypertension, diabetes and stroke to coronary heart disease risk factors in their adult progeny. Am J Epidemiol 113:290, 1981.

55. Connor, WE, et al: Plasma lipids, lipoproteins and diet of Tarahumara Indians of Mexico. Am J Clin Nutr 31:1131, 1978.

56. Voors, AW, et al: Smoking, oral contraceptives, and serum lipid and lipoprotein levels in youths of a total biracial community. Prev Med 11:1, 1982.

57. Freedman, DS, et al: Cigarette smoking initiation and longitudinal changes in serum lipids and lipoproteins in early adulthood: The Bogalusa Heart Study. Am J Epidemiol 124:207, 1986.

58. Morrison, JA, et al: Cigarette smoking, alcohol intake and oral contraceptives: Relationships to lipids and lipoproteins in adolescent school children. Metabolism 28:1166, 1979.

59. Wahl, P, et al: Effect of estrogen/progestin potency on lipid/lipoprotein cholesterol. N Engl J Med 15:862, 1983.

60. Friedman, M, et al: Coronary-prone individuals Type A behavior pattern: Some biochemical characteristics. JAMA 212:1030, 1970.

61. Hunter, SM, et al: Type A coronary-prone behavior pattern and cardiovascular risk factor variables in children and adolescents: The Bogalusa Heart Study. J Chron Dis 35:613, 1982.

62. Farris, RP, et al: Influence of milk source on serum lipids and lipoproteins during the first year of life: The Bogalusa Heart Study. Am J Clin Nutr 35:42, 1982.

63. Fomon, SJ: Infant Nutrition, ed 2. WB Saunders, Philadelphia, 1974.

64. Nicklas, TA, et al: Dietary factors relate to cardiovascular risk factors in early life: The Bogalusa Heart Study. Arteriosclerosis 8:193, 1988.

65. Frank, GC, Berenson, GS, and Webber, LS: Dietary studies and the relationship of diet to cardiovascular risk factor variables in 10-year-old children: The Bogalusa Heart Study. Am J Clin Nutr 131:328, 1978.

66. Weidman, WH, et al: Nutrient intake and serum cholesterol level in normal children 6 to 16 years of age. Pediatrics 61:354, 1978.

67. Glueck, CJ, et al: Relationships of nutrient intake to lipids and lipoproteins in 1234 white children. Arteriosclerosis 2:523, 1982.

68. Frank, GC, et al (eds): Dietary Data Book: Quantifying Dietary Intakes of Infants, Children and Adolescents: The Bogalusa Heart Study, 1973–1983. Monographs of the Planning and Analysis Core Components of the National Research and Demonstration Center—Arteriosclerosis (NRDC-A). Louisiana State University Medical Center, New Orleans, Library of Congress Catalog Card No. 86-51215, 1986.

69. Fomon SJ: Reflections on infant feeding in the 1970s and 1980s. Am J Clin Nutr 46:171, 1987.

70. Frank, GC, et al: Sodium, potassium, calcium, magnesium and phosphorus intakes of infants and children: The Bogalusa Heart Study. J Am Diet Assoc 88:801, 1988.

71. Nicklas, TA, et al: Cardiovascular disease risk factors from birth to seven years of age: The Bogalusa Heart Study. V. Dietary intakes. J Pediatr 80(Suppl 5, Part 2):797, 1987.

72. Nicklas, TA, Webber, LS, and Berenson, GS: Persistence of levels for selected dietary components during the first four years of life: The Bogalusa Heart Study. Submitted for publication.

73. Frank, GC, et al: Dietary intake as a determinant of cardiovascular risk factor variables—Part A: Observations in a pediatric population. In Berenson, GS (ed): Causation of Cardiovascular Risk Factors in Children: Perspectives on Cardiovascular Risk in Early Life. Raven Press, New York, 1986.

74. Dietary Intake Source Data: United States 1976–1980, Vital and Health Statistics, U. S. Department Health and Human Services, Public Health Service National Center for Health Statistics series 11, No. 231, publication (PHS) 83-1681. US Gov't Printing Office, 1983.

75. Dietary Intake Findings, United States 1971–74. Data from the National Health Survey. DHEW Publ. No. (HRA) 77-1647, 1977.

76. Peterkin, BB: Nationwide food consumption survey, 1977–78. In Nutrition in the 1980s. Constraints on Our Knowledge. Alan R. Liss, Inc., New York, 1981.

77. Morrison, JA, et al: Nutrient intake: Relationships with lipids and lipoproteins in 6–19 year old children. Metabolism 29:133, 1980.

78. Friend, B, Page, L, and Martson, R: Food consumption patterns in the United States: 1909–13 to 1976. In Levy, R. and Rifkind, B. (eds): Nutrition, Lipids and Heart Disease. Raven Press, New York, 1979.

79. Call, DL and Sanchez, AM: Trends in fat disappearance in the United States, 1909–65. J Nutr 93:1, 1967.

80. Dromer, GW: Fats and oils: Natural and processed foods. In White, PO, Fletcher, DC, and Ellis M (eds): Nutrients in Processed Foods-Fats-Carbohydrates. Publishing Sciences Group, Aston, MA, 1975.

81. Cresanta, JL, et al: Trends in fatty acid intakes of 10-year-old children, 1973 to 1982. J Am Diet Assoc 88:178, 1988.

82. Weidman, W Jr, et al: AHA committee report—Diet in the healthy child: Task Force Committee of the Nutrition Committee and the Cardiovascular Disease in the Young, Council of the American Heart Association. Circulation 67:1411A, 1983.

83. Anderson, JW, et al: Hypocholesterolemic effects of oat-bran or bean intake for hypercholesterolemic men. Am J Clin Nutr 40:1146, 1984.

84. Singleton, SP, et al: Cholesterol reduction among volunteers in a health promotion project. Am J Health Promotion 2:5, 1988.
85. Downey, AM, et al: Development and implementation of a school health promotion program for the reduction of cardiovascular risk factors in children and prevention of adult coronary heart disease: "Heart Smart." In Hetzel, BS and Berenson, GS (eds): Cardiovascular Risk Factors in Childhood: Epidemiology and Prevention. Elsevier Science Publishers, Amsterdam, 1987.
86. Downey, AM, et al: Implementation of "Heart Smart": A cardiovascular school health promotion program. J Sch Hlth 57:98, 1987.
87. Berenson, GS, et al: Heart Smart Cardiovascular Health Curriculum for Elementary School Children. Copyright Reg. TXu 304 257, 1987.
88. Nicklas, TA, et al: Heart Smart School Lunch Program: A vehicle for cardiovascular health promotion. Am J Hlth Prom. In press.
89. Serpas, DC, et al: Comparison of a personalized fitness module to a traditional fitness unit on knowledge, attitude, and cardiovascular endurance of fifth grade students: "Heart Smart." J Teach Phys Educ. Submitted for publication.
90. Hunter, SM, et al: Inoculation against learned helplessness: Implications for adopting healthy lifestyles in children: Heart Smart. In press.
91. Nicklas, TA, et al: "Heart Smart" Program: A family intervention program for eating behavior of children at high risk for cardiovascular disease. J Nutr Educ 20:128, 1988.
92. Johnson, CC, et al: The "Heart Smart" family health promotion program. In press.
93. Nicklas, TA, et al: A family approach to cardiovascular risk reduction through diet. J Nutr Educ Great Educational Material (GEM) 19:302A, 1987.
94. Johnson, CC, et al: Cardiovascular risk in parents of children with elevated blood pressure: "Heart Smart" Family Health Promotion. J Clin Hypertens 3:559, 1987.

PART 2

Cardiovascular Risk Factors: Blood Pressure, Blood Vessels, and the Heart

CHAPTER 3

Hypertension as a Risk Factor

Edward J. Roccella, Ph.D., M.P.H.
Ann E. Bowler, M.S.

Good health has been one of the most sought after goals of humans for all of recorded history. However, what constitutes the status of good health has remained elusive. A recently suggested definition has expanded the earlier perception of health from being merely the absence of disease to including being free from risk of disease and untimely death.[1] This broadened concept of good health recognizes the importance of avoiding or eliminating the risk of disease. By definition, an expression of risk represents the probability of changing health status over a period of time. Factors associated with the occurrence of a disease are considered to be risk factors for that specific disease condition, and factors that increase the probability of the occurrence of a disease state are suspected of causing the change in health status.

For over 60 years, the importance of hypertension as a cardiovascular risk factor has been mentioned in the medical literature. As early as 1925, the Society of Actuaries published a study based on life insurance company records of 560,000 men showing that hypertension was associated with untimely deaths and suggesting that elevated blood pressure constituted a health risk.[2] A clinical study monitoring the range of blood pressures in 11,383 individuals during the 1930s led investigators to express the opinion that the determination of blood pressure gives more information concerning the future prognosis of a patient than any other commonly used test.[3]

Mortality studies carried out in the 1940s and 1950s were instrumental in identifying groups at high risk of dying from cardiovascular sequelae. Thus, the initial stage of development in the effort to prevent or reduce coronary heart disease (CHD) was the identification of risk factors. In the 1940s, this pursuit instigated the initiation of the Framingham Heart Study, which even today is the best source of data on cardiovascular risk factors.

MEASURING RISK

Studies that obtain evidence of risk directly from the experience of human population cohorts, such as the Framingham study, are observational rather than experimental in design. This means there is no opportunity in the study to hold constant factors other than the exposure of interest. This nonexperimental, non-randomized design makes it mandatory to adhere to the prescribed rules of evidence before accepting conclusions based on observations.

The population is examined initially to screen out persons who may already have the disease of interest. To measure the risk of cardiovascular morbidity associated with hypertension in the Framingham cohort, those free of CHD or target-organ damage were initially classified into two subgroups: those exposed to the risk factor, that is, hypertensives, and those whose blood pressures were in the normal range. Both groups now have been followed prospectively for over 35 years to determine which individuals experienced cardiovascular events and which individuals did not. At prescribed time intervals, the rate of cardiovascular sequelae occurring among the hypertensives was divided by the rate of identifiably defined cardiovascular disease (CVD) among those whose blood pressures remained in the normal range. This ratio is the *relative risk* of cardiovascular morbidity associated with hypertension, the quantitative measure that is often used when risks are calculated and compared.

Table 3–1 provides examples of the relative risk of having CVD associated with increasing levels of systolic blood pressure in middle-aged men who had no other major risk factors.[4] It should be noted that these figures are all relative to the risk associated with a reading of 120 mmHg systolic blood pressure (SBP) and as such have no intrinsic quantifiable value, unless one knows the risk that was set at 1.00 and used as a standard. In this example, the CVD incidence rate within 8 years of normotensive individuals in the Framingham study was 35 cases per 1000 individuals. Using this standard, analysts can calculate the increasing risk of probability of having CVD as systolic pressure rises. The risk almost doubles (68 per 1000) at 165 mmHg, a level that was considered to be of little clinical concern until revised guidelines were published in the 1984 report of the Joint National Committee for the Detection, Evaluation, and Treatment of High Blood Pressure.[5]

After calculating the risks associated with blood pressure levels from an obser-

Table 3–1. Relative Risks of Having Cardiovascular Disease Within 8 Years Associated with Systolic Blood Pressure Levels in a 45-Year-Old Man* Based on 18-Year Follow-up

Systolic Pressure (mmHg)	Relative Risk
120	1.00
135	1.23
150	1.54
165	1.94
180	2.40
195	2.86

*Nonsmoking, without glucose intolerance, with cholesterol of 210 mg/dl.

Data from The Framingham Study. An Epidemiological Investigation of Cardiovascular Disease. Section 31.

vational study, statistical tests are then applied to determine if the difference of disease occurrence in the subgroups with and without hypertension is by chance. Once the association between hypertension and CHD was established as a statistically significant relationship, several additional criteria needed to be analyzed before concluding that the association was causal in nature.

ESTABLISHING RISK FACTOR CAUSALITY

Establishing risk factor causality involves the inferential process of evaluating the association of the risk factor, in this case hypertension, with the cardiovascular event. In turn, this process involves assessing characteristics of the data that support the risk factor association, namely strength, consistency, and dose-response relationship as well as timing, biologic plausibility, specificity, and replication. This section demonstrates how analytical studies have determined that elevated blood pressure meets all these criteria and therefore has been established as a cause of cardiovascular morbidity and mortality.

STRENGTH, CONSISTENCY, AND DOSE-RESPONSE OF THE DATA

In judging the strength of the hypertension/CHD association from the data discussed in this section, it is helpful to know that guidelines suggested for interpreting the strength of associations list relative risk values between 1.7 and 2.9 as implying moderate risk, with any relative risk value greater than 3.0 considered to be high.[6]

Relative risks calculated from the Framingham study (18-year follow-up)[7] and the American Heart Association Pooling Project[8] have been strong and consistent. Table 3–2 presents the results of analyses from five prospective cohort studies that compose the Pooling Project: Framingham (11-year follow-up), Albany, Chicago Gas Company, Chicago Western Electric, and Tecumseh. These studies, with relatively minor exceptions, showed consistent dose-response increases in relative risk as diastolic pressures increased. The endpoint event in the five studies of the Pooling Project was death from CHD. The Framingham 18-year follow-up data were used to examine the incidence of stroke associated with rising blood pressures.[9] Tables 3–2 and 3–3 illustrate the consistency in the rise of the relative risk of death with increasing diastolic pressure, even though the mortality rates for normotensives at entry, used as a standard, differ considerably among the studies. The stroke data presented for both men and women illustrate the fact that relative risks for two cohorts can be quantitatively similar even when the absolute rates differ. A comparison of the risks of CHD experienced by men and women demonstrates that comparisons of relative risks can be deceiving unless the risks are calculated relative to the same standard rate.

A strong and consistent dose-response relationship between stystolic blood pressure levels and cardiovascular morbidity also depicts the absolute risks associated with both systolic and diastolic pressures. Data from the Framingham Heart Study (Fig. 3–1) demonstrates that the absolute risk of cardiovascular sequelae increases in proportion to SBP at all levels of measurement.[4] The association is clear in both sexes from the lowest to the highest pressures observed. The curves graphically represent the point—already mentioned—that although the absolute

Table 3.2. Relative Risks of Coronary Heart Disease (CHD) Death in Relation to Diastolic Blood Pressure Levels at Entry. (Five Pooling Project Studies; White Men Aged 40–54 at Entry)

DBP (mmHg)	Framingham*				Albany†			
	No at Entry	CHD Deaths	Rate	R.R.	No. at Entry	CHD Deaths	Rate	R.R.
< 80	237	5	21.1	1.00	336	11	32.7	1.00
80–89	391	17	43.5	2.06	761	22	28.9	0.88
90–94	212	14	66.0	3.19	310	11	35.5	1.08
95–104	185	14	75.7	3.59	214	7	32.7	1.00
≥ 105	92	9	97.8	4.64	135	14	103.7	3.17

*Average follow-up: 11.5 yr.
†Average follow-up: 9.86 yr.
‡Average follow-up: 9.71 yr.
§Average follow-up: 8.52 yr.
‖Average follow-up: 8.05 yr.
Data from The Framingham Study. An Epidemiological Investigation of Cardiovascular Disease. Section 31.

risk for men is greater than that for women at any level of systolic pressure, the relative risk is as great in women as in men.

Figure 3–2 is an additional demonstration of how risk expressed as relative units rather than absolute units may be misleading.[10] When the association of mortality and blood pressure is shown by the relative risks of age-specific groups, the relative risk of all age-groups increases with increasing pressure. However, the gradient gets less steep as age advances. This seems plausible inasmuch as a systolic pressure of 160 mmHg is quite common in older men and not seen as often in younger men in whom it may seem more ominous. However, in the second chart of Figure 3–2, the same data are shown using a scale of the absolute risk of deaths

Table 3–3. Relative Risk of Stroke for Men and Women Aged 45–74 Years at Entry: 18-Year Follow-up

Diastolic Pressure (mmHg)	Men		Women	
	Rate*	R.R.	Rate*	R.R.
< 80	17.9	1.00	13.2	1.00
80–84	26.5	1.48	19.8	1.50
85–89	32.4	1.81	24.3	1.84
90–94	39.7	2.22	30.0	2.27
95–99	48.7	2.72	36.9	2.80
100–104	59.6	3.33	45.4	3.44
105–109	72.9	4.08	55.8	4.23
> 110	89.1	4.97	69.5	5.26

*per 10,000.
Data from The Framingham Study. An Epidemiological Investigation of Cardiovascular Disease. Section 30.

Table 3.2. Relative Risks of Coronary Heart Disease (CHD) Death in Relation to Diastolic Blood Pressure Levels at Entry. (Five Pooling Project Studies; White Men Aged 40–54 at Entry) (*continued*)

Chicago Gas‡				Chicago Western Electric§				Tecumseh‖			
No. at Entry	CHD Deaths	Rate	R.R.	No. at Entry	CHD Deaths	Rate	R.R.	No. at Entry	CHD Deaths	Rate	R.R.
311	9	28.9	1.00	355	6	16.9	1.00	141	4	28.4	1.00
388	19	49.0	1.69	702	22	31.3	1.85	186	6	32.2	1.14
149	10	67.1	2.32	398	12	30.2	1.78	114	4	35.1	1.24
60	4	66.7	2.31	269	10	37.2	2.20	81	5	61.7	2.17
28	2	71.4	2.47	134	11	82.1	4.86	50	8	160.0	5.63

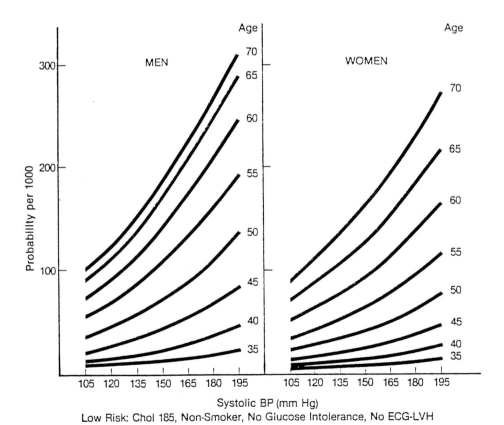

Figure 3–1. Probability of cardiovascular disease in eight years in low-risk subjects according to systolic blood pressure (mmHg) at specified ages in each sex: 18-year follow-up.
SOURCE: The Framingham Study.

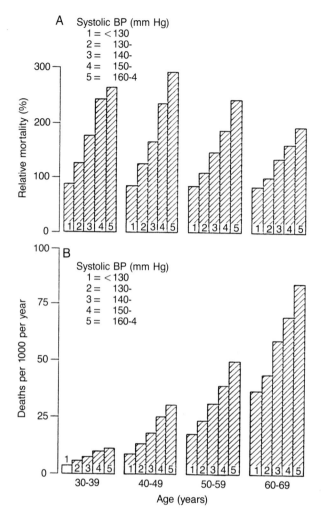

Figure 3–2. Age-specific mortality in men according to blood pressure and age, from life insurance data: (*A*) relative risk, and (*B*) absolute risk. (Adapted from Rose.[10])

per 1000 per year associated with systolic pressures. The pattern for increasing age intervals is quite different here, reflecting the fact that the absolute risk associated with elevated blood pressure is far greater in older men. Not only does risk increase with rising blood pressure, but it also increases with advancing age regardless of blood pressure. This explains why absolute numbers of deaths rather than relative risk are used to give a more accurate picture when making comparisons between subgroups of a population.

In recent years, the notion that diastolic pressure is the chief determinant of cardiovascular risk has been challenged. On re-examination of the early epidemiologic studies that first correlated cardiovascular complications and increasing blood pressures, analysts found these initial studies of actuarial data showed that for any level of diastolic pressure, the risk of mortality rose progressively and significantly with increasing increments in systolic pressure.[11] Moreover, results from the Chicago Stroke Study[12] and the Framingham study[13] indicate systolic pressure may actually be a better indicator of the risk of cardiovascular sequelae from hypertension than diastolic pressure, especially in the elderly, whose diastolic pressures are often less accurately determined. In any case, whether diastolic or systolic pressure is used, the dose-response characteristic of the association between blood pressure levels and CHD occurrence is consistent.

TIMING

The criterion of timing is also to be considered in the process of inferring a causal relationship between a risk factor and disease. As applied to hypertension, the timing of events involves considering that the elevation of blood pressure not only precedes its cardiovascular sequelae but also often does so with such an extended lag time that the association was not recognized until long-term data were studied. Moreover, the lack of symptoms accompanying a rise in blood pressure also may have impeded an earlier understanding of the importance of hypertension as a biologic marker of an increased cardiovascular risk. There is no question that the timing of the two events of the association is consistent with a causal relationship.

BIOLOGICAL PLAUSIBILITY

Although there is still much that is not understood about the cause of high blood pressure, the plausible biologic pathways for hypertension to bring on cardiovascular consequences have been described. A sustained elevation of blood pressure increases the pressure load of the heart and eventually causes hypertrophy of the left ventricle. Hypertrophy of the smooth muscle cells of the arteries also results from elevated pressure and may manifest in the kidney, leading to renal insufficiency. In the brain, the increased arterial pressure may cause arterial ruptures and subsequent hemorrhagic stroke. Furthermore, high blood pressure can accelerate the evolution of atherosclerosis and the multiple CHD repercussions of this additional risk factor.

SPECIFICITY

As a criteron for inferring causality, the specficity of an association refers to a situation in which the disease is limited to the subgroup of the population exposed to the risk factor. Although this situation greatly strengthens the argument for causation, the lack of specificity does not detract in cases with endpoints, such as CHD, in which it has been widely accepted that more than one risk factor for a disease exists and that one risk factor causes more than one disease. Hypertension and CHD exemplify both aspects of this multiple factor, multiple endpoint theory.

Since the early 1950s, epidemiologic investigators have been studying several cardiovascular risk factors to establish their relative importance. Major contributions to the understanding of the effects of multiple risk factors have been made by the Framingham study,[14] the Stockholm Prospective Heart Study,[15] the Multiple Risk Factor Intervention Trial,[16] and the Oslo Risk Reduction Study.[17] Table 3–4 lists the major risk factors for CHD in order of their relative importance as determined by the Framingham Heart Study.[18] Although age, sex, and genetic factors carry the highest risks, they cannot be altered, leaving three major modifiable risk factors: elevated blood pressure, elevated serum total cholesterol levels, and smok-

Table 3–4. Major Risk Factors for Coronary Heart Disease

Unmodifiable
  Increasing age
  Male sex
  Family history
Modifiable
  High blood pressure
  High plasma total cholesterol and low HDL* cholesterol levels
  Smoking
  Physical inactivity
  Diabetes
  Obesity

*HDL = high-density lipoprotein.
From Kannel et al.[14]

ing. Of these, elevated blood pressure is considered the most reliable predictor of CHD morbidity and mortality, especially for stroke and congestive heart failure.[19]

Several cardiovascular complications have been shown to be consequences of sustained elevation of arterial pressure. The Framingham Heart Study has shown that persons with hypertension have twice the incidence of peripheral vascular disease, sudden death, CHD, and myocardial infarction and four times the incidence of stroke as do those with normal blood pressure.[20] Moreover, hypertension interacts with other risk factors as a contributing cause of atherosclerosis, which in turn is a risk factor for pathologic developments in the heart, aorta, brain, and kidney. Additional examples of conditions that arise as a direct result of damage to vessels from elevated blood pressure are intracranial bleeding, aortic dissection, and renal insufficiency.[21]

An examination of hypertension within the context of multiple co-risk factors indicates an intricately interwoven web of causation leading to a variety of cardiovascular clinical manifestations.

REPLICATION

The replication of the finding of an association across studies is a crucial standard for inferring cause and effect. Studies of different designs, conducted by different investigators in different geographic locations, taking place at different time periods, have all documented the increased cardiovascular risk that is associated with rising levels of blood pressure. The 1979 Blood Pressure Study of Life Insurance Data,[2] the Framingham Heart Study,[4] the Oslo Study,[17] the Bogalusa Heart Study,[22] and the Muscatine Study of Coronary Heart Disease Factors in Children,[23] all large cohorts followed over long time periods, revealed consistent findings—replication in its fullest form.

Thus, the rules of evidence establishing a causal link between hypertension and CHD have all been met, some to a greater extent than others. By analyzing the data and expressing the findings as quantitative expressions of the risk associated with hypertension, the first stage in the investigation of the development of CHD was completed.

REVERSING THE RISK

Studies of population cohorts have documented the risks associated with elevated blood pressure, resulting in the identification of hypertension as a causal risk factor for CHD. However, it was unknown whether lowering blood pressures would decrease risk or prolong life. The need to find the answer to this second question motivated investigators to initiate the second stage in the campaign to reduce cardiovascular morbidity and mortality, namely to implement randomized, controlled trials evaluating the benefit of hypertension treatment.

The first controlled clinical trial demonstrating the benefits of lowering blood pressure was the Veterans Administration Cooperative Group Study on Antihypertensive Agents, conducted in the 1960s.[24,25] This trial established that lowering diastolic blood pressures (DBP) that initially were in the range of 90 to 129 mmHg reduced the rates of nonfatal and fatal events. Substantial reduction in risk was shown by intervening with drug treatment for the groups with moderately and severely elevated pressures (DBP 115 to 129 mmHg), and some benefit also was shown in those with milder elevations (90 to 114 mmHg). This reduction in risk in the latter group, however, appeared to apply chiefly to those with pressures of 105 mmHg or greater.

With risk reduction through treatment clearly established for patients with moderately and severely elevated pressures, a great deal of effort since the time of the Veterans Administration studies has gone into measuring the benefit of drug treatment for patients with diastolic pressures in the mild range (90 to 104 mmHg). Over 70 percent of all hypertensives fall within this category. More than half the excess deaths attributable to hypertension come from this milder hypertension range.

Even though the absolute risks for stroke and for CHD in individuals with hypertension in the mild range may not seem as threatening as in the moderate and severe ranges (see Tables 3–2 and 3–3), clinical trial data revealed that when blood pressure elevations in the mild range are not controlled, there is considerable likelihood that in a relatively short period of time the blood pressure will move out of the mild range and into the greater danger zone of moderate or severe high blood pressure. When the Hypertension Detection and Followup Program (HDFP) rescreened men and women who three years earlier had an initial screening of diastolic levels of 95 mmHg or over but did not enter the program because their second screening pressures were under 90 mmHg, the investigators found that diastolic pressure in 11.8 percent of these individuals had already risen to levels of 105 mmHg or higher.[27] Data from other studies support this observation of the risk of rising to higher elevations in those with mild hypertension. The significant rises in blood pressure shown in Table 3–5 occurred in trials in which, except for HDFP, persons with cardiovascular complications were excluded. With each incremental increase in the severity of hypertension, the risks of target-organ damage, morbidity, and death all rose.

In addition to the risk of progression of blood pressure levels, evidence is available from several randomized controlled drug trials that indicates some benefit from treating hypertensives in the 90 to 104 mmHg, or mild, range. Table 3–6 shows the results of four placebo-controlled trials. Because the numbers were too small to test the efficacy of reducing the risk of each endpoint separately, the combined endpoint of all fatal and nonfatal events was established. Specific endpoint

Table 3–5. Risk of Marked Rise in Blood Pressure in
Patients with Uncontrolled Mild Hypertension

Study	Duration of Follow-up (Yr)	Increase Observed (%)
USPHS	7–10	12.2 with DBP* 131+
HDFP	3 (substudy)	11.8 with DBP 105+
Australian Trial	3	6.0 with DBP 110+
Oslo Trial	5	17.2 with DBP 110+

*DBP = Diastolic blood pressure.

Based on the data of Smith[28]; Hypertension Detection and Follow-up Program Cooperative Group[29]; Australian National Blood Pressure Study Committee[30]; and Helgeland.[17]

events included death, nonfatal stroke, myocardial infarction, other ischemic heart disease, transient ischemic attack, congestive heart failure, aortic aneurysm, retinopathy, encephalopathy, and renal failure. The incidence of these combined endpoints was reduced by 19 to 35 percent in the drug versus placebo patients in these trials of mild hypertension.

These findings were confirmed and extended in the much larger HDFP.[27] More than half of the HDFP participants had blood pressures in the mild (diastolic blood pressure 90 to 104 mmHg) range. A main finding of this trial was a 20 percent lower all-cause death rate at the 5-year point for those in the Stepped Care (SC) group vigorously treated with antihypertensive drug therapy compared with those in the Referred Care (RC) group who received the prevailing care of the community. Reduction of risks and mortality rates was observed at *all* levels within the mild range (Table 3–7). Stepped-care patients with mild hypertension also had lower rates for combined fatal and nonfatal events, including stroke, myocardial infarction, angina pectoris, and left ventricular hypertrophy.

Recently, 8.3-year survival data have been published on HDFP participants, and the absolute difference between the Stepped Care and Referred Care death rates was greater than at the close of the 5-year trial.[31] For those within the mild high blood pressure (HBP) range, the 8.3-year mortality rates were 112.9 per 1000 participants in the SC group and 135.4 per 1000 participants in the RC group, indicating that the absolute mortality advantage found at five years persisted and increased with time even though the SC program was discontinued after five years of treatment.

Table 3–6. Effect of Antihypertensive Drug Treatment on Mild
Hypertension: Fatal Plus Nonfatal Endpoints

Trial	N	Treated	Placebo	Difference Treated vs. Placebo
VA (90-104)	170	14	21	−34.8
USPHS	389	56	29	−37.0
Oslo	785	25	34	−31.0
Australian	3427	138	168	−19.2

Based on the data of Helgeland[17]; Veterans Administration Cooperative Study Group on Antihypertensive Agents[24]; Smith[28]; Australian National Blood Pressure Study Committee. [30]

Table 3-7. Five-Year Mortality Among Participants with Entry
Diastolic Blood Pressure (DBP) 90-104 mmHg, Stepped Care (SC)
vs. Referred Care (RC): Hypertension Detection and Follow-up
Program (HDFP)

Entry DBP (mmHg)*	Stepped Care			Referred Care			Reduction in Mortality SC vs RC
	N	Deaths	Death Rate† per 100	N	Deaths	Death Rate per 100	
90-104	2,906	154	5.6	2,954	195	7.2	21.9
90-94	1,127	54	4.9	1,120	70	6.6	25.6
95-99	1,027	47	4.8	992	63	7.0	31.1
100-104	752	53	7.1	842	62	8.0	11.3

*Not receiving treatment at entry.
°Death rate adjusted by age-sex-race, using as the common standard population all HDFP participants.
From Hypertension Detection and Follow-up Program Cooperative Group.[29]

The British Research Council Trial was another large trial that examined the benefits of lowering mild hypertension.[32] This trial compared drug treatment with placebo. Over 17,000 participants were involved, although, unlike the HDFP, persons with cardiovascular complications were excluded. Therefore, overall mortality and morbidity were lower, and, consequently, comparisons of specific endpoints were less likely to be conclusive in this trial. However, for the main trial endpoint, stroke, a significant reduction of 45 percent was observed for those treated with drugs compared with those in the placebo group.

Although there are extensive data available from numerous well-designed randomized clinical trials, the ability of drug treatment of mild hypertension to reduce the risk of the development of coronary artery disease and its complications is a critical but yet-unanswered question. Analysis of the findings suggests that the benefits of drug treatment on the incidence of fatal or nonfatal myocardial infarctions or on mortality related to coronary artery disease are modest at best. Data from these trials show a trend of reduced mortality from coronary artery disease in the intervention groups; however, the difference does not reach statistical significance.

The point made previously, that most trials show larger reductions in stroke than in coronary artery disease, is not surprising. The progression of atherosclerotic disease may occur over a longer time period than that available in a clinical trial. In addition, it is well known that in those with increased levels of blood pressure, the risk of stroke rises more steeply than the risk of coronary artery disease. The multiplicity of risk factors, modifiable and unmodifiable, that are associated with atherosclerosis lessens the potential impact that blood pressure reduction can achieve on the composite risk.

There is no question, however, that the combined results from the various trials emphasize that effective management of hypertension can reduce mortality for large numbers of people. There is strong evidence that reduction of elevated blood pressure reduces risk and prolongs life, even for persons with lower levels of hypertension.

RISK AND THE IMPLICATIONS FOR HIGH BLOOD
PRESSURE CONTROL PROGRAMS

Risk measurement can provide the basis for identifying hypertension as a causal factor for CHD and for documenting the efficacy of blood pressure reduction. Moreover, additional methods of measuring risk also play an important part in the third phase of the campaign against CHD: the implementation of high blood pressure–control programs.

A method of quantitatively expressing risk is the concept of *attributable risk.* This method is useful in targeting resources in the subsets of the populations that have the greatest need for program activities. This method of measuring risk is derived by subtracting the death rate in hypertensives from the death rate among normotensives. In this manner, the mortality rate that can be attributed to hypertension for both systolic blood pressure and diastolic blood pressure was determined in a 1961 study of the 40 to 69-year-old population of Evans County, Georgia. Table 3–8 presents the results of 10-year follow-up for the four race/sex groups.[33] The difference in 10-year survival rates for hypertensives (defined for SBP as > 139 mmHg and for DBP as > 89 mmHg) and for normotensives was calculated to determine the increased risk of death in each of the population subgroups. This calculation measures hypertension attributable risk. The population attributable risk was determined by multiplying the hypertension attributable risk for each race/sex group by the prevalence of hypertension in that population subgroup. As shown in Table 3–8, the data for Evans County indicate that although the hypertension attributable risk was highest for white men, the population attributable risk tended to be higher for blacks, especially black women. Thus, the higher hypertensive prevalence rates found in blacks leads to higher population attributable risk, a quantitative measure of the larger burden that hypertension places on that race group. Similarly, the population attributable risk may be used as a measure of

Table 3–8. Risks of Mortality Associated with Systolic and Diastolic Blood Pressures

Race/Sex	Systolic Blood Pressure						
	Survival Rates		*Hypertension Attributable Risk*	*Prevalence*	*Population Attributable Risk*	*Mortality Rate*	*Population Attributable Fraction*
	<139	*>139*					
White men	0.85	0.69	0.16	0.54	0.09	0.24	0.36
White women	0.93	0.85	0.08	0.60	0.05	0.12	0.42
Black men	0.85	0.68	0.17	0.71	0.12	0.26	0.45
Black women	0.92	0.78	0.14	0.81	0.12	0.19	0.61
	Diastolic Blood Pressure						
	<94	*>94*					
White men	0.81	0.67	0.14	0.36	0.05	0.24	0.21
White women	0.89	0.84	0.05	0.33	0.02	0.12	0.15
Black men	0.80	0.69	0.11	0.63	0.07	0.26	0.26
Black women	0.89	0.76	0.14	0.67	0.09	0.19	0.47

Based on the data of Deubner et al.[33]

improvement that could be accomplished by eliminating or reducing the problem of hypertension and its sequelae from that population. This becomes a useful figure in measuring program impact.

The fraction of all deaths attributed to hypertension in a population (population attributable fraction) is determined by dividing the population attributable risk by the overall death rate for that population. The fraction of all deaths that represents excess deaths associated with hypertension is considerably higher in black women, approximately 50 percent, than in the three other groups (see Table 3–8). The population attributable fraction emphasizes the importance of targeting hypertension control programs to black women, the subgroup with the highest population attributable risk.

The importance of distinguishing between *relative risk, hypertension attributable risk, prevalence,* and *population attributable risk* and *fraction* becomes apparent when comparing the significance of hypertension among different race and sex subgroups. For example, it has been argued that the black man with any given level of elevated blood pressure is more likely to suffer fatal complications than the white man with similar blood pressures. However, the basis for this type of comparison should be the hypertension attributable risk for the respective race-sex subgroup in question. In the Evans County experience, the hypertension attributable risk was similar or higher for white men than for black men, depending on whether systolic or diastolic pressures were used in the calculation. However, a planning decision that sets priorities for hypertension control efforts should consider the population attributable risk levels for these same race-sex subgroups. Population attributable risk includes hypertension prevalence rates in their calculation and thus are higher for black men. The crucial determinant in the planning decision is where the intervention potentially has the greatest impact, and this is determined not only by comparing the risk of mortality for a given hypertensive but also by comparing the likelihood of hypertension occurring in subgroups.

SUMMARY

Hypertension has been demonstrated to be a clear risk factor for CHD. The finding that hypertension is a risk factor has been demonstrated in observation studies, actuarial data and clinical trials. The relationship between blood pressure and CHD is strong. As blood pressure rises, risk for cardiovascular events increases. This is true for both sexes, for blacks and whites, and for all age categories.

Clinical trials, both large and small, have demonstrated that lowering blood pressure can reverse the risk and reduce morbidity and mortality. This cause-and-effect relationship has been replicated consistently, and there is not one well-controlled trial of adequate size that has failed to show this finding.

It is important to know which concept of risk to use in developing hypertensive programs. The concept of relative risk is useful to determine whether a public health program is needed within a population, but it has less value in identifying which subset of the population in which to intervene. In essence, relative risk is used to mandate a program but cannot determine where the program should be directed. Hypertension attributable risk describes which individuals are at greatest risk and serves to guide planners as to which groups have the greatest mortality once blood pressure becomes elevated. Population attributable risk becomes the most useful tool in identifying or locating those communities of highest-risk individuals.

REFERENCES

1. Stokes, J III, Noren, J, and Shindell, S: Definition of terms and concepts applicable to clinical preventive medicine. J Comm Health 8:33, 1982.
2. Blood pressure study 1979. Societies of the Association of Life Insurance Medical Directors and the Society of Actuaries, November 1980.
3. Robinson, SC and Brucer, M: Range of normal blood pressure: A statistical and clinical study of 11,383 persons. Arch Intern Med 64:409, 1939.
4. Kannel, WB: Some lessons in cardiovascular epidemiology from Framingham. Am J Cardiol 37:269, 1976.
5. The 1984 Report of the Joint National Committee on Detection, Evaluation, and Treatment of High Blood Pressure. Arch Intern Med 144:1045, 1984.
6. Daniels, SR, Greenberg, RS, and Ibrahim, MA: Etiologic research in pediatric epidemiology. J Pediatrics 102:494, 1983.
7. The Framingham Study: An epidemiological investigation of cardiovascular disease. Section 31. The results of the Framingham Study applied to four other U.S.-based epidemiological studies of cardiovascular disease. National Heart, Lung, and Blood Institute, Bethesda, Md, 1976. DHEW publication no. (NIH)76-1083.
8. The Pooling Project Research Group. Relationship of blood pressure, serum cholesterol, smoking habit, relative weight and ECG abnormalities in incidence of major coronary events: Final report of the pooling project. Dallas: American Heart Association, Dallas, 1978. Monograph no. 60.
9. The Framingham Study: An epidemiological investigation of cardiovascular disease. Section 30. Some characteristics related to the incidence of cardiovascular disease and death: Framingham Study, 18-year followup. National Heart, Lung, and Blood Institute, Bethesda, Md, DHEW publication no. (NIH)74–599.
10. Rose, G: Strategy of prevention: Lessons from cardiovascular disease. Br Med J 282:1847, 1981.
11. Grubner, RS: Systolic hypertension: A pathogenetic entity: Significance and therapeutic considerations. Am J Cardiol 9:773, 1962.
12. Shekelle, RB, Ostfield, AM, and Klawans HL Jr: Hypertension and risk of stroke in an elderly population. Stroke 5:71, 1974.
13. Kannel, WB, Dawber, TR, and McGee, DL: Perspectives on systolic hypertension: The Framingham Study. Circulation 61:1179, 1980.
14. Kannel, WB, McGee, D, and Gordon, T: A general cardiovascular risk profile: The Framingham study. Am J Cardiol 38:46, 1976. .
15. Bottiger, LE and Carlson, LA: Risk factors for ischemic vascular death in men in the Stockholm Prospective Study. Atherosclerosis 36:389, 1980.
16. Multiple Risk Factor Intervention Trial Research Group: Multiple risk factor intervention trial. JAMA 248:1465, 1982.
17. Helgeland, A: The Oslo Study: Treatment of mild hypertension: A five-year controlled drug study. Am J Med 69:725, 1980.
18. Superko, HR, Wood, PD, and Haskell, WL: Coronary heart disease and risk factor modification. Am J Med 78:828, 1985.
19. Whelton, PK: Blood pressure in adults and the elderly. In Bulpitt, CJ (ed): Handbook for Hypertension. Amsterdam, Elsevier Science Publishers B.V., 1985.
20. Kannel, WB and Sorlie, P: Hypertension in Framingham. In Paul, O (ed): Epidemiology and Control of Hypertension. New York, Symposia Specialists, 1975.
21. Leitschuh, M and Chobanian, A: Vascular changes in hypertension. In Bulpitt, CJ (ed): Handbook of Hypertension. Amsterdam, Elsevier Science Publishers B.V., 1985.
22. Voors, AW, et al: Studies of blood pressure in children ages 5–14, in a total biracial community: The Bogalusa Heart Study. Circulation 54:319, 1976.
23. Lauer, RM, et at: Coronary heart disease factors in school children: The Muscatine Study. J Pediatr 86:697, 1975.
24. Veterans Administration Cooperative Study Group on Antihypertensive Agents: Effects of treatment on morbidity in hypertension: Results in patients with diastolic pressures averaging 115 through 129 mmHg. JAMA 202:128, 1967.

25. Veterans Administration Cooperative Study Group on Antihypertensive Agents. Effects of treatment on morbidity in hypertension. II. Results in patients with diastolic blood pressures averaging 90 through 114 mmHg. JAMA 213:1143, 1970.
26. Stamler, J, et al: Hypertension screening of 1 million Americans: Community Hypertension Evaluation Clinic (CHEC) Program. JAMA 235:2299, 1976.
27. Apostolides, AY, et al: Three-year incidence of hypertension in thirteen U.S. Communities. Prev Med 11:487, 1982.
28. Smith, WM: Treatment of mild hypertension results of a ten-year intervention trial. Circ Res Suppl I40:98, 1977.
29. Hypertension Detection and Follow-up Program Cooperative Group: Five-year findings of the Hypertension Detection and Follow-up Program. I. Reduction in mortality in persons with high blood pressure, including mild hypertension. JAMA 242:2562, 1979.
30. Australian National Blood Pressure Study Committee: The Australian therapeutic trial in mild hypertension. Lancet 1:1261, 1980.
31. Hypertension Detection and Follow-up Program Cooperation Group: Persistence of reduction in blood pressure and mortality of participants in the Hypertension Detection and Follow-up Program. JAMA 259:2113, 1988.
32. Medical Research Council Working Party: MRC trial of treatment of mild hypertension: Principal results. Br Med J 291:97, 1985.
33. Deubner, DC, et al: Attributable risk, population attributable risk, and population attributable fraction of death associated with hypertension in a biracial population. Circulation 52:901, 1975.
34. Lenfant, C and Roccella, EJ: Trends in hypertension control in the United States. Chest 86:459, 1984.

CHAPTER 4

Systolic Hypertension in the Elderly: Controlled or Uncontrolled

Jeffrey L. Probstfield, M.D.
Curt D. Furberg, M.D., Ph.D.

Systolic hypertension was suggested to be a significant pathogenetic entity in 1962 by Gubner.[1] Most physicians had not acknowledged it, and in 1960 Schettler[2] had stated that systolic or atherosclerotic hypertension was a form that was of no particular interest from either a practical or a clinical point of view.

Gubner's conclusion was based on analyses of the Build and Blood Pressure Study conducted by the Society of Actuaries.[3] This study pooled the experience of 26 insurance companies in the United States and Canada and described findings from approximately 3,900,000 people who were policy holders and an experience of 102,000 deaths. The study included all individuals between the ages of 15 and 65 issued ordinary life insurance contracts during the years 1935 through 1953. All were traced to the anniversary dates of their policies in 1954. Although this was a very large data set, the information on individuals with systolic blood pressures (SBP) in the strata 168 to 177 mmHg and 178 to 192 mmHg was insufficient to make statistically valid conclusions regarding mortality.[4] Regardless, Tables 4–1 and 4–2, taken from Gubner's 1962 publication, clearly demonstrated two key points: (1) the risk of death for increasing systolic pressures notwithstanding diastolic pressure strata was an ever-increasing one, and (2) the increased risk for the examined strata showed a more pronounced increase associated with SBP than for diastolic blood pressure (DBP). This led Gubner to make the following statement:

> The conclusion seems inescapable that moderate elevation of systolic pressure, which has generally been viewed indifferently by physicians as a passive accompaniment of diastolic hypertension, has a decidedly adverse significance of its own.[1]

Since that time, the examination of the various aspects of pathophysiology, epidemiology, risk assessment, and treatment of sustained isolated systolic hypertension (ISH) has increased steadily. These lines of investigation have now matured

Table 4-1. Ratio of Actual to Expected Mortality (Males, Policy Issue Ages 50–59)*

Systolic Blood Pressure (mmHg)	Diastolic Blood Pressure (mmHg)				
	68 to 82 (%)	*83 to 87* (%)	*88 to 92* (%)	*93 to 97* (%)	*98 to 102* (%)
98–127	83	98	102	—	—
128–137	105	108	111	166	—
138–147	140	140	153	195	178
148–157	144	177	200	213	193
158–167	206	183	214	254	367

*1959 Build and Blood Pressure Study, Society of Actuaries.[3]
(From Gubner,[1] with permission.)

into a randomized controlled, double-blind trial that seeks to evaluate the preventive effect of antihypertensive drug treatment and the potential alteration of natural history of ISH. These topics are reviewed in this chapter.

PREVALENCE

Prevalence estimates for ISH are available from several studies. For example, the Chicago Stroke Study (N = 2772) reported that for individuals between the ages of 65 and 74, the prevalence was 7.3 percent, with ISH defined as SBP $\geq$ 160 and DBP $\leq$ 80 mmHg.[5] The HDFP program reported a prevalence of 6.8 percent in 158,906 screenees between 60 and 69 years of age and SBP $\geq$ 160 and DBP < 90 mmHg.[6] In the Rancho Bernardo Study of 2636 persons, the prevalence of ISH was 3.3 percent in individuals between the ages of 60 and 64 and increased to 10.9 percent for those above 75 years of age.[7] The Systolic Hypertension in the Elderly Program (SHEP) pilot data from screenees showed for individuals between 60 and 69 years, 70 and 79 years, and 80 and above, 7 percent, 13 percent, and 20 percent, respectively, as the prevalence of ISH (Table 4–3).[8] The National Health

Table 4-2. Ratio of Actual to Expected Mortality (Males, Policy Issue Ages 15–69)*

Systolic Blood Pressure (mmHg)	Diastolic Blood Pressure (mmHg)				
	68 to 82 (%)	*83 to 87* (%)	*88 to 92* (%)	*93 to 97* (%)	*98 to 102* (%)
98–127	83	103	109	—	—
128–137	106	116	137	160	160
138–147	136	144	166	194	208
148–157	150	185	189	231	272
158–167	211	180	215	249	307

*1959 Build and Blood Pressure Study, Society of Actuaries.[3]
(From Gubner,[1] with permission.)

Table 4–3. Prevalence of Isolated
Systolic Hypertension* in SHEP Pilot
Study

	Age 60–69 %	Age 70–79 %	Age 80+ %
Female			
White	8	14	21
Nonwhite	10	14	22
Male			
White	6	11	17
Nonwhite	10	9	18
Total	7	13	20

*Systolic blood pressure $\geq$ 160 mmHg and diastolic blood pressure <90 mmHg

and Nutrition Examination Survey also demonstrated an increasing prevalence with age[9] (Table 4–4). These last two studies also clearly demonstrated a higher prevalence in women than in men. Finally, the SHEP pilot showed a slightly higher prevalence of ISH among nonwhites (mainly blacks) compared with whites[8] (Table 4–3). This confirmed an earlier observation of the HDFP. There is, however, some evidence that the prevalence of ISH in the United States may be decreasing with time.[10]

ETIOLOGY AND PATHOPHYSIOLOGY

Although a direct causal relationship between specific anatomic or biochemical phenomena and the attendant altered physiology of ISH is yet to be established, there is a clear and strong negative correlation between large vessel compliance and a systolic hypertension in older individuals.[11] This is at least in part related to a decrease in connective tissue elasticity and the more frequent occurrence of atherosclerosis in this age group.[12-15] Furthermore, these phenomena are known to be

Table 4–4. Prevalence of Isolated
Systolic Hypertension by Age and Sex,
National Health and Nutrition
Examination Survey (NHANES I),
1971–75*

	55–64	65–74
Men	2.6	10.3
Women	5.2	11.8

*Percent with isolated systolic hypertension (systolic blood pressure $\geq$ 160 mmHg and diastolic blood pressure <90 mmHg).

Adapted from Hypertension in Adults 25–74 Years of Age, United States, 1971–75. Vital and Health Statistics Series 11, no. 221, National Center for Health Statistics, US Dept of Health and Human Services, 1981.

related to the increase in aortic impedance and in peripheral vascular resistance that occurs with age. Finally, a decrease in aortic compliance results in increased resistance to systolic ejection and is frequently associated with a disproportionate change in SBP.[15-17]

Changes in a number of biochemical and cellular elemental structures have been associated with aging, but their exact role in the development of or maintenance of a hypertensive state, and specifically ISH in the elderly, is not established. Among these changes are increased circulating levels of catecholamines[18] and a decreased level of beta-adrenergic sensitivity (decreased receptor affinity for the agonist).[19] Alpha-[20] and beta-adrenergic[21] receptor numbers and alpha-adrenergic[20] sensitivity are unchanged with increasing age. Not specifically related to the aforementioned findings is a clear age-associated reduction in glomerular filtration rate and renal function.[22] A role for any or all of these in ISH is unclear.

Rowe and Troen[59] have speculated that a decrease in tonic inhibitions of the brain stem vasomotor centers owing to diminished baroreceptor activity may result in an exaggerated level of activity in the sympathetic nervous system. Regardless, it is clear that hypertension has an age-independent effect in reducing baroreflex sensitivity.[23,24] Furthermore, sustained elevations or reductions in blood pressure result in a resetting of baroreflex sensitivity, which can be lost if the vascular changes of aging or chronic hypertension become fixed.[25] It remains to be demonstrated whether or not these changes can be reversed by antihypertensive therapy, with appropriate reduction of blood pressure.

RISK IMPLICATIONS

SYSTOLIC VERSUS DIASTOLIC BLOOD PRESSURE

Curiously, at some distant time point, DBP took on greater clinical and pathophysiologic significance than SBP. In 1985, Fisher[26] suggested three reasons:

1. Physiology textbooks note that the walls of the blood vessels are subjected to a constant pressure equal to that of DBP.[27]
2. In acute hypertensive encephalopathy, diastolic pressure is markedly elevated with attendant arteriolar damage.
3. In early essential hypertension and in certain cases of glomerulonephritis in which there is cardiac weakness, blood pressure elevation is entirely manifest in the diastolic reading.[28]

Although Fisher pointed out in the early 1960s that systolic pressure elevations with normal diastolic pressures were not uncommon in patients with intracerebral hemorrhage, the data from the Build and Blood Pressure Study[3] previously discussed and from the Framingham Study convincingly documented the prognostic significance of both blood pressure readings in the prediction of cardiovascular sequelae.[29] If anything, coronary heart disease (CHD) and stroke have been demonstrated to be more closely associated with an elevation of SBP than DBP. This has been subsequently corroborated by Colandrea and colleagues.[30] Garland and coworkers[7] demonstrated an increased risk for both men and women with SBP > 160 mmHg and DBP <90 mmHg for total mortality and stroke but not for ischemic heart disease. Furthermore, Curb and colleagues[6] have reported an increase in total mortality in those individuals above age 30 with SBP ≥160 mmHg and DBP <90 mmHg. This rate increased with age. In the Veterans Administration study, when both the effects of SBP and DBP on morbidity and mortality were analyzed, there was no evidence for the greater impact of DBP.[31] More recently, the data from the 317,871 Multiple Risk Factor Intervention Trial screenees corroborate the increased risk associated with ISH and a greater risk with an increase in SBP than with increases in DBP.[32] In summary, in every study in which the relative effects of systolic and diastolic pressure have been compared, SBP elevation has been associated with a greater impact on total and cause-specific mortality and morbidity.

WHAT IS THE RISK OF AN INCREASED SYSTOLIC PRESSURE?

In childhood and adolescence, elevated SBP almost certainly represents a hyperdynamic circulation.[33] However, as early as the fourth decade, epidemiologic data demonstrate a direct association between SBP and the incidence of stroke and ischemic heart disease and an increase in all-cause mortality.[34] Data from the Framingham Study show a doubling of the stroke incidence for men over age 65 years, comparing those with SBP between 160 and 169 mmHg to those with SBP below 110[35] (Table 4–5). Women over age 65 have more than a tripling of stroke incidence for the same blood pressure comparison. The Honolulu Heart Study shows a doubling of age-adjusted incidence of hemorrhagic stroke comparing those with SBP below 121 mmHg to those with pressures above 150 mmHg and nearly a quadrupling in thrombotic stroke for the same groups[36] (Fig. 4–1).

The observed 20-year incidence of cardiovascular disease (CVD) for those over age 55 from the Framingham Study with SBP above 160 mmHg and DBP below 95 mmHg is 3.5 (men) and 3.8 (women) times greater than for those who have SBP <110 mmHg[24] (Table 4–6).

Additionally, the Framingham data show that total mortality in those women who have SBP above 160 mmHg and DBP below 95 mmHg is 2.5 times that of normotensive women. Men with the same blood pressure and age characteristics have approximately twice the mortality risk of their normotensive counterparts[8] (Fig. 4–2).

Increases in risk (3.0) for death from stroke have been reported in white men among the MRFIT screenees; also, increases in the risk of premature death from

Table 4–5. The Framingham Study Average Annual Incidence of Stroke per 10,000 Persons

Selected Systolic Blood Pressure Levels* (mmHg)	Men 65–74 yr	Women 65–74 yr
<110	42	26
120–129	56	39
140–149	74	58
160–169	97	87
180–189	129	129
190+	148	157

*Does not consider level of diastolic blood pressure.
SOURCE: The Framingham Study: Some characteristics related to the incidence of cardiovascular disease and death, 18-year follow-up. Section 30. NIH 74-599, 1973.

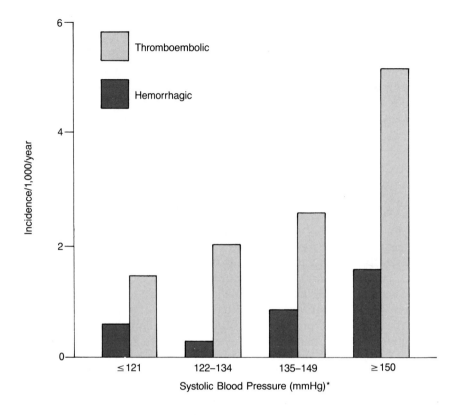

Figure 4–1. Annual incidence of stroke by systolic blood pressure. Age-adjusted 6-year follow-up: men 45–68 years of age at entry. (From the Honolulu Heart Study,[36] with permission.)

any cause or from CHD have been demonstrated.[32] These data demonstrate convincingly that in both men and women increases in SBP place individuals at increased risk of stroke, CVD, and premature death compared with their normotensive counterparts. Moreover, the risk is greater for nonwhites than whites (Table 4–3).

Table 4–6. Two-Year Incidence of Cardiovascular Disease Among Persons 55–74 Years of Age with Isolated Systolic Hypertension* by Sex

Sex	Incidence Rate per 1000	Relative Risk Compared with Normotensives
Male	113.0	3.5
Female	50.3	3.8

*Systolic blood pressure ≥160 mmHg and diastolic blood pressure <95 mmHg.
SOURCE: The Framingham Study: 20-year follow-up.[35]

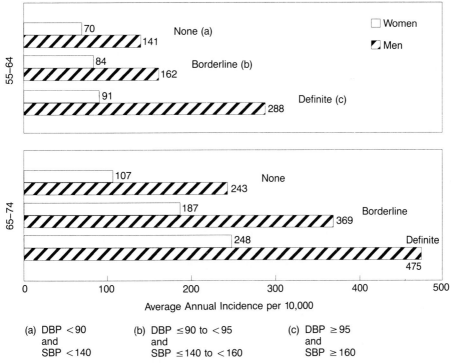

Figure 4–2. Mortality rate (per 10,000) by blood pressure status: (*a*) DBP <90 and SBP <140; (*b*) DBP ≤90 to <95 and SBP ≤140 to <160; (*c*) DBP ≥95 and SBP ≥160: 18-year follow-up. SOURCE: The Framingham Study,[29] with permission.

CAN ISOLATED SYSTOLIC HYPERTENSION BE CONTROLLED?

A preferred approach to therapeutic control of an altered physiologic process begins with an understanding of the basic mechanisms involved. In a previous section, some of the proposed altered anatomic and physiologic processes associated with the expected aging process and those related to ISH have been described. This information makes clear the notion that targeted therapy for hypertension in the elderly, and particularly ISH, demands the so-called low and slow approach to adjustments in the treatment regimen. This jargon terminology serves as a reminder to clinicians that reduced baroreflex sensitivity, reduced beta-adrenergic sensitivity, and reduced renal clearance of parent drugs and active metabolites contribute to impaired blood pressure homeostasis in the face of powerful therapeutic agents. Furthermore, age-related changes in cerebral autoregulation ironically may exacerbate or promote new symptoms when antihypertensive therapy is initiated. Recent findings suggest that a gradual approach to blood pressure reduction may partially correct abnormalities in blood pressure regulation.[37]

One very important consideration for control is what is the goal to be attained. The current Joint National Committee (JNC) guidelines recommend that the long-term goal of all blood pressure control, regardless of age, be SBP of <140 mmHg and DBP of <90 mmHg.[38] In some patients who have extreme elevations of SBP, this may not be possible, but SBP reductions of at least 20 mmHg should be attainable in all individuals without inducing intolerable side effects. This may require several changes in regimen along with the low and slow approach.

Most randomized clinical trials have focused on the treatment of diastolic hypertension, and the data demonstrate that when treatment is instituted, there is a roughly equivalent relative reduction in both SBP and DBP. However, data from trials in ISH now clearly indicate that initiation of treatment results in a disproportionate decrease in SBP without inducing diastolic hypotension. One-year data in the SHEP pilot study showed a treatment differential of 17 mmHg (12 percent) in the SBP with only a 6 mmHg (9 percent) reduction in the DBP.[39] These reductions were achieved over the first 3 months of therapy, and most of the change occurred in the first month. Moreover, this reduction in blood pressure was accomplished in 88 percent of people with single-drug therapy. Of those requiring a second drug, approximately half reached the arbitrary therapeutic goal of a 20 mmHg reduction in SBP.[40] Although dose one and dose two of the Step 1 drug in the SHEP pilot were 25 and 50 mg of chlorthalidone respectively, unpublished data from the SHEP pilot actually show 81.6 percent of participants controlled on 12.5 mg of chlorthalidone during the second and third year of follow-up in a dose-reduction study.[41] The answer to the question posed is a resounding yes. ISH can be controlled and with relatively low doses of therapeutic agents. The concomitant side effects are described subsequently.

DETECTION AND EVALUATION

Although the recommended methods for detection of abnormal blood pressure in the elderly are similar to those for the remainder of the population, there are several general and specific guidelines to keep in mind so that detection of ISH in this group may be valid and reliable.

General issues include the following:

1. Cuff size is important.
2. Multiple measurements are necessary (at least three) on several different occasions.
3. Indirect measurement of SBP is more accurate than that of DBP and is as reliable as the direct measurement of SBP.[42-44]
4. SBP is no more unstable than DBP.[45]

Specific issues include the following:

1. Blood pressure measurement (especially SBP) in the postprandial period is inaccurate (usually substantially lower).[46]
2. Blood pressure measurements in both the sitting and standing positions before and during drug therapy are very important because of the possibility of orthostasis.
3. An occasional elderly patient has pseudohypertension because of severe medial sclerosis of the brachial artery.[47,48] Patients with extreme blood pressures but no end-organ damage should be suspected of having this entity.[49]

Evaluation for secondary causes of blood pressure elevation in this group is unwarranted, unless the blood pressure levels are refractory to usual forms of therapy.

NONPHARMACOLOGIC APPROACH TO THERAPY

Specific investigation of the nonpharmacologic approaches in patients with ISH is meager. Trials in adults using a nonpharmacologic approach to blood pressure control, however, have consistently shown reduction in both SBP and DBP.

The current JNC guidelines recommend the following nonpharmacologic approaches to the control of hypertension and specifically suggest that these methods should be used as initial therapy for those who have ISH.[38]

1. Weight reduction—to within 15 percent of desirable weight.
2. Restriction of alcohol—not to exceed 1 oz of ethanol per day (corresponds to 2 oz of 100-proof whiskey, 240 ml or 8 oz of wine, or 720 ml or 24 oz of beer).
3. Sodium restriction—70 to 100 mEq per day (equals 1.5 to 2.5 g of sodium or 4 to 6 g per day of salt).
4. Potassium ion supplementation in those with normal renal function—>80 mEq or 3 to 4 g per day, for example, 1 cup raisins equals 30 mEq; 1 baked potato equals 20 mEq; 1 cup stewed prunes equals 25 mEq; 1 banana equals 10 mEq; 8 oz orange juice equals 10 mEq.
5. Tobacco avoidance—continued smoking may reduce the effect of certain pharmacologic agents, specifically beta-blockers.
6. Biofeedback and relaxation—to be used particularly in conjunction with pharmacologic therapy.
7. Exercise—regular aerobic exercise program (for example, walking, cycling, jogging, or swimming).

PHARMACOLOGIC APPROACH TO THERAPY

Although all antihypertensive drugs have been shown to be effective in the elderly and particularly in those with ISH, the JNC guidelines recommend that diuretics, beta-blockers, calcium channel blockers, and angiotensin converting enzyme (ACE) inhibitors be considered for use as monotherapy or Step 1 agents.[38] Central and peripherally acting adrenergic inhibitors should be considered for addition to the recommended agents for monotherapy as Step 2 treatment. Any drug for use as a monotherapeutic agent can be used also as a Step 2 drug.

A complete review of the pharmacologic properties of antihypertensive agents is beyond the scope of this chapter. However, a selected review of the chlorthalidone data, which has particular relevance to ISH, follows.

Although elderly patients may be particularly sensitive to volume depletion, the thiazides and their close relatives, the quinazolines (for example, chlorthalidone), are known to exert antihypertensive activity by another mechanism. In addition to the evidence already cited for blood pressure control in the SHEP pilot, very important publications by Materson and colleagues[50] and Morledge and colleagues[51] have demonstrated that blood pressure control is possible using much smaller doses of chlorthalidone than were originally believed necessary. The first study done in mild hypertensives demonstrated considerable efficacy without tachyphylaxis for up to 12 weeks in patients using doses as low as 12.5 mg of chlorthalidone. In the second study, Morledge and colleagues specifically investigated a group of 172 ISH patients (SBP ≥160 mmHg, DBP <90 mmHg) 60 years or older for 12 weeks, using doses of 12.5, 25, or 50 mg of chlorthalidone in a double-blind,

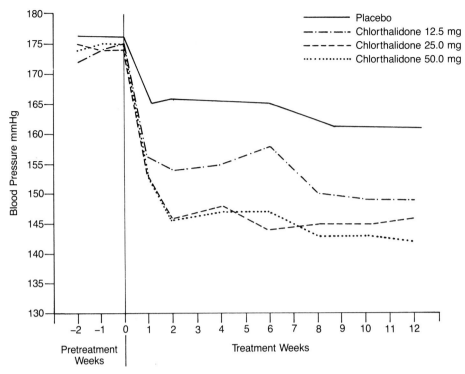

Figure 4–3. Mean sitting systolic blood pressure during the 12-week treatment period in each of the four groups. At all treatment visits (weeks 1, 2, 4, 6, 8, 10, and 12), the three chlorthalidone groups were significantly different from placebo (P <.05). At weeks 2, 4, 6, 8, 10, and 12, the chlorthalidone 25.0- and 50.0-mg groups were significantly different from the chlorthalidone 12.5-mg group (P <.05). (Adapted from Morledge, et al.[51])

placebo-controlled trial. Figure 4–3 shows the effect of the treatment regimens on SBP. Comparing Figure 4–3 with Figure 4–4 demonstrates the disproportionate reduction for SBP. Furthermore, Table 4–7 shows that at 12 weeks, 63 percent of patients had reached the goal of greater than or equal to 20 mmHg reduction. With the 25 and 50 mg doses, the percentages were 70 percent and 81 percent respec-

Table 4–7. Study of Isolated Systolic Hypertension: Therapeutic Success* Rate at the End of Weeks 1, 6, and 12

	Week		
Group	*1*	*6*	*12*
Placebo	26%	26%	22
Chlorthalidone 12.5 mg	47%	49%	63%*
Chlorthalidone 25.0 mg	50%	80%†	70%†
Chlorthalidone 50.0 mg	55%	78%†	81%†

*Sitting systolic blood pressure of less than 140 mmHg or decreased by greater than or equal to 20 mmHg or both.

†Significantly different from placebo (P <.01).

(Adapted from Morledge, et al.[51])

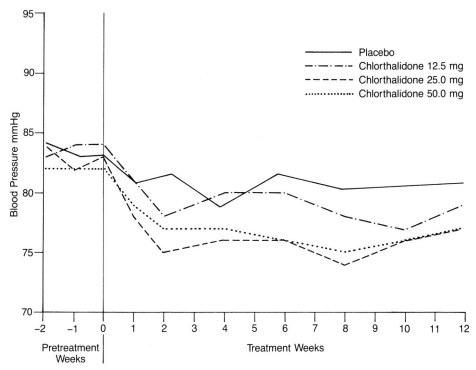

Figure 4–4. Mean sitting diastolic blood pressure during the 12-week treatment period in each of the four groups. At weeks 2, 4, and 6, the chlorthalidone 25.0- and 50.0-mg groups were significantly different from the placebo and chlorthalidone 12.5-mg groups (P<.05). At weeks 8, 10, and 12, the chlorthalidone 25.0- and 50.0-mg groups were significantly different from the chlorthalidone 12.5-mg group and all three chlorthalidone groups were significantly different from placebo (P <.5). (Adapted from Morledge, et al.[51])

tively. Finally, Table 4–8 describes the mean reduction in 3 SBP strata (160 to < 170, 170 to <180, ≥180 mmHg) for the various therapeutic regimens. The data clearly show a substantial reduction in SBP in all strata, even with 12.5 mg chlorthalidone. Although some additional blood pressure lowering occurs at the higher doses, only in patients with SBP equal to or greater than 180 mmHg does 50 mg of chlorthalidone appear to have substantial additional benefit over either 12.5 mg

Table 4–8. Study of Isolated Systolic Hypertension:
Blood Pressure Decreases in Each of the Treatment Groups
Stratified by Baseline Pressure

	Decrease (Mean ± SD) from Baseline to Week 12 (mmHg) Baseline Sitting Systolic Blood Pressure		
Group	*160–<170*	*170–<180*	*≥180*
Placebo	5.3 ± 11.6	8.2 ± 8.8	20.8 ± 9.2
Chlorthalidone 12.5 mg	21.6 ± 10.9	22.5 ± 15.7	28.4 ± 13.3
Chlorthalidone 25.0 mg	25.7 ± 12.9	28.2 ± 14.8	32.9 ± 19.4
Chlorthalidone 50.0 mg	26.4 ± 7.5	27.8 ± 11.4	38.4 ± 13.6

(Adapted from Morledge, et al.[51])

or 25 mg. These data clearly show the benefit of low-dose chlorthalidone therapy for the majority of patients with ISH.

SHOULD ISOLATED SYSTOLIC HYPERTENSION BE TREATED?

Gifford[52] cited several reasons why physicians and their patients may be reluctant to initiate treatment of systolic hypertension in the elderly, including the following:

1. Systolic hypertension in the elderly may be a manifestation merely of atherosclerosis of the aorta, and it may be this phenomenon rather than the hypertension that confers the increased risk for cerebrovascular and cardiovascular death.
2. There is an ill-founded fear that the treatment of ISH results in an equal reduction of both SBP and DBP, leading to arterial diastolic hypotension.
3. Intolerance to antihypertensive therapy in the elderly is thought to be prevalent.
4. There are no data from well-controlled trials that support a decreased risk for those individuals who have their ISH treated and controlled.

However, these issues may be responded to as follows: The epidemiologic data support a clear role for elevated SBP in the subsequent development of stroke and other cardiovascular events, both fatal and nonfatal. Data from several sources suggest that a disproportionate decrease in SBP occurs for those who have ISH, and arterial hypotension does not play a significant role. Although regular doses and dosing of antihypertensive medications promote untoward symptoms in the elderly, lower doses of antihypertensive medications at less frequent intervals can be shown to control SBP effectively. Finally, the lack of prospective randomized controlled data demonstrating a reduced risk for those treated for sustained ISH is recognized and would appear to be the only scientifically substantive reason for withholding therapy in those patients with ISH.

As early as 1973, intervention on hypertension in the elderly was identified as an important research issue. The United States Public Health Service and Veterans Administration Cooperative Studies programs each sponsored trials in the early 1970s investigating mild hypertension.[31,53] Investigators from both these studies had considered separate trials of hypertension in the elderly. An investigator-initiated grant application from a consortium of these investigators was submitted in 1978 to the National Heart, Lung, and Blood Institute and the National Institute on Aging proposing a clinical trial in predominantly systolic hypertension or ISH in an elderly population to investigate the treatment effect on fatal and nonfatal strokes as well as cause-specific and total mortality and major morbidity. The focus was later changed to that of ISH specifically. The pilot study was funded in 1979 and the full-scale study in 1983.

SHEP PILOT[39]

The specific objectives of the SHEP Pilot Study were to test methods of recruitment, enrollment, adherence, and efficacy of antihypertensive medication for lowering SBP in a population with ISH. Additionally, it was to assess the evaluation instruments used to determine the incidence of dementia and depression and to assess side effects of the drug-treatment regimens.

In a randomized double-blind, placebo-controlled design, the Step 1 medication was chlorthalidone; the Step 2 drug on the basis of a randomized design was a beta-blocker (metoprolol), reserpine, or hydralazine for those participants requiring a second medication.

The five centers screened 27,199 persons and enrolled 551 participants during a one-year recruitment period. Adherence to the treatment regimen was excellent among active participants, with over 90 percent of both the prescribed Step 1 and Step 2 medications taken according to a system of self-report. However, 18.5 percent of the participants stopped taking the SHEP medication during the first year. Regardless, 75 percent of participants reached goal SBP at 3 months on Step 1 medication alone, and this result was sustained throughout the remainder of the study. Troublesome or intolerable symptoms of a variety of types were reported prior to randomization in about one third of the participants; small increases occurred during the trial, but little could be ascribed directly to the active study medication regimen. All the objectives of the pilot study were met, and the decision to go to the full-scale study was made in the fall of 1983.

SHEP Main Trial[54]

The SHEP main trial is a randomized double-blind, placebo-controlled trial to determine whether antihypertensive treatment of sustained ISH (SBP ≥ 160 mmHg and DBP <90 mmHg) reduces the 5-year incidence of fatal and nonfatal stroke. It has 16 clinical centers and a coordinating center (Table 4–9). Important secondary endpoints include cause-specific and total mortality and such selected morbid endpoints as multi-infarct dementia, clinical depression, deterioration of cognitive function, and quality of life. Recruitment was demanding; however, 4736 persons (target 4800) with ISH, age 60 years and over, were enrolled (1 percent of those initially contacted) between March 1, 1984, and January 15, 1988. This sample size, with allowance for 16 percent dropouts and 19 percent crossover, will have 90 percent power with a 2-sided alpha of 0.05 to detect a 32 percent effect on the primary endpoint.

Potential participants were those who met blood pressure criteria and those taking antihypertensive medication and without documented diastolic hypertension who had their medication tapered and discontinued with consent obtained from the participant and primary care physician and who then met blood pressure criteria. Eligible participants were randomized to stepped-care therapy with chlorthalidone (12.5 and 25 mg per day) followed by atenolol (25 and 50 mg per day) (alternative, reserpine, 0.05 and 0.1 mg per day) or matching placebos as first and second steps. They are being followed quarterly. Sixty-six percent of participants were not on antihypertensive medication prior to randomization. The group is 38.6 percent nonblack male, 47.5 percent nonblack female, 4.5 percent black male, and 9.3 percent black female. At baseline, the age-range distribution was 41 percent, 60 to 69; 45 percent, 70 to 79; and 14 percent, 80 and over (mean 71.6). The cohort's SBP range distribution was 57 percent, 160 to 169 mmHg; 27 percent, 170 to 179 mmHg; and 16 percent, 180 mmHg and over (mean 170.3); the mean DBP was 76.6 mmHg. Of participants, 59.8 percent had codeable baseline electrocardiographic abnormalities. The trial is jointly sponsored by the National Heart, Lung,

Table 4–9. SHEP Investigators

Institution	Principal Investigator
Albert Einstein College of Medicine	M. Donald Blaufox, M.D., Ph.D.
Emory University School of Medicine	W. Dallas Hall, M.D.
Kaiser Permanente Center for Health Research	Thomas Vogt, M.D., M.P.H.
Medical Research Institute of San Francisco	W. McFate Smith, M.D., M.P.H.
Miami Heart Institute	Jeffrey Raines, Ph.D, F.A.C.C.
Northwestern University Medical School	David Berkson, M.D.
Pacific Health Research Institute	Helen Petrovitch, M.D.
Robert Wood Johnson Medical School	John B. Kostis, M.D.
University of Alabama, Birmingham	Harold W. Schnaper, M.D.
University of California, Davis	Nemat O. Borhani, M.D., M.P.H.
University of Kentucky Medical Center	Gordon Guthrie, M.D.
University of Minnesota	Richard H. Grimm, Jr., M.D., Ph.D.
University of Pittsburgh	Robert McDonald, M.D.
University of Tennessee	William A. Applegate, M.D., M.P.H.
Washington University	H. Mitchell Perry, Jr., M.D.
Yale University	Henry Black, M.D.
University of Texas/Health Sciences Center	C. Morton Hawkins, Sc.D.
Mayo Clinic (Steering Committee Chairman)	Kenneth G. Berge, M.D.
National Heart, Lung, Blood Institute Project Office	Jeffrey L. Probstfield, M.D.
National Heart, Lung, Blood Institute	Eleanor Schron, R.N., M.S.
National Institute on Aging	J. David Curb, M.D., M.P.H.
National Institute on Aging	Lot B. Page, M.D.

and Blood Institute and the National Institute on Aging. The trial is now in follow-up phase with scheduled termination in 1991.

What Treatment While We Wait for SHEP?

A recent report on hypertension in the elderly cited no clinical trial evidence of benefit in patients treated for ISH;[55] furthermore, the Joint National Committee on Detection, Evaluation, and Treatment of High Blood Pressure guidelines published in 1984[56] and 1988[38] differ very little in their recommendations on the treatment of ISH. Several points are made in the current JNC document, including the following:

1. Sustained elevation of SBP must be documented before treatment is contemplated or indicated.
2. Treatment must be individualized on a case-by-case basis because clinical trial results that might give a more general approach await the results of SHEP
3. A hygienic approach is indicated first. A general list of nonpharmacologic approaches enumerated in a previous section is appropriate for intervention in hypertension, and it is suggested that any and all should be attempted to achieve potential benefit.
4. Several antihypertensive drugs have been shown to be effective and relatively nontoxic when used cautiously in the elderly with ISH. Particular notice must be taken of sensitivity to volume depletion and sympathetic inhibition in this group.

Table 4–10. SHEP Pilot Study: Prevalence of Symptoms Characterized as Troublesome or Intolerable at Baseline and During Follow-Up by Study Group

	Baseline			1 Month			1 Year*		
	Chlorthalidone (n = 443) (%)	Placebo (n = 108) (%)	Significance of Difference	Chlorthalidone (n = 443) (%)	Placebo (n = 108) (%)	Significance of Difference	Chlorthalidone (n = 423) (%)	Placebo (n = 107) (%)	Significance of Difference
Cardiopulmonary									
Faintness on standing	3	4		3	5		5	7	
Heart beating faster or skipping	3	0	p = 0.08	2	1		3	7	p = 0.05
Chest pain or heaviness	3	2		2	2		4	4	
Unusual shortness of breath	2	3		2	2		5	3	
Unusual tiredness	5	3		7	5		7	9	
Cold or numb hands	2	2		1	0		5	7	
Ankle swelling	5	2		2	1		4	7	
Psychosocial									
Depression that interfered with activities	1	2		2	1		4	6	
Nightmares	1	1		1	0		1	2	
Problems in sexual function	1	1		2	1		2	0	
Problems in sleeping	8	7		3	6		10	10	
Unusual worry or anxiety	5	3		3	3		7	10	
Loss of appetite	0	0		2	1		2	2	
Other									
Nausea or vomiting	2	0		5	2		2	2	
Skin rash or bruising	3	2		1	1		5	7	
Unusual joint pain	10	14		4	7		12	18	
Severe headaches	3	1		3	1		3	3	
Excessive thirst	1	0		1	0		1	1	
Stuffy nose	5	5		4	4		8	9	
Other	3	5		10	11		11	18	
Summary Status									
Any of above	30	33		34	31		44	48	p = 0.06
Any of above characterized as intolerable	2	3		2	2		3	6	

*The number of observations at 1 year is larger than the number attending the 1-year clinic visit because it includes persons who were queried by telephone about these symptoms.

(From Hulley, et al,[39] with permission.)

79

Table 4–11. Study of Isolated Systolic Hypertension: Summary of Adverse Reactions

Group	N	No. of Patients		
		Had AR (%)	*Had Drug-Related AR (%)*	*Discontinued Due to AR (%)*
Placebo	39	21 (54)	2 (5)	5 (13)
Chlorthalidone 12.5 mg	47	22 (47)	4 (9)	3 (6)
Chlorthalidone 25.0 mg	43	23 (53)	10 (23)	4 (9)
Chlorthalidone 50.0 mg	47	31 (66)	12 (26)*	7 (15)
Total	176	97	28	19

*Significantly different from placebo (P < .05)
AR = Adverse reactions.
Adapted from Morledge, JH, et al.[51]

ADVERSE REACTIONS TO DRUG THERAPY

The largest single group of ISH patients followed for the longest period of time were in the SHEP pilot study.[39] In Table 4–10, information is given on adverse effects in that trial. At baseline, 30 percent of those assigned to chlorthalidone had any of the list of symptoms used to assess adverse effect to study medication; 33 percent of those assigned to placebo gave comparable data. Two and three percent respectively reported these symptoms as intolerable. One year after initiation of therapy, 44 percent and 48 percent respectively, reported any symptoms in the chlorthalidone and placebo groups respectively; 3 percent and 6 percent respectively, of these symptoms were described as intolerable. These data indicate that the symptoms ascertained in the SHEP pilot are common among the elderly, and that there is no evidence that they were induced by chlorthalidone. Table 4–11 gives complementary data from the Morledge study.[51] The number of adverse reactions in all groups (placebo and three active drug doses) was relatively comparable. The number ascribed to the drug appeared to be drug-related and dose-related.

The SHEP pilot showed changes in the chlorthalidone-treated group at one year for the following serum measurements: potassium, creatinine, and uric acid. Small and insignificant changes in glucose were found. No change in total serum cholesterol was noted.[39]

One fifth of the chlorthalidone-treated patients had serum potassium levels below 3.5 mEq per liter, and the clinician elected to supplement these with oral potassium. Potassium levels below 3.0 mEq per liter were rare. One case of acute gout was observed in the study. The minor increase in serum creatinine is of uncertain clinical importance.

The report of Morledge and colleagues[51] showed the expected dose-dependent decrease in serum potassium with chlorthalidone; those at higher doses of active drugs were given potassium supplements more often. Findings with regard to uric acid, creatinine, glucose, and cholesterol were similar to the pilot SHEP experience.

SPECIFIC RECOMMENDATIONS

Four current publications that review the management of hypertension in the elderly, including ISH, call for caution in the initiation of therapeutic management.[38,49,56,58] These cautions are raised not because ISH cannot be controlled or because the patients have adverse effects from the therapeutic agents. The genuine concern is that clinicians and patients may take it for granted that successful control of ISH will necessarily mean that the attendant risk of ISH has been reduced or eliminated. The answer to this question awaits the conclusion of the SHEP main trial.

While waiting for the SHEP results, it is certainly prudent in those patients with consistent systolic pressure readings ≥ 160 mmHg to implement hygienic measures as outlined in the nonpharmacologic approach. Furthermore, if the decision is made to implement therapy, a specific goal should be kept in mind. The Working Group on Hypertension in the Elderly[49] suggested that systolic blood pressure for those with ISH be lowered to between 140 and 160 mmHg while diastolic pressure is maintained above 70 mmHg. If the hygienic approach proves unsuccessful, the decision to implement pharmacologic therapy must remain for each physician to make in the context of an individual patient's characteristics. For those who have a "high cardiovascular risk burden" or who have unusually high blood pressure readings or profound symptoms associated with hypertension, the physician may choose to implement drug therapy. This must be done using the low and slow approach. The data support low-dose chlorthalidone as an effective agent. A more limited data set supports low-dose hydrochlorothiazide as a useful agent.[58]

The recent publication by The Working Group on Hypertension in the Elderly[49] states that monotherapy with beta-blockers in the elderly is less successful in blood pressure control. In those who have a contraindication or intolerance to diuretics, a calcium channel blocker or an ACE inhibitor may be the initial therapy. However, published data on the efficacy of these agents in ISH are lacking.

For those who require additional therapy, a beta-blocker, reserpine, methyldopa, or clonidine may be added as a second agent. If additional therapy is required, hydralazine is recommended as a Step 3 drug.

Perhaps as important in therapeutic management are the drugs that should be avoided. Any agents or doses of agents that are likely to provoke hypotension should not be used. This list of agents specifically includes guanethidine, prazosin, pargyline, and guanadrel.

Finally, the elderly patient, although wanting to comply with the physician's

Table 4–12. The Working Party on Hypertension in the Elderly: Psychosocial Factors in the Elderly That May Alter Adherence or Response to Treatment

1. Transportation problems are frequent.
2. Diets of elderly may be deficient in fruits and vegetables, leading to hypokalemia.
3. Wife is frequently the medical caregiver; widowers may be without help.
4. Impediments in hearing and eyesight may require special consideration.
5. Mental confusion may lead to improper diet or neglect of medications.
6. Safety caps are difficult for elderly to manipulate.
7. Living alone with little contact may hinder adherence.
8. Low, fixed income may limit prescription acquisition and keeping physician appointments.
9. Over-the-counter preparations frequently used by elderly may lead to drug interactions.
10. Institutionalized patients must have supervision if therapy for isolated systolic hypertension is to be started.
11. The presence of dementia or depression may limit opportunity for therapy.

recommendations, may have a variety of psychosocial factors that may alter the adherence pattern or the response to therapy. These issues were discussed in detail by the Working Group on Hypertension in the Elderly;[49] they have been adapted into a tabular form in Table 4–12.

SUMMARY

ISH is a distinct pathogenetic entity defined by SBP readings of ≥ 160 and DBP <90 mmHg. The etiology, although not well understood, is in some manner related to a reduction in connective tissue elasticity of large blood vessels and an increase in aortic impedance or a decrease in aortic wall compliance. The pathophysiologic consequences include an increased resistance to systolic ejection of blood and a disproportionate increase in SBP. Although not directly related, there is an important increase in peripheral vascular resistance.

The prevalence of ISH in several studies is about 7 percent in those over age 60 and increases with age to nearly 20 percent in those over age 80. There is higher prevalence in females and nonwhites. The guidelines for detection of ISH are similar to those for blood pressure evaluation in general. Precautions for detection and evaluation in the elderly include multiple blood pressure measurements in the fasting state and sitting and supine blood pressure measurements before and during therapy. Pseudohypertension, although rare, should be kept in mind. There is a clear risk associated with ISH for stroke, CVD, and premature death, which increases with age and rising levels of SBP.

ISH can be controlled effectively with pharmacologic therapies. A reasonable goal is a 20 mmHg reduction in systolic pressure. *Proof of reduced risk for stroke, CHD, and death in those with controlled ISH remains to be demonstrated. The SHEP pilot study has demonstrated feasibility of addressing this issue. The full-scale SHEP study addresses this issue and has completed recruitment of the desired sample size and is in follow-up phase. Scheduled completion is in 1991.*

While we wait for the SHEP full-scale trial results, the prudent approach is for nonpharmacologic therapy and use of pharmacologic agents in that group of patients who demonstrate a large cardiovascular risk burden or increasing symptoms specifically associated with hypertension. The decision to treat must be on an individual patient basis. Pharmacologic therapy is possible in most patients with few or no adverse effects. The "low and slow" approach to therapy is helpful in minimizing these adverse effects. Low-dose diuretics have been documented to be effective in blood pressure control. Chlorthalidone, 12.5 or 25 mg per day, is suggested. Other agents, such as beta-blockers, reserpine, ACE inhibitors, and calcium channel blockers, are best used as Step 2 agents.

REFERENCES

1. Gubner, RS: Systolic hypertension: A pathogenetic entity. Am J Cardiol 9:773, 1962.
2. Schettler, G: Prevention and treatment of "atheromatous complications" of hypertension. In Bock, KD and Cottier, PT (eds): Hypertension: An International Symposium. Springer-Verlag, Berlin, 1960.
3. Build and Blood Pressure Study. Society of Actuaries, Chicago, 1959.
4. Gubner, RS: Life expectancy of the young hypertensive. In Brest, AN and Moyer, JH (eds): Hypertension: Recent Advances. Lea & Febiger, Philadelphia, 1961.

5. Shekelle, RB, Ostfeld, AM, and Klawans, HL Jr: Hypertension and risk of stroke in an elderly population. Stroke 5:71, 1974.
6. Curb, JD, et al: Isolated systolic hypertension in 14 communities. Am J Epidemiol 121:362, 1985.
7. Garland, C, et al: Isolated systolic hypertension and mortality after age 60 years. Am J Epidemiol 118:365, 1983.
8. The SHEP Pilot Study: Unpublished material, 1986.
9. Roberts, J and Rowland, J: National Center for Health Statistics. Hypertension in Adults 25–74 years of age, United States, 1971–1975. Vital and Health Statistics. Series 11, no. 221, DHHS pub. no. (PHS) 81-1671 Public Health Service, U.S. Government Printing Office, Washington, DC, 1981.
10. McClellan, W, et al: Isolated systolic hypertension: Declining prevalence in the elderly. Prev Med 16:686, 1987.
11. Simon, AC, et al: Systolic hypertension: Hemodynamic mechanism and choice of antihypertensive treatment. Am J Cardiol 44:505,1979.
12. Hallock, P and Benson, IC: Studies on the elastic properties of human isolated aorta. J Clin Invest 16:595, 1937.
13. Kannel, WB, et al: Systolic blood pressure, arterial rigidity, and risks of stroke. JAMA 245:1225, 1981.
14. Chobanian, AV: Pathophysiologic considerations in the treatment of the elderly hypertension patient. Am J Cardiol 52:49D, 1983.
15. Tarazi, RC, Martini, F, and Dustan, HP: The role of aortic distensibility in hypertension. In Milliez, P and Sasar, M (eds): International Symposium on Hypertension. Monaco, Boehringer Ingelheim, 1975.
16. Tarazi, RC: Regression of left ventricular hypertrophy by medical treatment: Present status and possible implications. Am J Med 78:80, 1983.
17. Koch-Weser, J: Correlation of pathophysiology and pharmacotherapy in primary hypertension. Am J Cardiol 32:499, 1973.
18. Ziegler, MG, Lake, CR, and Kopin, IJ: Plasma noradrenaline increases with age. Nature 261:333, 1976.
19. Feldman, RD, et al: Alterations in leukocyte β-receptor affinity with aging: A potential explanation for altered β-adrenergic sensitivity in the elderly. N Engl J Med 310:815, 1984.
20. Abrass, IB, Ko, T, and Scarpace, PJ: Platelet alpha-adrenergic receptor function in aging (abstract). Clin Res 32:479a, 1984.
21. Abrass, IB, and Scarpace, PJ: Human lymphocyte beta-adrenergic receptors are unaltered with age. J Gerontol 36:298, 1981.
22. Rowe, JW, Andres, R, Tobin, JD, et al: The effect of age on creatinine clearance in men: A cross-sectional and longitudinal study. J Gerontol 31:155, 1976.
23. Mancia, G, et al: Blood pressure variability in man: Its relation to high blood pressure, age, and baroreflex sensitivity. Clin Sci 59:401s, 1980.
24. Gribbin, B, et al: Effect of age and high blood pressure on baroreflex sensitivity in man. Circ Res 29:424, 1971.
25. Brown, AM: Receptors under pressure: An update on baroreceptors. Circ Res 46:1, 1980.
26. Fisher, CM: Point of view: The ascendency of diastolic blood pressure over systolic. Lancet 2:1349, 1985.
27. West, JB (ed): Best and Taylor's Physiological Basis of Medical Practice, ed 11. Williams and Wilkins, Baltimore, 1985.
28. Fishberg, AM: Hypertension and Nephritis. Lea & Febiger, Philadelphia, 1930.
29. Kannel, WB and Dawber, TR: Hypertension as an ingredient of a cardiovascular risk profile. Br J Hosp Med 11:508, 1974.
30. Colandrea, MA, et al: Systolic hypertension in the elderly. Circulation 41:239, 1970.
31. Veterans Administration Cooperative Study Group on Antihypertensive Agents: Effects of treatment on morbidity in hypertension. II. Results in patients with diastolic blood pressure averaging 90 through 114 mm Hg. JAMA 213:1143, 1970.
32. Rutan, GH, et al: Mortality associated with diastolic hypertension and isolated systolic hypertension among men screened for the Multiple Risk Factor Intervention Trial. Circulation 77:405, 1988.
33. Adamopoulos, PN, Chrysanthakopoulis, SK, and Frohlich, ED: Systolic hypertension: Non-homogeneous diseases. Am J Cardiol 36:697, 1975.
34. Kannel, WB, et al: Epidemiologic assessment of the role of blood pressure in stroke: The Framingham Study. JAMA 214:301, 1970.

35. Kannel, WB, Dawber, TR, and McGee, DL: Perspectives on systolic hypertension: The Framingham Study. Circulation 61:1179, 1980.
36. Kagan, A, Popper, JS, and Rhoads, GG: Factors related to stroke incidence in Hawaiian Japanese Men: The Honolulu Heart Study. Stroke 11:14, 1980.
37. Lipsitz, LA: Abnormalities in blood pressure homeostasis associated with aging and hypertension: Clinical implications and research needs. NIH Blood Pressure Regulation and Aging: Proceedings from a Symposium. 201, 1986.
38. The 1988 Report of the Joint National Committee on Detection, Evaluation, and Treatment of High Blood Pressure. Arch Intern Med 148:1023, 1988.
39. Hulley, SB, et al, for the SHEP Research Group: Systolic Hypertension in the Elderly Program (SHEP): Antihypertensive efficacy of chlorthalidone. Am J Cardiol 56:913, 1985.
40. Perry, HM, et al: Morbidity and mortality in the Systolic Hypertension in the Elderly Program (SHEP) Pilot Study: A randomized clinical trial. Stroke 20:4, 1989.
41. Systolic Hypertension in the Elderly Program Pilot Study: Unpublished material, 1986.
42. Littler, WA, et al: Continuous recording of direct arterial pressure in unrestricted patients: Diagnosis and management of high blood pressure. Circulation 51:1101, 1975.
43. Van Bergen, FH, et al: Comparison of indirect and direct methods of measuring arterial blood pressure. Circulation 10:481, 1954.
44. Mutch, LMM, et al: Perinatal mortality and neonatal survival in Avon: 1976–79. Br Med J 282:119, 1981.
45. Jorde, LB and Williams, RR: Innovative blood pressure measurements yield information not reflected by sitting measurements. Hypertension 8:252, 1986.
46. Lipsitz, LA, et al: Intraindividual variability in postural blood pressure in the elderly. Clin Sci 69:337, 1985.
47. Spence, JD, Sibbald, WJ, and Cape, RD: Pseudohypertension in the elderly. Clin Sci Mol Med 55:399, 1978.
48. Messerli, FH, Ventura, HO, and Amodeo, C: Osler's maneuver and pseudohypertension. N Engl J Med 312:1548, 1985.
49. The Working Group on Hypertension in the Elderly. Statement on hypertension in the elderly: Special communication. JAMA 256:70, 1986.
50. Materson, BJ, et al: Dose response to chlorthalidone in patients with mild hypertension: Efficacy of a lower dose. Clin Pharmacol Ther 24:192, 1978.
51. Morledge, JH, et al: Isolated systolic hypertension in the elderly: A placebo-controlled, dose-response evaluation of chlorthalidone. JAGS 34:199, 1986.
52. Gifford, RW Jr: Isolated systolic hypertension in the elderly: Some controversial issues. JAMA 247:781, 1982.
53. Smith, WM, for the US Public Health Service Hospitals Cooperative Study Group: Treatment of mild hypertension: Results of a ten-year intervention trial. Circ Res (Suppl) 40:I-98, 1977.
54. The Systolic Hypertension in The Elderly Program (SHEP) Cooperative Research Group: Rationale and design of a randomized clinical trial on prevention of stroke in isolated systolic hypertension. J Clin Epidemiol 41:1197, 1988.
55. Davidson, RA and Caranasos, GJ: Should the elderly hypertensive be treated? Evidence from clinical trials. Arch Intern Med 147:1933, 1987.
56. The 1984 Report of the Joint National Committee on Detection, Evaluation, and Treatment of High Blood Pressure. Arch Intern Med 144:1045, 1984.
57. Gifford, RW Jr: Management of isolated systolic hypertension in the elderly. JAGS 34:106, 1986.
58. Vardan, S, et al: Systolic hypertension in the elderly: Hemodynamic response to long-term diuretic therapy and its side effects. JAMA 250:2807, 1983.
59. Rowe, JW and Troen, BR: Sympathetic nervous system and aging in man. Endocr Rev 1:167, 1980.

CHAPTER 5

Left Ventricular Hypertrophy: An Independent Factor of Risk

Edward D. Frohlich, M.D.

A clinically or physiologically identifiable variable that imparts independent and statistically significant chances for increased morbidity and mortality has been termed a "factor of risk."[1] This term, "risk factor," which was coined by the investigators of the Framingham study and employed validly or not by others, has been of great value for fundamental investigative and public health purposes in the area of cardiovascular diseases.

Implied, but by no means true, is the concept that once the presence of the independent risk factor has been identified epidemiologically, clinically, and with biostatistical confidence, its elimination or reversal will improve or enhance the likelihood for reduction of the morbidity or mortality rates related to that factor. The truth is that imparting significant increased risk related to that factor is one thing, but the demonstration of reversal of that risk by eliminating the factor is yet another issue. This chapter concerns the independent risk associated with the establishment of the presence of left ventricular hypertrophy (LVH) and explores the nature of that risk and the present evidence (in 1989) that this risk may be reduced by its so-called reversal.

CARDIOVASCULAR RISK FACTORS

As a result of a number of outstanding, prospectively designed and well-conducted epidemiologic studies, a number of cardiovascular factors that impart a significantly greater risk of increased morbidity and mortality for coronary heart disease (CHD) and sudden death have been identified (Table 5–1). Several of these CHD risk factors are, by definition, nonmodifiable and include advancing age of the individual, male gender (particularly under 50 years of age), and the race of the individual (particularly in those who are black).[1-8] Fortunately, there are a number of other CHD risk factors that can be modified, and their associated risk for increased morbidity and mortality can be reduced by their reversal. These factors include diastolic hypertension; hyperlipidemia, and, more specifically, high total

85

Table 5–1. Cardiovascular Risk Factors

Nonmodifiable
  Advancing age
  Male gender
  Black race
Modifiable (With Likely Reduction in Risk; Demonstrated)
  Diastolic hypertension
  Hyperlipidemia (i.e., high total and LDL cholesterol)
  Diabetes mellitus
  Obesity
  Smoking
Modifiable (With Reduction in Risk Not Yet Demonstrated)
  Systolic (isolated) hypertension
  Left ventricular hypertrophy
  Hyperuricemia
  Physical inactivity
  Personality (Type A)

and the low-density lipoprotein fraction of serum cholesterol (and, also likely, hypertriglyceridemia); diabetes mellitus; exogenous obesity (especially of truncal distribution); and smoking.[9-16] The question of isolated systolic hypertension, particularly in the elderly patient, is under active study (see Chapter 4), and answers should be forthcoming in the relatively near future. The physically inactive individual and the so-called Type A hard-driving personality probably impart increased risk, but reversal of the associated morbidity and mortality risk with exercise or with behavioral modification still requires documentation. The risk associated with elevated serum uric acid levels and then reduction of these levels may be still harder to show. The independent risk associated with LVH is clear;[17-20] the following discussion concerns its development, the associated clinical complications that confound the problem, the possible mechanisms that may underlie the risk of LVH, and the evidence supporting improvement or reduction of that risk by certain clinical interventions.

LEFT VENTRICULAR HYPERTROPHY

DEVELOPMENT

Over the years, a considerable and compelling body of evidence has shown that the LVH that results from systemic arterial hypertension, and other pressure-overload diseases, is an adaptive structural phenomenon. Thus, LVH accompanies and reflects the progressively rising arterial pressure and left ventricular afterload that is associated with the parallel increase in total peripheral resistance, the hemodynamic hallmark of systemic arterial hypertensive vascular disease.[21-27] This development of concentric LVH associated with pressure overload[28] provides the structural physical forces that are necessary to maintain left ventricular pump performance[29,30] and the systemic perfusion of vital organs. As such, it is an adaptive phenomenon that serves pathophysiologically to delay the ultimate development of cardiac failure[31] if therapeutic control of the hypertensive disease is not achieved.[9-13] When this pump performance can no longer be maintained as arterial pressure, total peripheral resistance, and left ventricular impedance rise unchecked clinically and therapeutically; left ventricular failure supervenes,[23-25,32] indicating inability of the heart to adapt further to the progressive ventricular overload.

In addition to the hemodynamic factor of pressure-overload, in some individuals with hypertension there is a coexistent volume overload. As already indicated, pressure overload ventricular hypertrophy is concentric in nature;[28] the ventricular chamber adapts structurally by enlarging in all directions. When the ventricular chamber enlarges in response to a volume overload, the hypertrophy is inappropriate or eccentric in its dimensional alterations.[28] Volume overload may be found as a result of exercise—a so-called physiologic hypertrophy. However, volume overload hypertrophy may also occur in patients with volume overload due to exogenous obesity[16] and perhaps in certain so-called volume-dependent forms of hypertension. When pressure and volume overload coexist in hypertension, and also with certain valvular heart diseases, the structural adaptation is dimorphic.[33] This, perhaps, explains why patients with coexistent systemic arterial hypertension and exogenous obesity are at enhanced risk for development of congestive heart failure.[1,4,8]

NONHEMODYNAMIC FACTORS

In recent years, studies have indicated that the height of arterial pressure does not always correlate with the magnitude of the increased ventricular mass in hypertension.[23-25] For example, our studies with the naturally developing genetic hypertension in the rat—spontaneous hypertension—indicated that left ventricular mass increased independent of the rise of arterial pressure and, in fact, continued to increase even after arterial pressure no longer rose.[34-36] Indeed, our studies with patients with essential hypertension failed to demonstrate a close correlation between increased left ventricular mass and arterial pressure.[37] By contrast, a significant correlation could be demonstrated between pressure and mass in other forms of experimental and clinical hypertension.[38,39] Although it is conceivable that the pressure overload may not be operative to the same extent in all forms of hypertension,[23-25,34-36] it seemed to us that other factors—nonhemodynamic in character—could also participate in the development of the hypertrophy.[23-25,39-41] Among these nonhemodynamic factors were: circulating levels of humoral agents (for example, norepinephrine, angiotensin), intramyocytic agents (growth and autocrine/paracrine), factors relating to the gender and race of the patient, coexisting diseases with hypertension (for example, exogenous obesity, coronary arterial disease, tobacco addiction, diabetes mellitus, and so on), factors relating to the aging process itself, and even the pharmacologic agents to which the patients had been subjected.[23-25,35,36,39-41] Not only do these factors relate to the increased ventricular mass, but also by virtue of their coexistence and association, each may confer an independent factor risk to the hypertrophic process that may be totally independent from the pressure (or even volume) overload.[42]

LVH: POTENTIAL MECHANISMS OF RISK

At the outset of this discussion it must be emphasized that the underlying explanation for the enhanced and independent risk associated with LVH is not known precisely. Several explanations or mechanisms are possible (Table 5–2).

Table 5–2. Potential Mechanisms That May Explain the Increased Cardiovascular Risk in Hypertensive Patients with Left Ventricular Hypertrophy

---

Hypertension-accelerated atherogenesis
Myocardial fibrosis
Coronary arterial insufficiency
Enhanced likelihood of cardiac dysrhythmias
Predisposition to sudden death
Reduced cardiac functional reserve
Transformation to less functional cardiac muscle (e.g., related to hypertension, antihypertensive therapy)
Deposition of amyloid and other substances
Altered release of endothelial relaxing or dilating substances

---

It is well-known that patients with hypertension are predisposed to the enhanced development of atherosclerosis and coronary arterial disease.[43,44] It would follow, therefore, that hypertensive patients with LVH should have higher arterial pressures than patients without hypertrophy, and, hence, their predisposition for associated atherosclerosis would be greater.[45] Indeed, this relationship may explain the increased frequency of coronary insufficiency, myocardial infarction, and sudden death in these patients. It also would explain the greater likelihood of myocardial fibrosis and the prevalence of symptomatic coronary arterial insufficiency in these patients.

Coronary insufficiency in patients with LVH is explicable on both functional as well as structural grounds: As Laplace's law states, the tension of a chamber (such as the heart) is directly related to the diameter of that chamber as well as the pressure within the chamber. In this respect, investigators have clearly shown that it is the tension of the ventricle that is the main determinant of oxygen consumption.[46] Thus, in patients with hypertension *and* LVH, both variables on which myocardial oxygen demand and consumption are based are present. This explains why angina pectoris may be present in patients with hypertension and normal coronary arteries. It may be solely the consequence of the elevated arterial pressure and the presence of coexistent LVH.

In addition to atherosclerosis and tension-related factors, other hemodynamic factors are possible, that is, other factors associated with severe hypertension (independent of atherosclerosis) that may damage the endothelium or coronary arteries. As a consequence of this endothelial damage, there may be impaired formation and release of the endothelium-derived relaxing factor (EDRF), the endothelium-derived constricting factor (EDCF or endothelin), or the release of other factors that may result in temporary or more prolonged coronary vasoconstriction.[36] This, in fact, may result in collagen deposition and myocardial fibrosis, which are frequently associated with LVH.

It follows then that the patient so predisposed to coronary arterial insufficiency (functional or organic) or myocardial fibrosis is at greater risk for the development of cardiac dysrhythmias and sudden death. In recent years, a number of retrospective and prospective studies have supported this contention,[17–20,47–49] and elsewhere in this text there is a separate discussion of the evidence for the various mechanisms and cardiac abnormalities that have been implicated.[50]

Given the greater likelihood for cardiac dysrhythmias and sudden death in patients with LVH, it follows that if certain antihypertensive agents enhance the risk for these adverse electrical phenomena, the interaction of both would enhance the risk. At present, controversy surrounds the role of diuretics and secondary hypokalemia in producing cardiac dysrhythmias and sudden death in patients with hypertension.[51-55] Until this controversy is resolved, it seems reasonable to suggest that hypokalemia should be prevented or corrected in a patient with hypertension, especially if these patients have LVH.

Furthermore, inasmuch as patients with LVH have already demonstrated evidence of myocardial adaptation to the pressure overload, it follows that these patients have already used a significant degree of their adaptive reserve.[42,56] This reserve may be expressed in terms of the reduced coronary arterial reserve that has been found with LVH[57] as well as the reserve pumping ability of the left ventricle. For these reasons, these patients may be at greater risk for development of congestive heart failure or acute pulmonary edema.

In recent years, experimental studies have demonstrated the existence of several different forms of myosin in the myocardium.[58] Some have suggested that certain types of myosin are more physiologic than others, implying that those "non-physiologic" myosins are pathologic and may not function normally.[59] Other studies have demonstrated a transformation in the types of myosin with certain antihypertensive drugs.[60] Whether these changes occur in man, whether they occur in patients with hypertension, or whether they are the result of antihypertensive drug therapy are subjects of speculation. Clearly, their implications are very important, and, no doubt, in the next several years the answers should be forthcoming. At present, we are left with a number of attractive possibilities to explain the enhanced risk of LVH in patients with hypertension.

REGRESSION OF LVH

Of obvious importance are the implications of therapeutic reduction of left ventricular mass with pharmacologic compounds and, in particular, the antihypertensive agents. In this regard, the current cardiovascular and hypertensive literature is replete with reports that certain agents *regress* LVH, whereas others do not. Implied in many of these reports are several points: (1) that there is an actual reversal of LVH to the normal myocyte; (2) that the risk attributable to LVH is reversed; and (3) that, more subtly, those agents that do not diminish left ventricular mass have less beneficial effects on the heart than those that do. The fact of the matter is that none of these conclusions are justified.

"REVERSAL" OF LVH

The term *regression* implies, as already indicated, that there is an actual reversal of the hypertrophy of the left ventricle. In actuality, there is no study in human beings that has reported this reversal of hypertrophy. Clinical studies have demonstrated reversal of the electrocardiographic[61,62] as well as the echocardiographic[61-68] changes. Animal studies have demonstrated reduction in the mass of the left ventricle.[69,70] These changes have been associated with normal contractile function and performance of the left ventricle in human beings when at rest and at the pharmacologically-induced normotensive pressures in human beings[62-68] and experimental hypertensive animals.[71,72] However, there is little or no information that is available concerning the performance of the left ventricle with *reversed* or *regressed* LVH at pretreatment hypertensive pressures. When arterial pressure is abruptly elevated to pretreatment levels in treated hypertensive animals with reduced cardiac mass, pumping ability of the heart may be impaired.[73,74] Moreover, no study to date has demonstrated normal performance. This is not to say that normal performance is not possible, but these assertions reflect the present state of our knowledge (in 1989).

Nevertheless, certain classes of antihypertensive agents have been associated with diminished left ventricular mass with treatment periods as short as 3 weeks in experimental hypertension[69-74] and 4 to 12 weeks in patients with essential hypertension.[62-68] Other studies involving prolonged periods of treatment (in human beings and animals) have shown reduction in cardiac mass with even those agents that have been said not to reduce cardiac mass.[75,76] This has suggested that there is a definite dissociation between the hemodynamic and nonhemodynamic effects of these pharmacologic agents.[41,42]

To summarize our present knowledge, centrally active adrenergic inhibiting agents (the prototype of which is methyldopa), angiotensin converting enzyme inhibitors, and probably calcium antagonists have been shown to reduce left ventricular mass in hypertensive patients and animals.[63-74] The data are somewhat confusing with respect to beta-adrenergic receptor blocking drugs, which probably demonstrate reduced mass in patients with hypertension[38] but not in all hypertensive animals. This disparity might be related to age, sex, or type of experimental hypertension.[35,36,77] Even centrally acting adrenergic inhibitors underscore this confusion of the dissociation between hemodynamic and nonhemodynamic factors. For example, at equivalent antihypertensive doses, clonidine did not reduce cardiac mass, but when the dose was increased threefold, cardiac mass was indeed reduced.[69] However, at that dosage the agent produced a peripheral agonistic effect on alpha-adrenergic receptors, increasing arterial pressure and vascular resistance. Furthermore, some drugs that reduce cardiac mass in animals with LVH may also reduce nonhypertrophied right or left ventricular mass in normotensive and hypertensive rats.[70,74]

In contrast to those agents that diminish left ventricular mass, direct-acting smooth muscle vasodilators, diuretics, and alpha-adrenergic receptor blocking agents do not diminish cardiac mass. They may even increase the mass of the left ventricle[69] (Table 5–3).

Table 5–3. Effects of Antihypertensive Agents on Left Ventricular Mass in Short-Term Studies

No Effect
Diuretics
Direct-acting smooth muscle vasodilators (i.e., hydralazine, minoxidil)
Alpha-adrenergic receptor inhibitors (i.e., prazosin, terazosin, indoramine)
Reduction in Cardiac Mass Demonstrated
Centrally active adrenergic inhibitors (e.g., methyldopa)
Angiotensin converting enzyme inhibitors
Calcium antagonists (verapamil, diltiazem, nitrendipine)
Conflicting Reports
Centrally acting adrenergic inhibitors (e.g., clonidine)
Beta-adrenergic receptor blockers

"REVERSAL" OF RISK

As already discussed, it is known that LVH is indeed an independent cardiovascular risk factor, although we do not understand the precise mechanism of the risk. Because the risk may be independent of the height of arterial pressure,[20] it is not enough to demonstrate efficiency of reduced risk via antihypertensive action alone. Prospective and well-controlled studies are essential in this regard, and, for this reason and at this time, it is inappropriate to ascribe benefit from the pharmacologic reduction of cardiac mass. Arguments to the contrary may be just as valid. It follows, therefore, that to ascribe increased risk when drugs do not reduce cardiac mass is also invalid.

SUMMARY

Left ventricular hypertrophy imposes a definite risk of increased cardiovascular morbidity and mortality. This increased risk is independent of other risks (including that of hypertension). The precise mechanism or mechanisms that account for this risk are not known, although several possible factors have been identified. A variety of antihypertensive agents have been shown to decrease the mass of hypertrophied left ventricle, although some may also diminish the mass of the normal ventricle. No study to date has demonstrated improvement in the risk from LVH with so-called reversal of LVH with pharmacologic agents.

REFERENCES

1. Kannel, WB, et al: Factors of risk in the development of coronary heart disease: Six years' follow-up experience. Ann Intern Med 55:33, 1961.
2. Build and Blood Pressure Study 1959. Vols I and II. Society of Actuaries, Chicago, 1959.
3. Gordon, T: Blood pressure of adults by race and area. United States 1960–62. National Center for Health Statistics, Hyattsville, Maryland, 1964; DHEW Publication No. (PHS) 1000 (series 11; no. 5).
4. Kannel, WB, et al: Relation of adiposity to blood pressure in the development of hypertension: The Framingham Study. Ann Intern Med 67:48, 1967.
5. Kannel, WB, et al: Role of blood pressure in the development of congestive heart failure: The Framingham Study. N Engl J Med 287:781, 1972.
6. Kannel, WB, Gordon, T, and Schwartz, MH: Systolic vs diastolic blood pressure and risk of coronary heart disease: The Framingham Study. Am J Cardiol 27:335, 1971.
7. Metropolitan Life Insurance Company: Blood Pressure: Insurance experience and its implications. Metropolitan Life Insurance Co, New York, 1961.
8. Stamler, J, et al: Multivariate analysis of relationship of six variables to blood pressure: Findings from Chicago community surveys. J Chronic Dis 28:499, 1975.
9. Veterans Administration Cooperative Study Group on Antihypertensive Agents: Effects of treatment on morbidity in hypertension. I. Results in patients with diastolic blood pressure averaging 115 through 129 mmHg. JAMA 202:1028, 1967.
10. Veterans Administration Cooperative Study Group on Antihypertensive Agents: Effects of treatment on morbidity in hypertension. II. Results in patients with diastolic blood pressure averaging 90 through 114 mm Hg. JAMA 213:1143, 1970.
11. Hypertension Detection and Follow-Up Program Cooperative Group: Five-year findings of the hypertension detection and follow-up program. II. Mortality by race, sex, age. JAMA 242:2572, 1979.
12. Multiple Risk Factor Intervention Trial Research Group: Baseline rest echocardiographic abnormalities, antihypertensive treatment and mortality in the Multiple Risk Factor Intervention Trial. Am J Cardiol 55:1, 1985.
13. Multiple Risk Factor Intervention Trial Research Group: Multiple Risk Factor Intervention Trial. Risk factor changes and mortality results. JAMA 248:1465, 1982.

14. Ostrander, LD Jr, et al: The relationship of cardiovascular disease to hyperglycemia. Ann Intern Med 62:1188, 1965.

15. Report of the National Cholesterol Education Program expert panel on detection, evaluation, and treatment of high blood cholesterol in adults. Arch Intern Med 148:36, 1988.

16. Frohlich, ED, et al: The problem of obesity and hypertension. Hypertension 5:III-71, 1983.

17. Kannel, WB, Gordon, T, and Offutt, D: Left ventricular hypertrophy by electrocardiogram. Prevalence, incidence and mortality in the Framingham Study. Ann Intern Med 71:89, 1969.

18. Anderson, KP: Sudden death, hypertension and hypertrophy. J Cardiovasc Pharmacol 6:S498, 1984.

19. Kannel, WB, et al: Precursors of sudden coronary death: Factors related to the incidence of sudden death. Circulation 51:606, 1975.

20. Kannel, WB and Sorlie, P: Left ventricular hypertrophy in hypertension: Prognostic and pathogenetic implications (the Framingham Study). In Strauer, BE (ed): The Heart and Hypertension. Springer-Verlag, Berlin, 1981.

21. Frohlich, ED: Haemodynamics of hypertension. In Genest, J, Koiw, E, and Kuchel, O (eds): Hypertension: Physiopathology and Treatment. McGraw-Hill, New York, 1977.

22. Frohlich, ED: Hemodynamic factors in the pathogenesis and maintenance of hypertension. Fed Proc 41:2400, 1982.

23. Frohlich, ED: The heart in hypertension. In Genest, J, et al (eds): Hypertension: Physiopathology and Treatment, ed 2. McGraw-Hill, New York, 1983.

24. Frohlich, ED: Hemodynamics and other determinants in development of left ventricular hypertrophy: Conflicting factors in its regression. Fed Proc 42:2709, 1983.

25. Frohlich, ED: Cardiac hypertrophy: Stimuli and mechanisms. In Sleight, P (ed): Scientific Foundations of Cardiology. William Heinemann, London, 1983.

26. Frohlich, ED, et al: Physiological comparison of labile and essential hypertension. Circ Res 27:55, 1970.

27. Dunn, FG, et al: Pathophysiologic assessment of hypertensive heart disease with echocardiography. Am J Cardiol 39:789, 1977.

28. Linzbach, AJ: Heart failure from the point of view of quantitative anatomy. Am J Cardiol 5:370, 1960.

29. Pfeffer, MA, Pfeffer, JM, and Frohlich, ED: Pumping ability of the hypertrophying left ventricle of the spontaneously hypertensive rat. Circ Res 38:423, 1976.

30. Pfeffer, MA, et al: Ventricular morphology and pumping ability of exercised spontaneously hypertensive rats. Am J Physiol 235:H193, 1978.

31. Meerson, FZ: The myocardium in hyperfunction, hypertrophy and heart failure. Circ Res 25(Suppl 2):1, 1969.

32. Frohlich, ED, et al: Mechanisms controlling arterial pressure. In Frohlich, ED (ed): Pathophysiology: Altered Regulatory Mechanisms in Disease, ed 3. JB Lippincott, Philadelphia, 1984.

33. Messerli, FH, et al: Dimorphic cardiac adaptation to obesity and arterial hypertension. Ann Intern Med 99:757, 1983.

34. Frohlich, ED, Pfeffer, MA, and Pfeffer, JM: Systemic hemodynamics and cardiac function in spontaneously hypertensive rats: Similarities with essential hypertension. In Strauer, BE (ed): The Heart in Hypertension. Springer-Verlag, Berlin, 1981.

35. Frohlich, ED: State of the art. The heart in hypertension: Unresolved conceptual challenges. Hypertension 11(Suppl I):19, 1988.

36. Frohlich, ED: State of the art. The first Irvine H. Page lecture: The mosaic of hypertension; past, present, and future. J Hypertension (in press).

37. Messerli, FH, et al: Clinical and hemodynamic determinants of left ventricular dimensions. Arch Intern Med 144:477, 1984.

38. Dunn, FG, et al: Racial differences in cardiac adaptation to essential hypertension determined by echocardiographic indexes. J Am Coll Cardiol 1:1348, 1983.

39. Frohlich, ED: The heart in hypertension. In Rosenthal, J and Chobanian, AV (eds): Arterial Hypertension, ed 2. Springer-Verlag, New York (in press).

40. Frohlich, ED and Tarazi, RC: Is arterial pressure the sole factor responsible for hypertensive cardiac hypertrophy? Am J Cardiol 44:959, 1979.

41. Tarazi, RC and Frohlich, ED: Is reversal of cardiac hypertrophy a desirable goal of antihypertensive therapy? Circulation 75(I):113, 1987.

42. Frohlich, ED: Left ventricular hypertrophy as a risk factor. Clin Cardiol 4:137, 1986.

43. Dustan, HP: Atherosclerosis complicating chronic hypertension. Circulation 50:871, 1974.

44. Wittels, EW and Gotto, AM Jr: Atherogenic mechanisms. In Frohlich, ED (ed): Pathophysiology: Altered Regulatory Mechanisms in Disease, ed 3. JB Lippincott, Philadelphia, 1984.
45. Dunn, FG and Frohlich, ED: Hypertension and angina pectoris. In Yu, PN and Goodwin, JF (eds). Lea & Febiger, Philadelphia, 1978.
46. Sarnoff, SJ, et al: Hemodynamic determinants of oxygen consumption of the heart with special reference to the tension time index. Am J Physiol 192:148, 1958.
47. Messerli, FH, et al: Hypertension and sudden death: Increased ventricular ectopic activity in left ventricular hypertrophy. Am J Med 77:18, 1984.
48. Savage, DD, et al: The spectrum of left ventricular hypertrophy in a general population sample: The Framingham Study. Circulation 75(I Pt 2):I26, 1987.
49. McLenachan, JM, et al: Ventricular arrhythmias in hypertensive left ventricular hypertrophy. N Engl J Med 317:787, 1987.
50. Dunn, FC: Prevention of sudden cardiac death. In Cardiovasc Clin (in press).
51. Holland, OB, Nixon, JV, and Kuhnert, L: Diuretic-induced ventricular ectopic activity. Am J Med 70:762, 1981.
52. Hollifield, JW and Slaton, PE: Thiazide diuretics, hypokalemia and cardiac arrhythmias. Acta Med Scand 647(Suppl):67, 1981.
53. Johansson, BW (ed): Electrolytes and cardiac arrhythmias. Acta Med Scand 647(Suppl):1, 1981.
54. Multiple Risk Factor Intervention Trial Research Group: Multiple Risk Factor Intervention Trial. Risk factor changes and mortality results. JAMA 248:1465, 1982.
55. Kannel, WB, Gordon, T, and Offutt, D: Left ventricular hypertrophy by electrocardiogram. Prevalence, incidence and mortality in the Framingham Study. Ann Intern Med 71:89, 1969.
56. Frohlich, ED: Potential mechanisms explaining the risk of left ventricular hypertrophy. Am J Cardiol 59(A):91, 1987.
57. Harrison, DG, et al: The effect of hypertension and left ventricular hypertrophy on the lower range of coronary autoregulation. Circulation 77(5):1108, 1988.
58. Umeda, PK, et al: Control of myosin heavy chain expression in cardiac hypertrophy. Am J Cardiol 59(A):49, 1987.
59. Schaible, TF, et al: Chronic swimming reverses cardiac dysfunction and myosin abnormalities in hypertensive rats. J Appl Physiol 60(4):1435, 1986.
60. Pauletto, P, et al: Propranolol-induced changes in ventricular isomyosin composition in rat. Am Heart J 109:1269, 1985.
61. Borhani, NO, et al: Incidence of coronary heart disease and left ventricular hypertrophy in the hypertension, detection, and follow-up program. Progr Cardiovasc Dis 29 (Suppl 1):55, 1986.
62. Dunn, FG, et al: Time course of regression of left ventricular hypertrophy in hypertensive patients treated with atenolol. Circulation 76:254, 1987.
63. Fouad, FM, et al: Reversal of left ventricular hypertrophy in hypertensive patients treated with methyldopa. Am J Cardiol 49:795, 1982.
64. Ventura, HO, et al: Cardiovascular effects and regional blood flow distribution associated with angiotensin coverting enzyme inhibition (captopril) in essential hypertension. Am J Cardiol 55:1023, 1985.
65. Dunn, FG, et al: Enalapril improves systemic and renal hemodynamics and allows regression of left ventricular mass in essential hypertension. Am J Cardiol 53:105, 1984.
66. Amodeo, C, et al: Immediate and short-term hemodynamic effects of diltiazem in patients with hypertension. Circulation 73:108, 1986.
67. Schmieder, RE, et al: Cardiovascular effects of verapamil in essential hypertension. Circulation 30:1143, 1987.
68. Grossman, E, et al: Systemic and regional hemodynamic and humoral effects of nitrendipine in essential hypertension. Circulation (in press).
69. Pegram, BL, Ishise, S, and Frohlich, ED: Effect of methyldopa, clonidine, and hydralazine on cardiac mass and hemodynamics in Wistar-Kyoto and spontaneously hypertensive rats. Cardiovasc Res 16:40, 1982.
70. Kobrin, I, et al: Reduced cardiac mass by nitrendipine is dissociated from systemic or regional hemodynamic changes in rats. Cardiovasc Res 3:158, 1984.
71. Spech, MM, Ferrario, CM, and Tarazi, RC: Cardiac pumping ability following reversal of hypertrophy and hypertension in spontaneously hypertensive rats. Hypertension 2:75, 1982.
72. Kuwajima, I, et al: Regression of left ventricular hypertrophy in two-kidney, one clip Goldblatt hypertension. Hypertension 4:113, 1982.

73. Natsume, T, et al: Ventricular performance in spontaneously hypertensive rats (SHR) with reduced cardiac mass. Cardiovasc Drugs Ther (in press).
74. Sasaki, O, et al: Left ventricular pumping ability and aortic distensibility after methyldopa in Wistar-Kyoto and spontaneously hypertensive rats. J Vasc Med Biol (in press).
75. Freis, ED and Ragan, DO: Relative effectiveness of chlorothiazide, reserpine, and hydralazine in spontaneously hypertensive rats. Clin Sci Mol Med 51:635s, 1976.
76. Pfeffer, JM, et al: Favorable effects of therapy on cardiac performance in spontaneously hypertensive rats. Am J Physiol 242(H):766, 1982.
77. Pfeffer, MA, et al: Development of SHR hypertension and cardiac hypertrophy during prolonged beta blockade. Am J Physiol 232(H):639, 1977.

CHAPTER 6

Prevention of Sudden Cardiac Death

Francis G. Dunn, M.B., Ch.B., F.R.C.P.

A 47-year-old male patient recently was referred to my clinic because he had been noted to have an abnormal electrocardiogram (ECG) at a health screening evaluation. The ECG revealed lateral myocardial ischemia, and the patient admitted on direct questioning to having mild retrosternal discomfort on effort. This had been virtually abolished by atenolol therapy. He was a nonsmoker and was normotensive. He did, however, demonstrate a mild elevation of serum cholesterol. An exercise test was undertaken, and the patient reached stage III of the full Bruce protocol, at which time he developed mild retrosternal discomfort and there was accentuation of the resting ECG abnormalities. Coronary arteriography was arranged, but prior to his admission for this study, the patient died suddenly at home.

Sudden, unexpected cardiac death is clearly a source of great distress to family, primary care physicians, and cardiologists alike. The distress is heightened by the fact that it seems to affect younger patients disproportionately, particularly when underlying coronary heart disease (CHD) is present.[1] The magnitude of the problem can be illustrated further by the fact that over 400,000 people die suddenly in the United States each year. This matter is of great concern when one considers the advances that have been made in all other fields of cardiovascular medicine. Despite this alarming figure, much information has accumulated in recent years with regard to the mechanisms and risk factors for sudden death (Table 6–1). This information has provided the basis for improvement in our ability to predict and hence to prevent this catastrophic complication of cardiac disease.

Definitions abound regarding sudden death. This is due at least in part to the different medical disciplines involved in the study of this condition. A generally accepted definition would be natural death due to cardiac causes initiated by abrupt loss of consciousness within one hour of the onset of the terminal symptoms, occurring in an individual who may or may not have recognized pre-existing heart disease, but in whom the time and mode of death are unexpected.[2] The arrhythmic mechanisms of sudden death have been elucidated from ambulatory monitoring at

Table 6–1. Risk Factors for Sudden Cardiac Death

Coronary artery disease
Left ventricular hypertrophy in hypertension
Hypertrophic and dilated cardiomyopathies
Wolff-Parkinson-White syndrome
Prolonged QT interval
Left ventricular dysfunction

the time of the acute event.[3] The underlying dysrhythmia leading to sudden cardiac death is ventricular fibrillation, preceded by ventricular tachycardia in the vast majority of patients.[3] Bradydysrhythmias may also cause sudden death, although in a much smaller percentage of cases. This chapter is directed, however, toward those situations in which ventricular fibrillation is the underlying rhythm preceding sudden death.

RISK FACTORS FOR SUDDEN CARDIAC DEATH AND THEIR MECHANISMS

CORONARY ARTERY DISEASE

Risk Factor

This condition is the major risk factor for sudden cardiac death (SCD).[4] The high early incidence of out-of-hospital SCD in patients with acute myocardial infarction (AMI) is well established, and it has been estimated that almost 50 percent of these patients die before they reach the hospital. In such cases, intraluminal thrombi have been found in 74 percent of patients dying suddenly on the basis of ischemic heart disease,[5] and a further 21 percent have plaque fissures.[5] Pathology evidence of AMI itself occurs in a much smaller percentage (27 percent).[4] This may be due partly to the fact that evidence of myocardial infarction may not have had time to develop in SCD patients. However, the low incidence of AMI may be a real phenomenon inasmuch as only a minority of patients surviving out-of-hospital cardiac arrest develop definite ECG and enzyme evidence of AMI.[6,7] Thus, although SCD is a common event in AMI, healed myocardial infarction is more common in SCD victims than AMI (44 percent versus 27 percent).[4] Sixty percent of all sudden death victims have three or more significantly obstructed vessels, 80 percent have at least two significantly stenosed vessels, and 94 percent have at least one significantly stenosed vessel.[4]

Mechanisms

A number of mechanisms contribute to SCD in patients with coronary artery disease (Table 6–2). Myocardial ischemia is likely to play an important role, and the high rate of acute coronary occlusion would be consistent with acute ischemic injury leading to ventricular tachycardia and fibrillation.[4] Valuable information has emerged from ambulatory monitoring performed prior to sudden death. In one study in 14 such patients, the incidence of patients experiencing more marked ST segment changes increased progressively until 3 hours preceding cardiac arrest, when most of the patients showed return of the ST segment toward normal.[3] It was

Table 6–2. Mechanisms for Sudden
Cardiac Death in Coronary Artery
Disease and in Left Ventricular
Hypertrophy

CAD	LVH
Myocardial ischemia	Myocardial ischemia
Scar tissue	Fibrous tissue
Left ventricular dysfunction	Left ventricular dysfunction
Coronary artery spasm	Hypertension
	Drug therapy

suggested in that study that the association of the return of the ST segment toward
normal with complex ventricular arrhythmias may have indicated reperfusion
arrhythmias. Acute ischemia, however, is unlikely to be the sole mechanism in view
of the high rates of previous myocardial infarction in SCD victims.[5]

Scar tissue has been shown to be an important substrate for ventricular tachycardia and ventricular fibrillation, both in healed myocardial infarction and in left
ventricular aneurysm.[8] Furthermore, resection of scar tissue or aneurysm may control these dysrhythmias.[8] Left ventricular dysfunction in patients with coronary
artery disease, with or without previous myocardial infarction, is also strongly associated with complex ventricular dysrhythmias, but it is not clear whether the ventricular dysrhythmias independently contribute to mortality when left ventricular
dysfunction is present.[9–11] Finally, coronary artery spasm may be a component in
SCD, and it is interesting to note in this regard that in Prinzmetal's original descrip-
tion, 50 percent of his patients had ventricular dysrhythmias with pain.[12]

LEFT VENTRICULAR HYPERTROPHY IN PATIENTS WITH HYPERTENSION

Risk Factor

The Framingham Study has shown that left ventricular hypertrophy (LVH) as
assessed by ECG is a risk factor for SCD.[13] This finding particularly applies to what
they describe as definite LVH (voltage plus ST-T wave changes), that is, LVH and
strain, and indeed this constitutes an independent risk factor for SCD in men.[13] In
women, definite LVH is an independent risk factor only in the absence of coronary
artery disease.[13] In order to assess further the importance of ECG LVH, multivar-
iant analysis was applied, controlling for age, systolic blood pressure, risk factors
for coronary artery disease, and ventricular dysrhythmias. This assessment revealed
that LVH remained a highly significant independent risk factor but only in men.
Our own data from the Glasgow Blood Pressure Clinic have demonstrated an independent contribution of LVH to coronary artery disease mortality, including SCD,
with a greater impact on men.[14]

Mechanisms

As with coronary artery disease, myocardial ischemia may be an important
mechanism for SCD in hypertensive patients with LVH (Table 6–2). Ischemia is
due to a combination of factors, including a reduction in maximal coronary vaso-

dilator capacity, an increase in coronary collateral resistance, and a reduction in subendocardial perfusion.[15] Furthermore, coexistent hypertension further distorts the myocardial oxygen supply-demand relationship by increasing oxygen consumption.

Coronary artery disease undoubtedly contributes to myocardial ischemia in a significant proportion of patients with LVH.[16] In addition, LVH makes the heart more vulnerable to ventricular fibrillation when coronary occlusion is produced.[15] It is likely also that in the presence of these abnormalities, coronary artery disease, which might otherwise be insignificant, becomes of pathophysiologic importance.

Another possible mechanism for SCD in LVH is that the hypertrophied myocardium forms a substrate for ventricular dysrhythmias, perhaps partly owing to fibrous tissue formation, which is frequently a part of the LVH process. Rats with spontaneous hypertension have a lower threshold for ventricular fibrillation than controls,[17] and after-potentials can be demonstrated in hypertrophied rat myocardium but not in normal rat myocardium.[18] In the clinical arena, a number of studies have demonstrated an increased prevalence of ventricular dysrhythmias in patients with hypertension and LVH and, in particular, nonsustained ventricular tachycardia.[19-22] This finding is in contradistinction to patients with hypertension without ventricular hypertrophy, in whom the presence of nonsustained ventricular tachycardia is a very rare finding.[19-22] The prevalence of nonsustained ventricular tachycardia varies considerably, being as high as almost 50 percent in one study.[19] Although these findings are of interest, it has not yet been shown that the presence of complex dysrhythmias in hypertension are in fact an important marker for subsequent SCD. Long-term follow-up of these patients will provide further information in this regard.

Although hypertension itself could contribute to the SCD in LVH, the risk cannot be explained solely by the blood pressure. It is likely, however, to play some contributory part,[15] as is left ventricular dysfunction. It is well established that in grade III or grade IV New York Heart Association cardiac patients, there is an increased rate of sudden death amounting to almost 15 percent per year.[23] Although no clear information is available on the relationship of milder degrees of left ventricular dysfunction to SCD, the abnormalities demonstrated in the hypertensive heart, particularly diastolic function abnormalities,[24] may be shown ultimately to be important in sudden death in these patients. Further study is needed in this area.

CARDIOMYOPATHIES

Both hypertrophic cardiomyopathy and dilated cardiomyopathy are associated with SCD. In particular, reports of an association between hypertrophic cardiomyopathy and SCD date back for 30 years.[25] Studies from the United Kingdom and the United States have confirmed these earlier reports and demonstrate a marked increase in ventricular dysrhythmias, especially ventricular tachycardia, in patients who subsequently die suddenly.[26,27] A number of different mechanisms are likely to contribute to SCD in hypertrophic cardiomyopathy, including hypertrophy itself, abnormalities of AV conduction, deterioration in left ventricular function, and increased outflow gradient with sudden decrease in cardiac output.[28]

The relationship between dilated cardiomyopathy and SCD is also well established.[28] As with hypertrophic cardiomyopathy, there is a high incidence of complex ventricular dysrhythmias and ventricular tachycardia.[29,30] Current evidence indicates that SCD cannot be predicted on the basis of these ventricular dysrhythmias, which appear to be associated more with left ventricular dysfunction.[30] The key factor in SCD in these patients appears to be the extent of cardiac failure.

CONDUCTION ABNORMALITIES

Less common but important risk factors for SCD are prolongation of the QT interval and Wolff-Parkinson-White syndrome. Prolongation of the QT interval may occur as an inherited syndrome or may be drug induced. Antiarrhythmic drugs, particularly those of class 1A, can give rise to prolongation of the QT interval with torsades de pointes ventricular tachycardia progressing to ventricular fibrillation. It should be emphasized that all antiarrhythmic drugs may have proarrhythmic effects, and therefore these agents should be used only when there is a clear indication. Wolff-Parkinson-White syndrome denotes an accessory pathway from the atrium to the left ventricule, which bypasses the AV node. Rapid atrial fibrillation with ventricular rates of 190 to 300 beats per minute may occur because of accelerated conduction down the accessory pathway. The rapid atrial fibrillation may degenerate into ventricular fibrillation.[31] Although this complication is unusual in patients with Wolff-Parkinson-White syndrome (around 1 percent), the patients in this group should be screened by 48-hour Holter monitoring and exercise testing. The presence of symptoms or supraventricular dysrhythmias indicates the need for electrophysiologic studies in these patients.

BIOCHEMICAL ABNORMALITIES

Hypokalemia is associated with SCD. This condition may be drug induced or may occur as a consequence of potassium-losing states, such as primary or secondary aldosteronism. However, no clear association has been demonstrated between ventricular extrasystoles, thiazide diuretics, and SCD.[32,33] Hyperkalemia also may be responsible for fatal ventricular dysrhythmias, most commonly as a consequence of renal failure or potassium-sparing drugs. Often, potassium-sparing agents may not cause hyperkalemia on their own, but when combined with other agents or conditions that reduce potassium excretion, a marked increase in potassium may occur. An example is the use of potassium-sparing agents with converting enzyme inhibitors. Hypomagnesemia also is well recognized now as providing a medium for complex ventricular dysrhythmias, and this biochemical abnormality too can be a consequence of drug therapy and, in particular, diuretics.

ADDITIONAL FACTORS

Age has an important influence on SCD.[13] Among sudden cardiac deaths, there is a progressive increase beginning in childhood.[34] Conversely, in coronary artery disease, there are more sudden deaths in percentage terms in younger patients,[1] so that whereas 76 percent of coronary artery disease deaths are sudden in the 20 to 39 age group, this percentage falls progressively with aging, so that in the 60 to 74 year age group, 40 to 50 percent die suddenly.

Sex differences are also important, with a considerable preponderance of SCD among men. This excess peaks in the age group 55 to 64, with a ratio of 7 to 1, and drops to 2 to 1 in the elderly.[1]

Obesity also must be regarded as an independent risk factor for SCD. The exact mechanism for this effect is unclear. It may be related to fatty infiltration of the myocardium or indeed to a specific type of cardiac hypertrophy, inasmuch as obesity almost certainly compounds the risk of SCD caused by hypertension, and the two conditions in concert result in a combination of eccentric and concentric cardiac hypertrophy.[35]

Differences are known to exist between blacks and whites in hemodynamics and in the cardiac adaptor responses to hypertension.[36] In particular, there seems to be a more direct relationship between arterial blood pressure level and the degree of cardiac hypertrophy among black patients. There is, however, no clear evidence to date of differences in the incidence of SCD between blacks and whites in the United States. In the black populations in Africa, SCD is thought to be uncommon, in most cases appearing not to be related to coronary artery disease.[37]

USEFULNESS OF CARDIAC STUDIES AS MARKERS FOR SUDDEN CARDIAC DEATH

ELECTROCARDIOGRAM

The ECG has been studied in considerable detail regarding its predictability for SCD. The Manitoba study of 3983 men who were apparently healthy revealed that the prevalence of any abnormal ECG finding was 72 percent in sudden death victims.[38] ST-T wave changes, ventricular extrasystoles, LVH, and left bundle branch block were all significant predictors of SCD. In particular, the combination of ventricular extrasystoles with ST-T wave changes or LVH substantially increased the risk of sudden death.[38] A study from the United Kingdom in patients with or without previous manifestations of coronary artery disease revealed that ventricular conduction abnormalities and ventricular extrasystoles were important predictors of sudden death only in patients with previous myocardial infarction or with symptoms of coronary artery disease.[39] These findings, however, were also predictive of nonsudden coronary deaths, and therefore the ECG could not predict in itself which patients were going to die suddenly.

ECG evidence of LVH and strain is independently associated with SCD in men with and without coronary artery disease and in women without coronary artery disease.[13] Myocardial infarction is also independently related to SCD but to a greater extent in men, and bundle branch block was an independent factor only if coronary artery disease was present. When additional factors, such as smoking, cholesterol, and cardiac failure, were taken into account, myocardial infarction remained an independent risk factor in men and women and LVH in men only.[13] The ECG is also the method for identifying Wolff-Parkinson-White syndrome, long QT interval, and patterns suggestive of cardiomyopathy. Thus, despite its low individual predictive power for SCD, the ECG is the most easily obtainable and worthwhile investigation currently available.

CHEST X-RAY

The chest x-ray is well known to be an insensitive method of detecting cardiac hypertrophy. Almost 50 percent of patients who have cardiac hypertrophy have a normal cardiac silhouette on the chest x-ray. However, the presence of cardiomegaly on the chest x-ray identifies the patient as being at a particularly increased risk of SCD and confirms pathology data relating increased cardiac mass to SCD.[40]

EXERCISE TESTING

The exercise test in symptomatic individuals is of key importance as a predictor of subsequent coronary events, including SCD. However, it is of limited value for identifying which patient is at risk of SCD, as distinct from other clinical syndromes associated with coronary artery disease. The development of ventricular tachycardia during exercise testing might be an important marker for SCD.

It is important also to consider whether the exercise test in symptom-free individuals might be a way in which sudden death can be predicted. Of relevance in this regard is a recent review by Epstein and associates.[41] Two studies of treadmill exercise testing[42-44] and risk factor analysis in symptom-free subjects were combined (Fig. 6–1). In a group of 10,000 patients, 9500 had a normal exercise test with normal risk factor analysis, whereas 500 did not. Of the 38 sudden cardiac deaths, 29 occurred in the normal group. (Thus although lower in percentage terms, more SCD occurred in those with a normal exercise test, and thus the majority would have been missed on the basis of this exercise screening program). Thus, exercise testing is not of predictive value in SCD in asymptomatic patients.

AMBULATORY ECG MONITORING

This technique has provided invaluable information regarding the changes in the ST segment and also the dysrhythmias that precede SCD.[3] In addition, the doc-

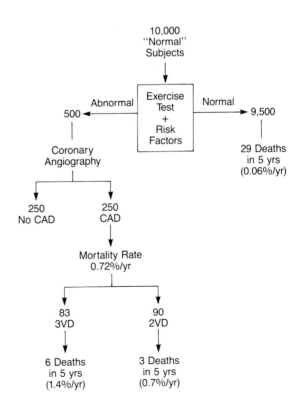

Figure 6–1. Practical implications of screening 10,000 subjects for asymptomatic coronary artery disease by means of exercise stress-testing and risk-factor assessment. These data are based on studies by Erikssen and Thaulow,[42] and Bruce, et al.[43,44] CAD denotes coronary artery disease, 3VD = three-vessel disease, and 2VD = two-vessel disease. (From Epstein, et al,[41] with permission.)

umentation of complex ventricular dysrhythmias has had important therapeutic and prognostic implications in patients with hypertrophic cardiomyopathy, Wolff-Parkinson-White syndrome, prolonged QT interval, and severe left ventricular dysfunction. Ambulatory ECG monitoring is therefore an integral part of the evaluation of such patients. It is also of value in the patient with a previous ventricular fibrillation episode to ensure efficacy of antiarrhythmic therapy. Ambulatory monitoring is not of value, however, for screening patients without clinical evidence of heart disease. The detection of even complex ventricular dysrhythmias by this method does not appear to be of prognostic importance unless accompanied by symptoms.[45] Even following myocardial infarction, it is debatable whether complex ventricular arrhythmias are an independent risk factor for SCD.[45] Left ventricular dysfunction appears to be more important as a predictor of SCD. An area of considerable interest recently has been that of silent myocardial ischemia and its possible role in SCD. At present there is no evidence that the finding of ischemic changes on ambulatory monitoring improves the prediction of SCD.

ECHOCARDIOGRAPHY

Inasmuch as the echocardiogram has been shown to be a more sensitive method of detecting LVH than the ECG, it might be expected to be more valuable as a marker for subsequent SCD. Although there have not been enough longitudinal data to indicate that echo LVH is a more sensitive marker, it has been shown recently that echocardiographic LVH is more sensitive in the detection of ventricular arrhythmias.[21] However, the results of long-term studies on the prognostic importance of echocardiographic LVH must be awaited before the importance of this technique in the prediction of SCD can be assessed.

CORONARY ARTERIOGRAPHY

There is no doubt that the presence of significant coronary artery disease, as demonstrated by coronary arteriography, is associated with an increased incidence of SCD. The standard indications for this procedure are well established. However, it may be justified also in patients who have hypertension and LVH and strain, and indeed significant coronary artery disease has been shown to occur in a high percentage of such patients, even in the absence of symptoms.[16] Our studies indicate that patients with hypertensive LVH and strain who have a positive exercise thallium scan, even if symptom-free, should be considered for coronary arteriography.[16] Clearly the invasive nature of this investigation does not permit it to be used in the population at large; however, the development of noninvasive ways of assessing the coronary circulation could make a substantial contribution to the prediction of SCD.

STRATEGY FOR PREVENTION

Major difficulties exist in mounting an effective prevention program because of the difficulty in predicting SCD on an individual basis. Furthermore, the results of risk factor intervention trials have been disappointing in their ability to reduce SCD, either by reducing cholesterol[46] or by lowering blood pressure.[33,47] A strategy for prevention should be directed first toward high-risk groups and second toward

Table 6–3. Strategy for Prevention of Sudden Cardiac Death

Patient Group	Management	Effect on Sudden Cardiac Death
Previous VF	Rule out CAD	Reduced
	EP testing	
	Appropriate antiarrhythmic therapy or AICD	
Post MI	Beta-adrenoreceptor blocking therapy	Reduced
	Aspirin	
HOCM	Ambulatory monitoring	Reduced
	Treat ventricular tachycardia	
WPW syndrome	Ambulatory monitoring and ETT	Reduced
	Evaluate dysrhythmias by EP testing	
	Appropriate drug therapy or surgery	
Prolonged QT interval	Evaluate symptoms and family history and drug therapy	Reduced
	Ambulatory monitoring and ETT	
	Treat symptomatic dysrhythmias	
LVH in hypertension	Avoid hypokalemia and hypomagnesemia	Not known
	Consider agents that regress LVH	
	Rule out coronary disease	
	Treat cardiovascular risk factors	
LV dysfunction	Ambulatory Monitoring	Not known
	? Antiarrhythmic therapy for ventricular tachycardia	
	Converting enzyme and inhibitors reduce mortality but not SCD	
General population	Basic screening with ECG and chest x-ray	Not known
	Treat risk factors	
	Community education in CPR	

VF = Ventricular fibrillation. MI = Myocardial infarction. HOCM = Hypertrophic obstructive cardiomyopathy. EP = Electrophysiological. CAD = Coronary artery disease. CPR = Cardiopulmonary resuscitation.

the population at large, in whom the great majority of sudden cardiac deaths will occur (Table 6–3).

PREVENTION IN HIGH RISK GROUPS

Survivors of Sudden Cardiac Death

Patients who have been successfully resuscitated from an episode of ventricular fibrillation, and who have not sustained a myocardial infarction, have an annual mortality thereafter of 15 to 30%.[48] The mortality in patients in whom the ventricular fibrillation is secondary to acute myocardial infarction is much lower, and the chance of recurrent ventricular fibrillation is not different from those sustaining a myocardial infarction without a cardiac arrest. In those patients in whom there has been no AMI, considerable attention has been directed toward preventing a second episode of ventricular fibrillation.

In the management of such patients, it is important first to rule out significant coronary artery disease, and therefore all these patients should have full noninvasive and invasive assessment. If this reveals that coronary artery disease is not the likely basis for the ventricular fibrillation, a detailed electrophysiologic assessment, including responses to routine antiarrhythmic drugs, should be undertaken. The electrophysiologic studies should be repeated after single and combined drug regimens, and if it is shown that the dysrhythmias are suppressed by drug therapy, that regimen should be continued under close monitoring on an outpatient basis. If, however, the ventricular dysrhythmias cannot be suppressed by drug therapy, more recent innovations, such as the automatic implantable cardioverter defibrillator (AICD), should be considered. Early studies with this device in over 1500 patients have demonstrated an annual death rate of less than 2 percent.[49] This represents a substantial reduction in the expected mortality in these patients. The AICD, therefore, represents a major thrust in the secondary prevention of ventricular fibrillation.

Post–Myocardial Infarction

For a number of years it has been evident that beta blocking agents reduce both morbidity and mortality following AMI.[50–52] This benefit, which includes a reduction in SCD, may persist for several years following myocardial infarction. More recently, aspirin has been shown to reduce SCD in the post–myocardial infarction patient,[53,54] and this is not surprising when one considers the work of Davies and Thomas, which shows the importance of thrombosis in patients with coronary artery disease who die suddenly.[5] Thus, aspirin is likely to exert its beneficial effect by prevention of platelet aggregation and consequent reduction of vasoactive substance release.

Another way in which SCD may be reduced is by coronary artery surgery. Thus, in the coronary artery surgery study (CASS), it was noted that surgery appeared to reduce the risk of SCD more than medical therapy.[55] Although this choice of therapy was not randomized, it was noted that the SCD rate was 1.8 percent in 129 surgically treated patients, as compared with 5.2 percent in 323 medically treated patients. The differences were more marked in patients in the highest quartile of risk. These data suggest that myocardial revascularization, presumably by reducing ischemic events and improving left ventricular function, may have advantages over medical therapy in preventing SCD.

Hypertrophic Obstructive Cardiomyopathy

There is now good evidence that marker dysrhythmias, especially nonsustained ventricular tachycardia, can predict SCD in patients with hypertrophic obstructive cardiomyopathy.[24,27] These ventricular tachycardias usually consist of six or more beats at a rate of greater than 120 beats per minute. It is noteworthy that treatment with amiodarone not only abolishes nonsustained ventricular dysrhythmias but also results in a reduction in SCD in this patient population.[56]

Wolff-Parkinson-White Syndrome

Clear guidelines are now being defined into ways of identifying those at risk of SCD. Any patient with Wolff-Parkinson-White syndrome who has palpitation should have maximum exercise testing and 48-hour ambulatory monitoring. If supraventricular dysrhythmias, and in particular rapid atrial fibrillation, are documented, full electrophysiologic testing is indicated. In particular, the refractory period down the accessory pathway should be documented, and appropriate therapy either with amiodarone or with ligation of the accessory pathway should be undertaken.

QT Prolongation

The basis for the QT prolongation should be established, and a detailed drug history should be taken from the patient. Coronary artery disease also may cause prolongation of the QT interval, but of particular relevance is the presence of the QT interval as part of a familial disorder. These patients are at an increased risk for sudden death, and, if symptomatic, members of the family should be screened for prolongation of the QT interval. The development of ventricular dysrhythmias during exercise and other situations of stress also should be assessed. Treatment for this condition depends on the presence or absence of syncope and the presence or absence of ventricular dyrsrhythmias on ambulatory monitoring.

Hypertensive LVH

To date there is no known intervention that reduces SCD in patients with hypertensive LVH. However, a number of guidelines in this patient population are worth considering. First, other risk factors for coronary artery disease should be identified and treated. Second, a choice of antihypertensive drugs for this population should take into account their ability to regress ventricular hypertrophy and the possible effects of drug-induced biochemical abnormalities on ventricular dysrhythmias. A case can be made for using agents such as converting enzyme inhibitors and beta-blocking agents, which regress LVH[57,58] without adversely altering ventricular function or the patient's electrolyte status. It should be emphasized that following regression of hypertrophy, cardiac function may be compromised if faced with a sudden acute increase in blood pressure.[59] Long-term studies are required to provide definitive evidence regarding the effects of converting enzyme inhibitors and beta blocking drugs on SCD in patients with hypertension and LVH. Finally, there would seem merit in preventing the development of LVH by early treatment of hypertension, rather than waiting for the hypertrophy to develop and then trying to reverse it.

Left Ventricular Dysfunction

Although this condition is known to be associated with a high incidence of SCD,[23] we still do not know how to approach the presence of ventricular dysrhythmias in this population. Clearly symptomatic episodes of ventricular tachycardia must be treated. Whether other complex dysrhythmias lead directly to SCD, or whether they simply reflect severe cardiac dysfunction, is not yet known. Mortality in patients with cardiac failure can be reduced by converting enzyme inhibition, but this improvement does not appear to be by a reduction in SCD.[60]

PREVENTION IN THE GENERAL POPULATION

Inasmuch as the great majority of SCD occurs in asymptomatic subjects, the impact from successful prevention would be encountered especially in this segment of the community. Unfortunately, there is no specific screening method that can successfully predict SCD. Despite this seemingly pessimistic situation, a number of measures merit consideration in the general population.

Cardiopulmonary Resuscitation (CPR)

Most hospitals now have a clearly defined policy for managing cardiac arrest, but it is outside the hospital environment that CPR has its major impact. Successful

CPR in the community is totally dependent on widespread training in basic life support. This requires a community-wide program such as that in Seattle, where resuscitation is initiated by a member of the lay population in as many as 35 percent of cases.[61] In those cases in which resuscitation was commenced by bystanders, the long-term survival was twice that of those cases in which resuscitation was delayed until the arrival of the specialist emergency team.[61] In one study among 352 consecutive victims of out-of-hospital cardiac arrest, 67 percent of those presenting with ventricular tachycardia survived to leave the hospital, and 23 percent of those with ventricular fibrillation survived to leave the hospital.[6] Clearly, without these measures, mortality in the latter group would have been 100 percent. The importance of early intervention can be further illustrated by data showing that patients resuscitated within 4 minutes have a 56 percent survival, in contrast to 17 percent in those in whom resuscitation was commenced after 8 minutes.[62] Thus, there is a considerable responsibility on the part both of the medical profession to institute training programs for cardiopulmonary resuscitation and of the lay population to respond in an enthusiastic and effective manner to this challenge.

Impact of Cardiovascular Risk Factor Assessment

The identification and treatment of cardiovascular risk factors in the symptom-free population is likely to result in the reduction of SCD in parallel with the other clinical sequelae of coronary artery disease. A good case can be made for a basic screening program for hypertension and lipid abnormalities in all men over the age of 30 and in women over the age of 40. This approach should include an unrelenting campaign against cigarette smoking. As part of the screening, clinical examination should focus on such abnormalities as aortic stenosis, LVH, hypertrophic cardiomyopathy, and the presence of left ventricular failure. ECG and chest x-ray should be included in this screening. Additional investigations would be indicated in people with a strong family history of cardiac death or with abnormalities on clinical examination, ECG, or chest x-ray.

CONCLUSION

The prevention of SCD remains one of the greatest challenges in the field of cardiovascular medicine today. Despite the difficulty in predicting which individuals are going to die suddenly, much knowledge has accumulated in recent years in regard to independent risk factors for SCD and their mechanisms. This has led to improved prophylaxis in a number of areas, particularly in the post–myocardial infarction patient and in those with hypertrophic cardiomyopathy, Wolff-Parkinson-White syndrome, and long QT syndrome. A number of questions remain unanswered, particularly in the field of hypertensive heart disease and in those with left ventricular dysfunction. Furthermore, a major challenge still exists in the prevention of SCD during the evolution of the first myocardial infarction. The question also remains why patients such as the one mentioned at the start of this chapter die suddenly, whereas others with similar profiles do not. Until the basic mechanisms leading to SCD are clearly understood, effective CPR, both within the hospital and within the community, will remain a fundamental part of our preventive strategy for SCD.

REFERENCES

1. Kannel, WB and Thomas, HE: Sudden coronary death: The Framingham Study. Ann NY Acad Sci 382:3, 1982.
2. Myerburg, RJ: Sudden death. J Cont Educ Cardiol 14:15, 1978.
3. Savage, HR, et al: Analysis of ambulatory electrocardiogram in 14 patients who experienced sudden cardiac death during monitoring. Clin Cardiol 10:621, 1987.
4. Libertson, RR, et al: Pathophysiologic observations in pre-hospital ventricular fibrillation and sudden cardiac death. Circulation 49:790, 1974.
5. Davies, MJ, and Thomas, A: Thrombosis and acute coronary artery lesions in sudden cardiac ischemic death. N Engl J Med 310:1137, 1984.
6. Myerburg, JR, et al: Clinical electrophysiologic and hemodynamic profile of patients resuscitated from pre-hospital cardiac arrest. Am J Med 68:568, 1980.
7. Cobb, LA, Werner, JA, and Trobaugh, GT: Sudden cardiac death. II: Outcome of resuscitation management and future directions. Mod Concepts CV Dis 49:31, 1980.
8. Zipes, DP: Management of cardiac arrhythmias. In Braunwald, E (ed): Heart Disease. WB Saunders, Philadelphia, 1984.
9. Luria, MH, Debanne, SM, and Osman, MI: Long-term followup after recovery from acute myocardial infarction: Observations on survival, ventricular arrhythmias, and sudden death. Arch Intern Med 145:1592, 1985.
10. Abjorn, C, Karlsson, E, and Sonnhag, C: Ventricular arrhythmias in acute myocardial infarction. Acta Med Scand 1201:119, 1977.
11. Lichtlen, PR, Bethge, KP, and Platiel, H: Incidence of sudden cardiac death in relation to left ventricular anatomy and rhythm profile. Z Kardiol 69:639, 1980.
12. Prinzmetal, M, Kennamer, R, Wada, T, et al: A variant form of angina pectoris. Am J Med 27:375, 1959.
13. Kreger, BE, Cupples, LA, and Kannel, WB: The electrocardiogram in prediction of sudden death: Framingham Study experience. Am Heart J 113:377, 1987.
14. Dunn, FG, Isles, CG, Brown, I, et al: The influence of left ventricular hypertrophy on mortality in the Glasgow Blood Pressure Clinic (abstr). Circulation 72(Suppl III):133, 1985.
15. Marcus, ML, et al: Alterations in the coronary circulation in hypertrophied ventricles. Circulation 75(Suppl I):I-19, 1987.
16. Dunn, FG and Pringle, SD: Left ventricular hypertrophy and myocardial ischemia in systemic hypertension. Am J Cardiol 60:23, 1987.
17. Versailles, JT, et al: Comparison between the ventricular fibrillation thresholds of spontaneously hypertensive and normotensive rats—investigations of antidysrhythmic drugs. J Cardiovasc Pharmacol 3:430, 1982.
18. Aronson, RS: Afterpotentials and triggered activity in hypertrophied myocardium from rats with renal hypertension. Circ Res 48:720, 1981.
19. McLenachan, JM, et al: Ventricular arrhythmias in patients with hypertensive left ventricular hypertrophy. N Engl J Med 317:787, 1987.
20. Messerli, FH, et al: Hypertension in sudden death. Am J Med 77:18, 1984.
21. Levy, D, et al: Risk of ventricular arrhythmias in left ventricular hypertrophy: The Framingham Heart Study. Am J Cardiol 60:560, 1987.
22. Pringle, SD, et al: Hypertensive left ventricular hypertrophy: Is there a high risk subgroup? (abst) J Am Coll Cardiol 9:114A, 1987.
23. Packer, M: Sudden unexpected death in patients with congestive heart failure: A second frontier. Circulation 72:681, 1985.
24. Hanrath, P, et al: Left ventricular relaxation and filling pattern in different forms of left ventricular hypertrophy: An echocardiographic study. Am J Cardiol 45:15, 1980.
25. Teare, D: Asymmetrical hypertrophy of the heart in young adults. Br Heart J 20:1, 1958.
26. Maron, BJ, et al: Sudden death in patients with hypertrophic cardiomyopathy: Characterization of 26 patients without functional limitation. Am J Cardiol 4:803, 1978.
27. McKenna, WJ, et al: Arrhythmia in hypertrophic cardiomyopathy: Exercise and 48-hour ambulatory electrocardiographic assessment with and without beta adrenergic blocking therapy. Am J Cardiol 45:1, 1980.
28. Brandenburg, RO: Cardiomyopathies and their role in sudden death. J Am Coll Cardiol 5:185B, 1985.

29. Huang, SK, Messer, JV, and Denes, P: Significance of ventricular tachycardia in idiopathic dilated cardiomyopathy: Observations in 35 patients. Am J Cardiol 51:507, 1981.

30. Van Olshausen, K, et al: Ventricular dysrhythmia in idiopathic dilated cardiomyopathy. Br Heart J 51:195, 1984.

31. Dreifus, LS, et al: Ventricular fibrillation: A possible mechanism of sudden death in patients with Wolff-Parkinson-White syndrome. Circulation 43:520, 1971.

32. Medical Research Council Working Party: On mild to moderate hypertension: Ventricular extra-systoles during thiazide treatment. Br Med J 287:1249, 1983.

33. Medical Research Council Working Party: MRC trial of treatment of mild hypertension. Br Med J 291:97, 1985.

34. Neuspiel, DR and Kuller, LH: Sudden and unexpected natural death in childhood and adolescence. JAMA 24:1321, 1985.

35. Messerli, FH, et al: Diamorphic adaptation to obesity and arterial hypertension. Ann Intern Med 99:757, 1983.

36. Dunn, FG, et al: Racial differences in cardiac adaptation in essential hypertension determined by echocardiographic indices. J Am Coll Cardiol 5:1348, 1983.

37. Lion, WN: Sudden unexpected and unexplained death. Accra Ghana Med J 7:170, 1968.

38. Rabkin, SW, Mathewson, FA, and Tate, RB: The electrocardiogram in apparently healthy men and the risk of sudden death. Br Heart J 47:546, 1982.

39. Pedoe, HDT: Predictability of sudden death from resting electrocardiogram: Effect of previous man-ifestations of coronary heart disease. Br Heart J 40:630, 1978.

40. Friedman, M, et al: Instantaneous and sudden death. JAMA 225:319, 1973.

41. Epstein, SE, Quyyumi, AA, and Bonow, RO: Myocardial ischemia—silent or symptomatic. N Engl J Med 318:1038, 1988.

42. Erikssen, J and Thaulow, E: Followup of patients with asymptomatic myocardial ischemia. In Rutishauser, W and Roskhamm, H (eds): Silent Myocardial Ischemia. Berlin, Springer-Verlag, 1984.

43. Bruce, RA, et al: Value of maximal exercise tests in risk assessment of primary coronary artery disease events in healthy men: Five years' experience of the Seattle Heart Watch Study. Am J Cardiol 46:371, 1980.

44. Bruce, RA, et al: Enhanced risk assessment for primary coronary heart disease events by maximal exercise testing: Ten years' experience of the Seattle Heart Watch Study. J Am Coll Cardiol 2:565, 1983.

45. Surawicz, B: Prognosis of ventricular arrhythmias in relation to sudden cardiac death. J Am Coll Cardiol 10:435, 1987.

46. The Lipid Research Clinics Coronary Primary Prevention Trial results: 1. Reduction in incidence of coronary heart disease. JAMA 251:351, 1984.

47. Multiple Risk Factor Intervention Trial Research Group: Multiple risk factor intervention trial. Risk factor changes and mortality results. JAMA 248:14677, 1982.

48. Schaffer, WA and Cobb, LA: Recurrent ventricular fibrillation and modes of death in survivors of out-of-hospital ventricular fibrillation. N Engl J Med 293:259, 1975.

49. Mirowski, M, et al: Mortality in patients with implanted automatic defibrillators. Ann Intern Med 98:585, 1983.

50. The Norwegian Multicenter Study Group: Timolol-induced reduction in mortality and reinfarction in patients surviving acute myocardial infarction. N Engl J Med 304:801, 1981.

51. β-Blocker Heart Attack Trial Research Group: A randomized trial of propranolol in patients with acute myocardial infarction: 1. Mortality results. JAMA 247:1707, 1982.

52. Hjalmarson, A, et al: Effect on mortality of metoprolol in acute myocardial infarction: A double-blind randomized trial. Lancet 2:823, 1981.

53. Aspirin Myocardial Infarction Study Research Group: A randomized controlled trial of aspirin in persons recovered from myocardial infarction. JAMA 243:661, 1980.

54. ISIS-2 Collaborative Group: Randomised trial of intravenous streptokinase, oral aspirin, both, or neither among 17,187 cases of suspected acute myocardial infarction. Lancet 1:349, 1988.

55. Holmes, DR Jr, et al: The effect of medical and surgical treatment and subsequent cardiac death in patients with coronary artery disease. Report from the Coronary Artery Surgery Study. Circulation 73:1254, 1986.

56. McKenna, WJ, Krikler, DM, and Goodwin, JF: Arrhythmias in dilated and hypertrophic cardio-myopathy. Med Clin North Am 68:983, 1984.

57. Dunn, FG, et al: Enalapril improves systemic hemodynamics and allows regression of left ventricular mass in essential hypertension. Am J Cardiol 53:105, 1984.
58. Dunn, FG, et al: Time course of regression of left ventricular hypertrophy in hypertensive patients treated with atenolol. Circulation 76:254, 1987.
59. Frohlich, ED: Hypertensive cardiovascular disease: A pathophysiological assessment. Hypertension 6:934, 1984.
60. Effects of enalapril on mortality in severe congestive cardiac failure: The Consensus Trial Study Group. N Engl J Med 316:1429, 1987.
61. Thomson, RG, Hallstrom, AP, and Cobb, LA: Bystander initiated cardiopulmonary resuscitation in the management of ventricular fibrillation. Ann Intern Med 90:7, 1979.
62. Eisenberg, M, Hallstrom, A, and Bergner, L: Long-term survival after out-of-hospital cardiac arrest. N Engl J Med 306:1340, 1982.

PART 3

Reversibility and Platelets

CHAPTER 7

Reversibility of Atherosclerosis*

Mark L. Armstrong, M.D.
Donald D. Heistad, M.D.
Marjorie B. Megan
J. Antonio G. Lopez, M.D.
David G. Harrison, M.D., Ph.D.

Atherosclerosis, which is the most common intimal arteriopathy in humans, is the principal cause of death in the United States and other industrial countries.[1]

Clinical manifestations of atherosclerosis usually appear suddenly, although the atherosclerotic process has been present for decades.[2,3] Identification of atherosclerosis in its latent, presymptomatic stage is an important goal in prevention of the symptomatic stage. The clinician today faces three questions about the control of atherosclerosis: (1) Is it practical to attempt detection of atherosclerosis in its presymptomatic stage? (2) If symptoms have already appeared, can further growth of lesions be arrested? (3) Can clinically important lesions be reversed?

Atherosclerosis may be detected at a presymptomatic stage in superficial arteries by ultrasound. Detection at a presymptomatic stage of coronary atherosclerosis, the greatest cause of morbidity and death, is not yet practical because detection is commonly done by arteriography. Detection of early lesions by arteriography is problematic, and both expense and risk are further deterrents to its use in unselected patients. Instead, the clinician categorizes patients in terms of the statistical probability of manifesting atherosclerosis rather than by actual detection of lesions. Statistical likelihood is expressed in terms of risk factors.

The importance of accurate identification of persons with increased risk stems from the recent evidence that reduction of excess risk leads to decreased morbid events.[4,5] Thus, some control of the atherosclerotic process is possible. We are now at the point at which the question, can the atherosclerotic process be reversed, is appropriate because it is now possible to reverse completely some putative risk factors. We would note, however, that when lesions are defined in terms of probability

*This work was supported by National Institutes of Health ASCOR HL 14320 and Program Project Grants HL 14388 and NS 24621.

113

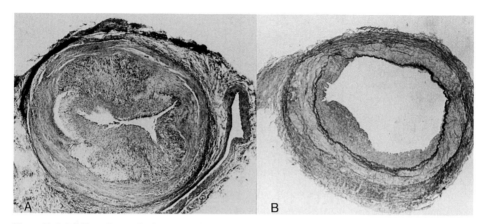

Figure 7–1. (*A*) Experimental atherosclerosis and regression in monkeys. Atherosclerotic coronary artery shows a stellate lesion with marked intimal proliferation, dense periluminal connective tissue, and prominent basal lipid and cell breakdown. Hematoxylin and orcein, × 60. (*B*) Regression artery shows an increase in lumen size and a residual intimal lesion that consists mainly of dense fibrosis, with marked loss of cellularity and visible lipid. Hematoxylin and orcein, × 60.

rather than observed directly, it is not possible to relate improvement in clinical outcomes after reduction of risk factors with any specific change in lesions. On the other hand, when significant reversal of the risk factor hypercholesterolemia is carried out in experimental settings, lesions also tend to improve. The actual size decreases (Fig. 7–1), and abnormal accumulations of some lesion components are depleted.[6]

We regard reversibility of atherosclerosis as a feasible concept. Evidence for reversal of structural and functional aspects of atherosclerosis in humans and other primates is summarized here. In this discussion, the term "regression" indicates decrease in lesion size, and the term "reversibility" refers to recovery of normal vascular function.

EVALUATING EXTENT OF ATHEROSCLEROSIS

PATHOLOGIC OBSERVATIONS

Only recently has atherosclerosis passed from a disease of unknown cause and apparently inexorable course to a disease in which the causes are partly known and in which the course can be ameliorated. The earliest examples of regression of

Table 7–1. Morphologic Studies of Regression of Atherosclerosis

Clinical Setting	Regression	Investigators
Wartime	+	Aschoff (1924)
	+	Variainen and Kanerva (1947)
Tuberculosis	arrest	McMeans (1916)
	+	Eilerson and Faber (1960)
Cancer	+	Wilens (1947)
	+	Wanscher (1951)
	+	Juhl (1957)

human lesions date from the period in which factors that contribute to the progression of atherosclerosis were unknown. Autopsy observations provided evidence for regression of atherosclerosis[7-13] in the setting of wasting conditions, such as wartime malnutrition, wide-spread cancer, and tuberculosis (Table 7–1). We agree with the usual interpretation of this information, that there is clear evidence that some decrease in lesion size occurred under conditions associated with a prolonged catabolic state of nutrition. When these observations were made, there was little evidence that lesion control was possible in less drastic metabolic conditions.

ARTERIOGRAPHIC STUDIES

Arteriography provided a powerful new tool for the evaluation of atherosclerosis. Many clinical studies were reported in which change in lumen appearance was interpreted to show progression, arrest, or occasionally regression of atherosclerosis (Table 7–2). Some attempt at reduction of risk factors was used to examine possible change in lesion size as shown by arteriography.[14-28]

Regression as defined by arteriography was infrequently found (Table 7–2). We believe that two factors account for the infrequency of regression. Some investigators simply ruled out the possibility of regression of lesions and categorically attributed increases in lumen size after treatment to lysis of overlying thrombi or disappearance of arterial spasm. A major reason, however, for the infrequent reporting of regression probably is that it occurred infrequently.

Nevertheless, there are important limitations in evaluating the significance of lesion size in angiographic studies.[29] The images reveal encroachment on the lumen and thus reflect the size of the lesion only indirectly. The time between arteriographic studies often is short, and the effectiveness of the antiatherosclerotic regi-

Table 7–2. Angiographic Studies of Regression

Status of Lesion	Investigator	Treatment
Improved (Cases/Total Cases)		
3/31	Öst (1967)[14]	
Case Report	DePalma (1970)[15]	
Case Report	Basta (1976)[16]	Diet/drug regimens
9/25	Barndt (1977)[17]	
15/94	Blankenhorn (1987)[18]	
2/2	Crawford (1979)[19]	
Case Report	Roth (1980)[20]	Life-style changes
Case Report	Starzl (1974)[21]	Portacaval shunt
3/22	Buchwald (1974)[22]	Ileal bypass
3/8	Thompson (1975)[23]	Plasma exchange
Unimproved (Total Cases)		
16	Cohn (1975)[24]	
25	Kuo (1979)[25]	
25	Nash (1982)[26]	Diet/drug regimens
71	Levy (1984)[27]	
39	Arntzenius (1985)[28]	Diet

mens in reducing risk factors often is modest and uncertain. Finally, a frequent question is whether regression consisted of resolution of overlying thrombus or a decrease in size of the plaque.

Several investigators cited in Table 7–2 gave detailed attention to these problems, including Blankenhorn and coworkers.[17,18] Moreover, in their study of coronary bypass patients,[18] they designed the study to rule out bias and to cause profound reduction of lipid risk factors. Under clearly specified details of observation, these investigators found evidence that lesion size could be arrested. The distribution of change in lesion size between groups supported the concept that actual regression of lesion size occurred after treatment of some patients with advanced coronary atherosclerotic disease.[18]

The overall results of arteriographic evaluations of effects of treatment on atherosclerosis suggest that little improvement in lesion size occurs in most patients, but a minority of patients show evidence of lesion regression. The combination of attention to pitfalls in technique and marked reduction of atherosclerotic risk factors[18,25,29] provides the best evidence from arteriographic studies that arrest of lesion size is possible, and even regression of lesions may occur if lipid risk factors are markedly reduced.[18]

PHYSIOLOGIC IMPROVEMENT

A third way in which lesions have been evaluated is in terms of functional improvement, with direct or indirect evidence for improvement in blood flow. Cardiac function often improves after coronary artery bypass grafting, but physiologic improvement is rarely evaluated after attempts to modify lesions by reduction of risk factors. In one study by Zelis and associates,[30] both claudication and peak hyperemic blood flow to the limbs were found to be improved after reduction of lipids in patients with type III hyperlipidemia. In a single case, Basta and associates[16] showed that reduction of lipids in a hypercholesterolemic patient who also had renovascular hypertension caused angiographic improvement in the renal arteries and reduced the renal venous renin tenfold to normal levels.[16] In the same patient, coronary lesions were minimally improved and bypass grafting was necessary, which illustrates that regression may be strikingly heterogeneous.

LESSONS FROM ANIMAL MODELS OF ATHEROSCLEROSIS AND REGRESSION

There are gaps in our knowledge of human atherosclerosis that can be filled provisionally with information from appropriate animal models. Experimental data are particularly useful in relating arterial hemodynamic and biochemical events to morphologic changes. Studies of experimental atherosclerosis in Old World monkeys have extraordinary value. Hypercholesterolemia in these animals produces multivessel atherosclerosis, with patterns of distribution and morphology that are very similar to those of human lesions.[31,32] This morphologic picture reflects the fact that as much as 92 percent of human DNA may be shared with Old World monkeys.[33] In this circumstance, the risks of tentative extrapolation of results into a clinical framework are probably less than the risk of foregoing valuable insights into the course and potential control of atherosclerosis in humans. For this reason, we cite observations of experimental regression that may parallel those that may be possible in human disease.

PLAQUE COMPONENTS AND THEIR POTENTIAL FOR REGRESSION

Regression of plaques cannot be considered *en bloc* because plaques have many components, and each of these components has a potentially distinct fate in response to dietary or other interventions. For some components (for example, lipid content), there is evidence that very significant depletion may occur when regression is attempted. For others (for example, calcification), the evidence is inconclusive. Evidence in relation to components that are common to all atherosclerotic lesions, including endothelial cells, intimal cells, lesion lipid, and the conective tissue matrix, is summarized. Responses of components that are associated primarily with larger, more advanced plaques, such as necrosis and calcification, neovascularization and hemorrhage, and mural fibrin and thrombosis, are then described. In considering whether components of human lesions improve, it should be remembered that except for lipid depletion, resolution of thrombi, and the episodic nature of mural hemorrhage, evidence about changes in individual components in human lesions is virtually nonexistent. Data from experimental atherosclerosis are used to provide evidence about the possibility of change but not the magnitude of change in components of human plaques.

ENDOTHELIUM

The endothelium is typically not denuded in the early phases of atherosclerosis,[34] but it is no longer as effective as a plasma filter. Endothelial cells are structurally altered in subtle ways, so that permeability to macromolecules is increased.[35,36] There is increased passage into the intima of atherogenic lipoproteins and probably platelet components and other molecules that have key roles in atherogenesis. As plaques enlarge and mature, endothelium may be lost and the centers of plaques may become bald expanses of subendothelium to further increase permeability.

In regression, the structure of endothelium becomes normal,[37] and permeability tends to return to normal levels. There is also evidence that bald patches of subendothelium are re-covered with endothelium.[37]

INTIMAL CELLS

The cells in the atherosclerotic intima are chiefly smooth-muscle cells and leukoyctes. The leukocytes are mainly macrophages,[38] but polymorphonucleated cells, lymphocytes, and even mast cells are seen. The presence of smooth-muscle cells in the intima is largely a response to factors that stimulate migration and mitogenesis. Leukocytes are recruited in an inflammation-like process that may be an important aspect of the genesis of the lesion. Cholesterol is delivered to the cells by lipoproteins, and the macrophages can engorge huge amounts of lipoprotein and thus acquire great intracellular stores of cholesterol. Macrophages also are centers of lytic activity for fibrous proteins of the extracellular matrix, and they probably have a role in the remodeling of small collagen strands and the development of fibrosis. Smooth-muscle cells can synthesize elastin,[39] and thus they may form the musculoelastic layers that are chacteristic of large plaques.

In regression, the intimal cells decrease in number,[40] and they no longer accumulate lipid.[41] Lipid-laden foam cells disappear from human[23] and experimental[42] lesions (Fig. 7–2). Macrophages and other leukocytes apparently leave lesion sites.[42]

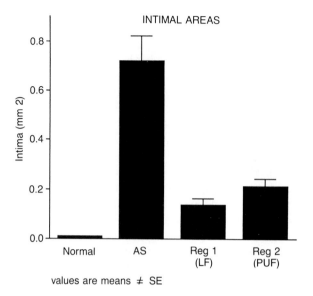

Figure 7–2. Coronary lesions after treatment of experimental atherosclerosis. Intimal mass was measured as area in histologic sections. In atherosclerosis (AS) the intima increased greatly because of lesions. After 18 months of dietary treatment (Reg 1 and Reg 2), there were marked reductions in intimal mass, with loss of foam cells and other components of lesions. Comparable regression was obtained with low-fat (LF) or polyunsaturated fat (PUF) diets. (From Armstrong, et al.[43])

Most of the remaining leukocytes perish without replacement, but many smooth-muscle cells survive and are transformed to a more uniform appearance as contractile-type cells.

LIPID CONTENT

Atherosclerotic lesions are by definition lipid-rich. Most of the excess lipid in lesions comes from low-density lipoprotein (LDL) molecules. Parts of the LDL molecules that are degradable or directly removable from the wall include protein, glycerol and fatty acids that compose triacylglycerols, and phospholipids. Removal of cholesterol and cholesteryl ester is much more limited. As atherosclerotic lesions develop, this differential removal leads to massive stores of intracellular cholesterol in intimal cells and large extracellular cholesterol pools that remain in the extracellular matrix of the intima. Extracellular cholesterol seems to be inert, but it has long been recognized that a slow turnover occurs,[44] even in severe lesions.[45] This turnover provides a possible mechanism of decreasing pool size in regression of lesions.

There is a consensus that lipid in lesions is one component that may be demonstrably depleted in regression (Fig. 7–3). Evidence for lipid depletion was noted in the early morphologic studies of regression in humans.[11] There may be vast losses from foam cell lesions.

It is less clear how much lipid may be lost from the extracellular matrix, particularly from necrotic pools (Fig. 7–4). There is little confirmatory evidence in man, and turnover of the extracellular lipid in humans is quite slow. In spite of this, it seems likely that some depletion of extracellular lipid may occur in humans, as in experimental regression in other primates.[47]

CONNECTIVE TISSUE

Part of a plaque is scar, characterized by connective tissue with prominent amounts of heavily cross-linked collagen and variable amounts of elastin. The part

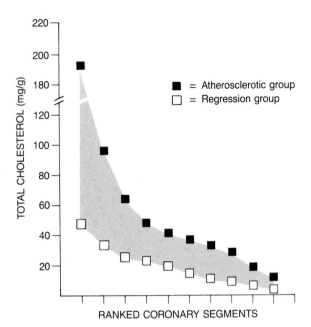

Figure 7–3. Effect of regression on total cholesterol content in coronary arteries in experimental atherosclerosis. The shaded area marks the difference in cholesterol content between the atherosclerotic and regression groups when the groups are ranked by cholesterol content of each animal's coronary artery segments. This finding shows the extensive lipid depletion that occurs in regression. (From Armstrong, et al.[46])

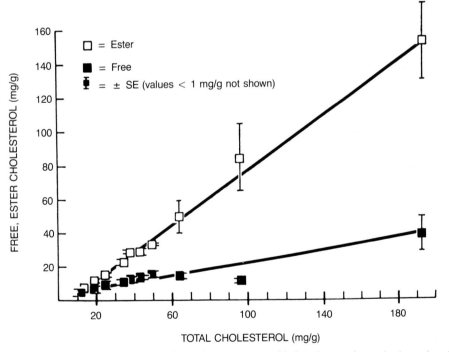

Figure 7–4. Effect of regression on cholesteryl ester content of lesions in experimental atherosclerosis. The tissue content of esterified and free cholesterol in the same coronary segments as those in Figure 7–3 is plotted against total cholesterol in the artery. There are striking linear correlations between total cholesterol and each fraction: the r value of cholesteryl ester is 0.99, and that of free cholesterol is 0.85. The slope for depletion of cholesteryl ester is several times greater than the slope for free cholesterol. The steep slope of cholesteryl ester is indicative of changes in cholesterol content secondary to foam cell depletion. The shallow slope of free cholesterol reflects the depletion rate that one might anticipate in the absence of foam cells. (From Armstrong, et al.[46])

of the connective tissue matrix that is not fibrous protein consists of proteoglycans, an interstitial filler of protein and mucopolysaccharides.

The proteoglycans readily undergo changes in mass and probably regress when lesion size decreases. It is not clear, however, whether the collagen mass of plaques can be reduced in regression. In principle, lysis of this matrix material might be possible, but the extent to which large dense scars might regress remains problematic.[48] Perhaps changes in collagen content in regression are similar to reductions found in simple granuloma systems.[49] The rate of collagen synthesis almost certainly decreases in regression, and collagen content may be reduced in late regression.[48] Increased intimal fibrosis is found nonetheless in almost all regression studies, including ours.[48,50] The key to fibrosis is cross-linking of collagen, and it seems likely that this process continues in regression as a dominant fact. Relatively small reductions in the number of collagen fibrils probably make little difference in a pervasive picture of ongoing fibrosis.

The fibrotic component of the lesion is probably the most important factor governing potential for regression of human plaques. If the plaques are rigid collagen shells, it seems unlikely that reduction in lesion size can occur. This view, however, may be an oversimplification. Lesions are created by hydraulic forces as well as by metabolic factors. If lesion content is reduced, a reshaping of plaque to a smaller size may be possible in time. Even old dermal scars, which are examples of dense fibrosis, often decrease in size after a decade of observation.[51]

NECROSIS AND CALCIFICATION

Cell death, particularly of foam cells, is very common in the abnormal milieu of the lesion. When this occurs, several constituents of the cell are removed. Cell-associated cholesterol, however, remains as a significant constituent of the lipid-rich necrotic pool. Thus, clumps of crystalline cholesterol found in lesions may be taken as evidence of prior cell breakdown. Cholesterol is highly fibrogenic,[52] and for this reason cholesterol crystals are most often found embedded in dense collagen. These areas are prone to calcification and even occasional cartilage or bone formation.[53] In other areas, cell fragments give rise to matrix vesicles, which, as in cartilage, acquire calcium salts and are the usual source of calcification in atherosclerotic lesions.[54]

The response of the various constituents of necrosis has been estimated in experimental studies of regression, and some depletion in humans seems likely. Based on studies in primates, it is likely that the cellularity of necrotic areas decreases, the lipid content slowly decreases, and even the crystalline cholesterol seen in histologic sections may diminish.[47] The connective tissue matrix shows inconsistent decreases, and the fate of dystrophic calcification is unclear, with clear evidence for its decrease in one model of regression[55,56] and our evidence that calcification failed to diminish in regression.[49] We interpret the net effect of regression as a real reduction in necrosis of the plaque, despite variable responses of the constituents of necrosis.

NEOVASCULARIZATION AND HEMORRHAGE

Atherosclerotic lesions lead to the formation of new microvessels (vasa vasorum) in the media and intima. These vessels probably arise from a combination of ischemia and inflammation.[57] Vasa probably have a protective role in the media, where they may help to prevent medial necrosis. In contrast, vasa in the intima are probably not protective. Flow through these channels is relatively low,[58] and intimal vasa may rupture, produce subintimal hemorrhage, and lead to increased encroachment of plaque into the lumen. If hemorrhage from vasa vasorum occurs near the endothelium, it may cause a thrombogenic milieu and lead to the formation of thrombi on the surface of the lesion.

A blueprint for sustained reversal of lesions would include regression of these potentially dangerous microvessels. There are no human data bearing on the fate of these lesions after regression regimens, but we have shown that neovascularization in atherosclerotic vessels in primates disappears in regression.[59]

FIBRIN AND THROMBUS

Human atherosclerotic lesions often contain large amounts of fibrinogen or fibrin.[60] This is degradable material and, if the endothelial defects that increase permeability in atherosclerosis[35] undergo regression, one would expect depletion of fibrin and fibrogen. Thrombus formation is fairly common on older plaques, and thrombi are a very common cause of clinical events in the coronary artery bed.

There is an important question about thrombi at a presymptomatic stage: Do microthrombi contribute to plaque growth? We believe that microthrombi, which are tiny clumps of platelets and fibrin, change plaques by intensifying the fibrotic reaction of collagen in plaques.[61] In addition, Duguid[62,63] has proposed that microthrombi become incorporated into lesions and thereby increase plaque size.

If microthrombi are found to be important in lesion growth, this concept would have a profound bearing on regimens designed to control plaque growth. The point is controversial, and the topic deserves attention beyond this brief mention. We would simply note that lesions with features of atherosclerosis often develop in many saphenous vein grafts after coronary bypass operations.[64] The use of antiplatelet agents (see Chapter 8) is successful in suppressing lesion formation in vein grafts.[65] We think that comparable mechanisms of lesion formation may operate in the native coronary bed.

VASCULAR RESPONSES IN ATHEROSCLEROSIS

Atherosclerotic arteries have a reduced capacity to dilate,[50] but constriction is often markedly increased.[66,68] These are cardinal points of arterial dysfunction that are found in prestenotic atherosclerosis, and these abnormalities should be considered separately from those associated with decreased perfusion because of stenosis of the lumen. The loss of dilator responses is partly due to functional changes in endothelium. The marked increase in constrictor responses in atherosclerosis relates both to changes in endothelial dysfunction and to changes in medial responsiveness in atherosclerosis.[68,69] Release of endothelium-derived relaxing factor is impaired in atherosclerosis.[69,71] After regression regimens, there is functional recovery of endothelium,[73] and dilator responses also reverse toward normal[72] (Fig. 7–5).

Arterial responses to a number of vasoconstrictor responses are potentiated in human atherosclerosis.[74–76] Exaggerated constrictor responses to a variety of agents may underlie the increased tendency to vasospasm that occurs in atherosclerosis,[77,78] and that may contribute to many episodes of clinical ischemia and death.

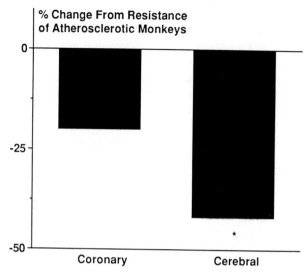

Figure 7–5. Reversal of impaired dilator function after treatment of experimental atherosclerosis. The vessel wall was fully dilated *in vivo* to calculate minimal resistance. Minimal resistance, which is a sensitive reflection of vascular structure, is increased by atherosclerosis. In monkeys with clear morphological evidence of regression of lesions, the coronary bed had only inconsistent reversal of impaired dilator capacity, and the cerebral bed had significant reversal of impaired dilator capacity. *p <0.05, compared with resistance in atherosclerosis. (From Armstrong, et al.[70])

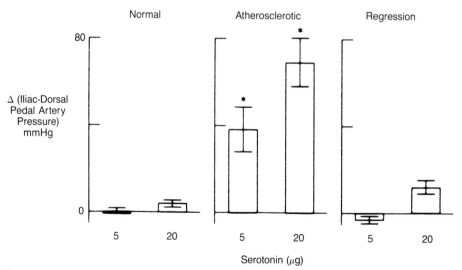

Figure 7–6. Vasoconstrictor response to serotonin. Serotonin caused marked increases in segmental pressure in atherosclerotic arteries (center panel), which indicates greater vasoconstrictor responses and probably greater suceptibility to vasospasm. After dietary treatment, there is modest reduction in lesion size and marked reversibility (right panel) of the exaggerated constrictor responses *p <0.05 atherosclerotic *vs.* normal and regression monkeys. (From Heistad, et al.[67])

After regression of experimental atherosclerosis, these abnormal constrictor responses are reversed to normal[67,73] (Fig. 7–6).

REVERSIBILITY AS A CENTRAL CONCEPT OF THERAPY

We have reviewed the evidence that lesions of human atherosclerosis may improve. The earliest evidence of improvement consists of observations that regression of lesions occurred during prolonged catabolic states (wartime malnutrition, tuberculosis, cancer). Subsequent evidence has shown that a general catabolic state is not necessary for lesion improvement, and that reduction of risk factors can lead to arrest of lesion growth and occasionally to actual regression of lesions.[18] We speculate that newer, more potent antilipidemic agents will further increase the frequency of regression. If microthrombi are a co-factor in enhancing lesion growth, antiplatelet measures might further restrain lesion growth and fibrosis. We consider lesion arrest a more realistic goal than regression for most atherosclerotic patients. For the near future, lesion regression will probably continue to be the exception rather than the rule.

The achievement of lesion arrest after reduction of risk factors has major implications. Arrested lesions probably undergo important functional improvements. It is plausible that these improvements include reversal of endothelial abnormalities that reduce dilator effects, recovery of a less thrombogenic vascular interface, reduction of the hazards associated with neovascularization of the wall, and reversal of exaggerated vasoconstrictor responses that may predispose the atherosclerotic artery to vasospastic episodes.

We propose that these functional improvements are intrinsic features of the arrest of lesion growth, which may start with retardation of plaque growth. If lesion arrest is achieved in the various arterial beds, clinical sequelae may be reversed to an important degree. It is possible that, even without reduction in the size of lesions, we can now reverse the course of atherosclerosis in a large number of afflicted patients.

REFERENCES

1. Inter-Society Commission for Heart Disease Resources: Optimal resources for primary prevention of atherosclerotic diseases. Circulation 70:153A, 1984.
2. McGill, HC, Geer, JC, and Strong, JP: Atherosclerosis and its origin. In Sandler, M and Bourne, GH (eds): Academic Press, New York, 1963.
3. McGill, HC Jr: Atherosclerosis: Problems in pathogenesis. In Paoletti, R and Gotto, AM Jr (eds): Atherosclerosis Reviews, Vol 2. Raven Press, New York, 1976.
4. Lipid Research Clinics Program: The Lipid Research Clinics Coronary Primary Prevention Trial results. I. Reduction in incidence of coronary heart disease. JAMA 25:351, 1984.
5. Frick, MH, et al: Helsinki Heart Study: Primary-prevention trial with gemfibrozil in middle-aged men with dyslipidemia: Safety of treatment, changes in risk factors, and incidence of coronary heart disease. N Engl J Med 317:1237, 1987.
6. Armstrong, ML: Regression of atherosclerosis. In Paoletti, R and Gotto, AM Jr (eds): Atherosclerosis, Vol 1. Raven Press, New York, 1976.
7. Aschoff, L: Lectures in Pathology (Delivered in the United States, 1924). Hoeber, New York, 1924.
8. Variainen, I and Kanerva, K: Arteriosclerosis and wartime. Ann Med Exper Biol Fenn 36:748, 1947.
9. McMeans, JW: Superficial fatty streaks: An experimental study. J Med Res 31:41, 1916.
10. Eilerson, P and Faber, M: The human aorta. Arch Pathol 70:103, 1960.

11. Wilens, SL: Resorption of arterial atheromatous deposits in wasting disease. Am J Pathol 23:793, 1947.

12. Juhl, S: Cancer and atherosclerosis. II. Applicability of postmortem statistics in the study of negative correlation. Acta Pathol Microbiol Scand 41:99, 1957.

13. Wanscher, O, Clemmesen, J, and Nielsen, A: Negative correlation between atherosclerosis and carcinoma. Br J Cancer 5:172, 1951.

14. Öst, CR and Stenson, S: Regression of peripheral atherosclerosis during therapy with high doses of nicotinic acid. Scand J Clin Lab Invest 19 (Suppl 99):241, 1967.

15. DePalma, RG, et al: Progression and regression of experimental atherosclerosis. Surg Gynecol Obstet 131:633, 1970.

16. Basta, LL, et al: Regression of atherosclerotic stenosing lesions of the renal arteries and spontaneous cure of systemic hypertension through control of hyperlipidemia. Am J Med 61:420, 1976.

17. Barndt, R, et al: Regression and progression of early femoral atherosclerosis in treated hyperlipoproteinemic patients. Ann Intern Med 86:139, 1977.

18. Blankenhorn, DH, et al: Beneficial effects of combined colestipol-niacin therapy on coronary atherosclerosis and coronary venous bypass grafts. JAMA 257:3233, 1987.

19. Crawford, DW, Sanmarco, ME, and Blankenhorn, DH: Spatial reconstruction of human femoral atheromas showing regression. Am J Med 66:784, 1979.

20. Roth, D and Kostuk, WJ: Noninvasive and invasive demonstration of spontaneous regression of coronary artery disease. Circulation 62:888, 1980.

21. Starzl, TE, et al: Portacaval shunt in hyperlipidaemia. Lancet 2:714, 1974.

22. Buchwald, H, Moore, RB, and Varco, RL: Surgical treatment of hyperlipidemia. Circulation 49 (Suppl 1):1, 1974.

23. Thompson, GR, Lowenthal, R, and Myant, MB: Plasma exchange in management of homozygous familial hypercholesterolemia. Lancet 1:1208, 1975.

24. Cohn, K, Sakai, FJ, and Langston, MF Jr: Effect of clofibrate on progression of coronary disease: A prospective, angiographic study in man. Am Heart J 89:591, 1975.

25. Kuo, PT, et al: Use of combined diet and colestipol in long-term treatment of patients with Type II hyperlipoproteinemia. Circulation 59:199, 1979.

26. Nash, DT, Gensini, G, and Esente, P: Effect of lipid-lowering therapy on the progression of coronary atherosclerosis assessed by scheduled repetitive coronary arteriography. Int J Cardiol 2:43, 1982.

27. Levy, RI, et al: The influence of changes in lipid values induced by cholestyramine and diet on progression of coronary artery disease: Results of the NHLBI type II coronary intervention study. Circulation 69:325, 1984.

28. Arntzenius, AC, et al: Diet, lipoproteins, and the progression of coronary atherosclerosis. The Leiden Intervention Trial. N Engl J Med 312:805, 1985.

29. Brown, GG, Bolson, EL, and Dodge, HT: Arteriographic assessment of coronary atherosclerosis: Review of current methods, their limitations, and clinical applications. Arteriosclerosis 2:2, 1982.

30. Zelis, R, et al: Effects of hyperlipoproteinemia and their treatment on the peripheral circulation. J Clin Invest 49:1007, 1970.

31. Armstrong, ML and Warner ED: Morphology and distribution of diet-induced atherosclerosis in Rhesus monkeys. Arch Pathol 92:395, 1971.

32. Armstrong, ML, Trillo, A, and Prichard RW: Naturally occurring and experimentally induced atherosclerosis in nonhuman primates. In Kalter, SS (ed): The Use of Nonhuman Primates in Cardiovascular Diseases. University of Texas Press, Austin, 1980.

33. Sibley, CG and Ahlquist, JE: DNA hybridization evidence of hominoid phylogeny: Results from an expanded data set. J Mol Evol 26:99, 1987.

34. Faggiotto, A and Ross, R: Studies of hypercholesterolemia in the nonhuman primate. II. Fatty streak conversion of fibrous plaque. Arteriosclerosis 4:341, 1984.

35. Schwartz, CJ, Gerrity, RG, and Lewis LJ: Arterial endothelial structure and function with particular reference to permeability. In Paoletti R and Gotto, AM Jr (eds): Atherosclerosis Reviews, Vol 3. Raven Press, New York, 1978.

36. Schwartz, CJ, et al: Arterial endothelial permeability to macromolecules. In Paoletti, R and Gotto, AM Jr (eds): Atherosclerosis Reviews, Vol 3. Springer-Verlag, New York, 1977.

37. Weber, G, et al: Regression of arteriosclerotic lesions in Rhesus monkey aortas after regression diet—Scanning and transmission electron microscope observations of the endothelium. Atherosclerosis 26:535, 1977.

38. Gown, AM, Tsukada, T, and Ross, R: Human Atherosclerosis. II. Immunocytochemical analysis of the cellular composition of human atherosclerotic lesions. Am J Pathol 125:191, 1986.
39. Ross, R and Klebanoff, SJ: The smooth muscle cell and in vivo synthesis of connective tissue protein. J Cell Biol 50:172, 1971.
40. Armstrong, ML and Megan, MB: Regression sequences after experimental atherosclerosis. In Gotto, AM Jr, Smith, LC, and Allen, B (eds): Atherosclerosis V. Springer-Verlag, New York, 1979.
41. Armstrong, ML: Atherosclerosis in Rhesus and cynomolgus monkeys. In Strong, JP (ed): Primates in Medicine. S. Karger, New York, 1976.
42. Stary, HC: Regression of early lesions in monkeys. In Schettler, G, Stange, E, and Wissler, RW (eds): Atherosclerosis — Is It Reversible? Springer-Verlag, New York, 1978.
43. Armstrong, ML, Warner, ED, and Connor, WE: Regression of coronary atheromatosis in Rhesus monkeys. Circ Res 27:59, 1970.
44. Gould, RG, Jones, RJ, and Wissler, RW: Lability of cholesterol in human atherosclerotic plaques. Circulation 20:967, 1959.
45. Katz, SS, et al: Cholesterol turn-over in lipid phases of human atherosclerotic plaque. J Lipid Res 23:733, 1982.
46. Armstrong, ML and Megan, MB: Lipid depletion in atheromatosis in coronary arteries in monkeys after regression diets. Circ Res 30:675, 1972.
47. Small, DM, et al: Physicochemical and histological changes in the arterial wall of nonhuman primates during progression and regression of atherosclerosis. J Clin Invest 73:1590, 1984.
48. Armstrong, ML and Megan, MB: Arterial fibrous proteins in cynomolgus monkeys after atherogenic and regression diets. Circ Res 36:256, 1975.
49. Armstrong, ML: Connective tissue in regression. In Paoletti, R and Gotto, AM Jr (eds): Atherosclerosis Reviews, Vol 3. Raven Press, New York, 1978.
50. Armstrong, ML, et al: Structural and hemodynamic responses of peripheral arteries of Macaque monkeys to atherogenic diet. Arteriosclerosis 5:336, 1985.
51. Warner, ED: Personal communication, 1975.
52. Abdulla, YH, Adams, CWM, and Morgan, RS: The reaction of connective tissues to implantation of purified sterol, sterol esters, phosphoglycerides, glycerides, and free fatty acids. J Pathol 94:63, 1967.
53. Armstrong, ML and Megan, MB: Responses of two Macaque species to atherogenic diet and its withdrawal. In Schettler, G and Weizel, A (eds): Atherosclerosis III. Springer-Verlag, New York, 1974.
54. Kim, KM: Calcification of matrix vesicles in human aortic valve and aortic media. Fed Proc 35:156, 1976.
55. Daoud, AS, et al: Regression of advanced swine atherosclerosis. Arch Pathol Lab Med 100:372, 1976.
56. Fritz, KE, et al: Regression of advanced swine atherosclerosis: Chemical studies. Arch Pathol Lab Med 100:380, 1976.
57. Barger, AC, et al: Hypothesis: Vasa vasorum and neovascularization of human coronary arteries. N Engl J Med 310:175, 1984.
58. Heistad, DD, Armstrong, ML, and Marcus, ML: Hyperemia of the aortic wall in atherosclerotic monkeys. Circ Res 48:669, 1981.
59. Williams, JK, Armstrong, ML, and Heistad, DD: Vasa vasorum in atherosclerotic coronary arteries: Responses to vasoactive stimuli and regression of atherosclerosis. Circ Res 62:515, 1988.
60. Smith, EB, Alexander, KA, and Massie, IB: Insoluble "fibrin" in human aortic intima: Quantitative studies on the relationship between insoluble "fibrin," soluble fibrinogen, and low density lipoprotein. Atherosclerosis 20:93, 1976.
61. Stary, HC: Evolution and progression of atherosclerosis in the coronary arteries of children and adults. In Bates, SR and Gangloff, EC (eds): Atherogenesis and Aging. Springer-Verlag, New York, 1987.
62. Duguid, JB: Thrombosis as a factor in the pathogenesis of coronary atherosclerosis. J Path Bact 60:207, 1946.
63. Duguid, JB: Thrombosis as a factor in the pathogenesis of aortic atherosclerosis. J Path Bact 60:57, 1948.
64. Campeau, L, et al: The relationship of risk factors to the development of atherosclerosis in saphenous-vein bypass grafts and progression of disease in the native circulation. N Engl J Med 311:1329, 1984.

65. Bonchek, LI, et al: Prevention of lipid accumulation in experimental vein bypass grafts by antiplatelet therapy. Circulation 66:338, 1982.
66. Heistad, DD, Breese, J, and Armstrong, ML: Cerebral vasoconstrictor responses to serotonin after dietary treatment of atherosclerosis: Implications for transient ischemic attacks. Stroke 18:1068, 1987.
67. Heistad, DD, et al: Dietary treatment of atherosclerosis abolishes hyperresponsiveness to serotonin: Implications for vasospasm. Circ Res 61:346, 1987.
68. Heistad, DD, et al: Augmented responses to vasoconstrictor stimuli in hypercholesterolemic and atherosclerotic monkeys. Circ Res 54:711, 1984.
69. Freiman, PC, et al: Atherosclerosis impairs endothelium-dependent vascular relaxation to acetylcholine and thrombin in primates. Circ Res 58:783, 1986.
70. Armstrong, ML, Heistad, DD, and Marcus, ML: Hemodynamic sequelae of regression of experimental atherosclerosis. J Clin Invest 104:113, 1983.
71. Harrison, DG, et al.: Alterations in vascular reactivity in atherosclerosis. Circ Res (Suppl 2) 61, 1987.
72. Forstermann, U, et al: Selective attenuation of endothelium-mediated vasodilation in atherosclerotic human coronary arteries. Circ Res 62:185, 1988.
73. Harrison, DG, et al: Restoration of endothelium-dependent relaxation by dietary treatment of atherosclerosis. J Clin Invest 80:1808, 1987.
74. Mudge, GH Jr, et al: Reflex increase in coronary vascular resistance in patients with ischemic heart disease. N Engl J Med 295:1333, 1976.
75. Winniford, MD, et al: Smoking induced coronary vasoconstriction in patients with atherosclerotic coronary artery disease: Evidence for adrenergically mediated alterations in coronary artery tone. Circulation 73:662, 1986.
76. Heusch, G and Deussen, A: The effects of cardiac sympathetic nerve stimulation on perfusion of stenotic coronary arteries in the dog. Circ Res 53:8, 1983.
77. Ginsburg, R, et al: Histamine provocation of clinical coronary artery spasm: Implication concerning pathogenesis of variant angina pectoris. Am Heart J 102:A19, 1981.
78. Waters, DD, et al: Comparative sensitivity of exercise, cold pressor, and ergonovine testing in provoking attacks of variant angina in patients with active disease. Circulation 67:310, 1983.

CHAPTER 8

Modification of Thrombogenic Factors in Cardiac Disease

Edward Genton, M.D.

Thrombosis is the formation of an intravascular mass from the constituents of blood due to activation of the hemostatic mechanism. It is a multifactorial reaction involving the intravascular lining, the blood platelets, and the coagulation system. The normal heart, similar to other endothelial surfaces, is seldom the site of thrombus formation. However, when any of the cardiac structures, whether myocardium, valves, or coronary arteries, become diseased, thrombosis involving that structure frequently occurs and dominates a part of the patient's course, contributing greatly to the morbidity and mortality associated with the condition. In caring for the patient with cardiac disease, it is imperative therefore that the likelihood of thrombosis is appreciated and methods for preventing or arresting the thrombotic process be understood and applied appropriately.

MECHANISM OF THROMBOSIS

Thrombosis in cardiac patients is usually triggered by disruption of the surface lining of intravascular structures (Fig. 8–1). Thrombosis in the coronary arteries may be the result of atherosclerosis altering endothelial cells; in the ventricular chambers, it may be the result of endocardial damage due to cardiomyopathies, myocardial infarction, and so forth; and on valve structures, it may be the result of chronic valve changes, such as are encountered in rheumatic valve disease, or may be associated with myxomatous degeneration in mitral valve prolapse, or may be the result of acute changes, such as with systemic lupus erythematosus or bacterial endocarditis. Exposure of blood to damaged vascular surface sets into motion the thrombotic process that stimulates platelet reactivity and activates the coagulation system.

The blood platelet contributes in several ways to thrombus formation.[1] Initially, when a vessel is injured, the blood platelet adheres to the injury site by interaction with exposed collagen. This leads to activation of the platelet, which results in change in the platelet shape to a more flattened and spread-out cell, followed by

THROMBOGENESIS

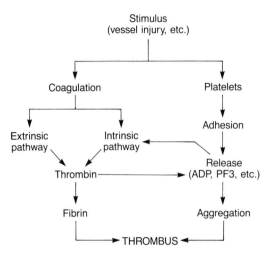

Figure 8-1. Schematic representation of thrombogenesis involving vessel damage, platelets, and coagulation.

release of contents of a variety of chemicals stored in platelet granules, including adenosine diphosphate (ADP), and release from the platelet membrane of products of prostaglandin activation, including thromboxane A_2 (TXA_2). The platelet-release reaction stimulates the building up of a platelet aggregate.

The coagulation system is activated by several stimuli associated with damage of vascular surface. This includes the effects of tissue thromboplastin released from injured tissue combining with coagulation factor VII, thereby activating the extrinsic thromboplastin pathway, and by activation of the intrinsic thromboplastin pathway when factor XII is activated on exposure to the site of damaged tissue. The intrinsic and extrinsic thromboplastin pathways result in sequential activation of coagulation factors and, thereby, generation of thrombin that converts fibrinogen to fibrin, which stabilizes the platelet thrombus and expands the thrombotic plug by incorporation of red cells into the fibrin lattice. Once formed, thrombin stimulates synthesis of more thromboxane A_2 and the release of platelet ADP from surrounding platelets, which further enhances thrombus formation.

METHODS FOR PREVENTION OR INHIBITION OF THROMBOSIS

Appreciation of the mechanism of thrombosis identifies several potential approaches to control of this process. Preventing damage to the vascular surface theoretically would be best, but methods for accomplishing this are usually not available, and the possibility of protecting endothelium or endocardium pharmacologically is not presently achievable. Therefore, methods must be used that inhibit the hemostatic mechanism by modifying platelet behavior or preventing thrombin generation and fibrin formation.

PLATELET INHIBITORS

Drugs that inhibit platelet reactivity may do so by interfering with one of several of the platelet reactions. This could include inhibition of arachidonic acid metabolism, increase in platelet adenosine monophosphate (cyclic AMP), or effects on other membrane activities. To date, aspirin and dipyridamole have produced positive results in clinical trials.

Aspirin

Aspirin affects platelet reactivity by irreversibly acetylating and, thereby, inhibiting platelet cyclo-oxygenase. This results in the prevention of thromboxane A_2 formation by preventing the conversion of arachidonic acid to intermediary endoperoxides, the precursors of TXA_2. This action does not affect platelet adhesion but does block the formation of platelet aggregates. Aspirin does not prevent release of ADP or thrombin mediating platelet aggregation and, therefore, would not block thrombus formation in circumstances in which thrombin is formed, which may be more important than ADP or TXA_2 in recruitment of circulating platelets.

Cyclo-oxygenase is inhibited in the platelet by even low doses of aspirin, and approximately 95 percent of cyclo-oxygenase synthesis is inhibited by 325 mg of aspirin daily. Because platelets cannot synthesize new cyclo-oxygenase, the inhibition is permanent for the life of the exposed platelets. Aspirin also blocks formation of PGI_2 from endothelial cells, which is probably undesirable. Because higher doses of aspirin are needed to inhibit cyclo-oxygenase in endothelial cells than in platelets, it is believed that the smallest dose of aspirin effective to inhibit cyclo-oxygenase should be used to avoid the undesirable inhibition of PGI_2 in patients with thrombotic disorders.

Dipyridamole

Dipyridamole is thought to affect platelet function by inhibiting platelet phosphodiesterase. This enzyme is involved with the breakdown of cyclic AMP and, when inhibited, maintains higher levels of cyclic AMP, which serves to inhibit platelet adhesion and aggregation.

ANTICOAGULANTS

Heparin and the coumarin derivatives (for example, warfarin) interfere with thrombin generation and fibrin formation and block formation of thrombi.[2]

Heparin

Heparin is a sulfonated mucopolysaccharide that complexes with antithrombin 3 and markedly enhances the effect of antithrombin 3 to inhibit serine proteinases, which includes a number of activated coagulation factors. Susceptibility to the heparin-antithrombin 3 complex varies with the different clotting factors, with some, such as factor Xa, being inhibited by low concentrations of the complex. Blocking activated factor X prevents the formation of thrombin and, therefore, prevents thrombosis. However, once thrombin has formed, larger amounts of heparin are necessary to inhibit that enzyme and arrest the thrombotic process.

Coumarin Derivatives

Coumarin derivatives act by inhibiting the vitamin K-dependent steps in the synthesis of several coagulation factors in the liver. This includes factors II, VII, IX, and X. Vitamin K functions as a cofactor in the conversion of glutamic acid residues into gamma carboxyglutamic acids. These are the reaction sites for the procoagulant proteins with calcium ions and phospholipids. Coumarins prevent the carboxylation of these proteins. They therefore serve as antithrombotic agents by leading to the formation of coagulation factors with reduced biologic activity.

THROMBOSIS AND ANTITHROMBOTIC THERAPY IN CLINICAL DISORDERS

VALVULAR HEART DISEASE

Valvular abnormalities involving either the left or the right side of the heart may be associated with development of thrombi on or around the valve. Mitral valve abnormalities have the highest frequency of thrombosis, especially mitral stenosis of rheumatic etiology; with mitral regurgitation, thrombosis occurs about one-half as often. With mitral disease, the two clinical factors that correlate with thrombosis and systemic embolization are advanced age and atrial fibrillation. Emboli are uncommon in patients under age 35, but after that age the incidence increases approximately 1.5 percent per patient year to an incidence of nearly 40 percent by the seventh decade. Atrial fibrillation is present in more than 75 percent of patients who develop emboli.

Once emboli develop, recurrence is frequent and occurs in more than 30 percent of patients over a 10-year period, with one-third of events occurring within the first month after the initial episode.

Degenerative changes in the mitral valve, such as occur with mitral valve prolapse or in patients with extensive mitral annulus calcification, are associated with some increase in thrombosis and embolization compared with normal valves, but, fortunately, the incidence is small.

The objective of treatment is to prevent initial emboli in high-risk cases or recurrence in patients following the first episode of systemic embolization. Adequate clinical trials are lacking in this patient population, but evidence from case series without concurrent controls leaves little doubt that long-term anticoagulant therapy controls valve thrombosis and embolization. It is suggested, therefore, that long-term warfarin therapy be employed in patients with valvular heart disease following systemic embolization or in patients with mitral stenosis with atrial enlargement in excess of 5.5 cm or when associated with atrial fibrillation. Platelet inhibitors used alone have not been adequately protective, but in patients on warfarin therapy who have breakthrough emboli, the action of dipyridamole may be beneficial. Aspirin also would afford protective effect but may increase likelihood of bleeding complications.

PROSTHETIC HEART VALVES

All available substitute valves are thrombogenic, with an approximate annual incidence of embolization of 3 percent from aortic valves and 15 percent from mitral valves. Bioprosthetic valves are much less thrombogenic, with an annual incidence of approximately one percent per year unless atrial fibrillation is present.

Warfarin anticoagulation has been documented to be effective in numerous clinical trials and reduces embolization by about two-thirds. It has been recommended that all patients with mechanical heart valves receive long-term anticoagulation. Patients with bioprosthetic valves should be treated for the first three months following surgery with warfarin anticoagulation and, thereafter, require anticoagulants only if chronic atrial fibrillation is present or atrial thrombi are documented. Platelet inhibitor therapy with dipyridamole may enhance warfarin effect and is indicated if breakthrough emboli occur. Platelet inhibitor drugs used alone are not adequate therapy for prophylaxis. It is not known whether platelet inhibitors are beneficial to patients with bioprosthetic valves who do not receive anticoagulation.

MYOCARDIAL ABNORMALITIES

Acute Myocardial Infarction

Thrombosis involving the endocardial surface of an infarcted ventricle frequently occurs in patients following acute myocardial infarction. The thrombogenic stimulus in such cases is probably damage to the endocardial surface, which regularly occurs with transmural infarctions. The true incidence of mural thrombi in patients with infarction varies with infarct location, infarct size, and whether an aneurysm develops. Patients with large anterior infarctions have mural thrombi in about one-third of cases, compared with an incidence of five percent with inferior infarction. The incidence of emboli into the systemic circulation is uncertain but in some series is reported in as many as 25 percent of patients and is most likely to occur when the thrombi are large and protrude with ragged surfaces into the ventricular cavity. Unfortunately, a high percentage of emboli enter the cerebral circulation and produce strokes. No measures other than anticoagulation prevent thrombus formation or arrest the process once it has developed. Heparin in low doses has not been effective. High-dose heparin followed by oral anticoagulation during the hospital phase, reduces embolization; studies have varied as to the degree that thrombi are prevented. It is likely that the stimulus for thrombus formation is so great in particular patients that clinical levels of anticoagulation will not prevent thrombi but may limit size of thrombus and likelihood for embolization.

It is recommended that patients who develop emboli have a several months' course of anticoagulants to prevent recurrence. Presently, it is uncertain which patients with infarction and mural thrombi documented by echocardiogram require anticoagulation to arrest the process and prevent embolization. Oral anticoagulants that follow heparin therapy reduce incidence of mural thrombi by at least 50 percent.

Cardiomyopathies

This category of heart disease includes a number of conditions of varied etiology. All have in common the damage of myocardial cells, with compromise of ventricular function. The incidence of mural thrombi varies with the different types of cardiomyopathies but occurs frequently in all; in some, such as alcoholic and postpartum cardiomyopathy, mural thrombi are found in nearly half of cases in ventricular or atrial chambers. Clinical embolic episodes are encountered in about one-third of cases. Although no adequately designed clinical trials have evaluated the effect of anticoagulants in such patients, it is reasonable to believe that they would effectively reduce the incidence of thrombosis and embolization. Chronic anticoagulation is probably indicated in these patients unless significant contraindication exists.

CORONARY ARTERY DISEASE

In coronary arteries affected with atherosclerotic lesions, the development of thrombotic occlusion frequently is the cause of change in clinical status. In unstable angina, studies have confirmed the presence of thrombosis in nearly half of patients if studied within 24 hours of symptoms. In the presence of acute myocardial infarction, it has been documented that in more than 85 percent of cases, thrombotic occlusion is present. In many patients with sudden cardiac arrest, platelet aggregates or platelet fibrin thrombi are found. The effect of antithrombotic therapy in coronary artery disease has been studied by clinical trials for years, initially with oral anticoagulants or heparin and more recently with platelet-inhibitor drugs.[3-6] Two well-designed clinical trials have evaluated the efficacy of aspirin treatment in patients with unstable angina, and both demonstrated approximately 50 percent reduction in the incidence of acute myocardial infarction or death. Similarly, heparin used intravenously in high dosage reduced by about 80 percent the mortality or acute myocardial infarction incidence in patients with unstable angina.

In patients who survive an acute myocardial infarction, aspirin therapy has been employed in seven controlled clinical trials and, overall, reduced the rate of reinfarction by approximately 20 percent and reduced the incidence of death by approximately 10 percent.

Recent attention has been turned to the use of aspirin for the primary prevention of coronary artery events, and in a group of more than 20,000 male physicians, it has been documented that there was reduction in the risk of myocardial infarction by 47 percent, although there was no statistical significance in the mortality incidence. It may be concluded that the majority of events in coronary disease patients are related to thrombosis and that platelet inhibitor therapy or heparin therapy may benefit outcome by inhibiting thrombus formation. It is generally accepted now that patients with unstable angina and those who have survived an acute myocardial infarction should receive aspirin therapy. Even after more than 25 years, however, the value of chronic oral anticoagulation therapy after myocardial infarction is unresolved.

SUMMARY

Thrombosis plays an important role in the development and course of most disorders affecting the heart. No effective methods are available to eliminate the thrombogenic stimulus for those conditions requiring the use of antithrombotic agents for prophylaxis or to arrest a thrombotic event. Available platelet and coagulation inhibitors are effective when properly selected and administered.

REFERENCES

1. Vermylen, J, Verstraete, and Fuster, V: Role of platelet activation and fibrin formation in thrombogenesis. J Am Coll Cardiol (Suppl B)8:2, 1986.
2. Wessler, S and Gitel, SN: Pharmacology of heparin and warfarin. J Am Coll Cardiol (Suppl B)8:10, 1986.
3. Harker, LA and Fuster, V: Pharmacology of platelet inhibitors. J Am Coll Cardiol (Suppl B)8:21, 1986.
4. Levine, HJ, Pauker, SG, and Salzman, EW: Antithrombotic agents in coronary artery disease. Chest (Suppl 98):95, 1989.
5. Stein, PD and Kantrowitz, A: Antithrombotic therapy in mechanical and biological prosthetic heart valves and saphenous vein bypass grafts. Chest (Suppl 102):95, 1989.
6. Resnekov, L, et al: Antithrombotic agents in coronary artery disease. Chest (Suppl 52):95, 1989.

PART 4

Behavioral Interventions
for the Cardiologist

CHAPTER 9

Psychosocial Factors in Coronary Heart Disease

Stephen M. Weiss, Ph.D.
Susan M. Czajkowski, Ph.D.
Sally A. Shumaker, Ph.D.
Roger T. Anderson, B.A.

Treatment and control of coronary heart disease (CHD), the leading cause of morbidity and mortality in the United States, absorb a considerable proportion of our health expenditures. As with other chronic diseases, research into those factors responsible for the development and progression of the disease process has produced a mosaic of potential etiologic agents. These agents include the basic biology of the cell and genetic, physiologic, biochemical, constitutional, and developmental variables, as well as psychophysiologic, psychosocial, sociocultural, and environmental factors. The relative importance of these factors, singly and in various combinations, forms the central debate surrounding the risk-factor controversy.

Research on psychosocial factors and CHD risk has recently gained impetus from advances in biotechnology and in data acquisition, analysis, and storage, which have provided an opportunity to obtain dynamic measurements of biologic processes *in vivo* as the organism acts on and reacts to its environment. This has opened up new vistas of scientific investigation in our efforts to understand how responses to environmental and psychologic challenges affect the physiologic integrity of organisms. By simultaneously manipulating the external environment while assessing the internal environment, researchers ultimately may come to understand both associational and causal relationships.

At present, the data concerning the role of cardiovascular response to environmental challenge in determining CHD risk are still preliminary. As noted in this chapter, considerable evidence supports the role of psychosocial factors contributing to, or being protective against, CHD. The unanswered questions concern the strength and *clinical* significance of these contributions and the potential for intervention strategies to meaningfully affect the disease process in the desired direction.

The entire body of research on psychosocial factors related to CHD is beyond the scope of this chapter; rather, it highlights three specific research topics that are representative: the *intra*personal, *inter*personal, and environmental areas of research.

Intrapersonal factors relate to those characteristics of the individual that may affect biologic and disease processes, such as behavioral or personality attributes, which we consider under the broad rubric coronary-prone behavior. We briefly review the data (and controversy) concerning Type A behavior, and the more recent research on hostility and anger.

The **interpersonal** domain concerns the role of social relationships (friends, family, co-workers) in the development and progression of CHD. The conceptual models of social support, social isolation, and social networks question whether specific characteristics or qualities of these relationships impact the disease process.

Finally, the **environmental** domain involves the broader context of individuals' lives, including work, home, social, and cultural settings, as well as climate, economic, political, and legal circumstances that may affect behavior in definable and predictable ways. Recent research on occupational stress is reviewed that provides valuable insights into such variables as environmental "demand" and "control" and how they may interact to enhance or inhibit CHD risk.

INTRAPERSONAL: CORONARY-PRONE BEHAVIOR AND CHD

The relationship between certain personality and behavioral characteristics and the clinical manifestation of CHD has been the subject of anecdotal reports for centuries.[1-3] The emotional and behavioral factors most often linked to CHD have included strong emotional states, such as anger, and personality characteristics, such as strong ambition or drive. Osler[4] considered "the robust, the vigorous in mind and body, the keen and ambitious man, the indicator of whose engine is always at full speed ahead" to be particularly "coronary-prone."

In the 1950s, Rosenman and Friedman[5,6] provided a formal label and a method for reliably assessing the constellation of competitive, hard-driving, time-urgent, and hostile behaviors thought to characterize the individual prone to heart disease. They defined this behavioral style, labeled the Type A Behavior Pattern (TABP), as "an action-emotion complex that can be observed in any person who is aggressively involved in a chronic, incessant struggle to achieve more and more in less and less time, and if required to do so, against the opposing efforts of other things or other persons." The method they developed to assess this pattern, the Structured Interview, consists of a series of challenging questions designed to elicit specific responses associated with this constellation of behaviors labeled *Type A*. Individuals labeled *Type B* are characterized by the relative absence of these behaviors.

Following several prevalence studies that showed an association between Type A behavior and CHD,[7,8] the TABP was shown to predict CHD incidence in the Western Collaborative Group Study (WCGS), a prospective study of 3,154 men who were free of CHD symptoms at intake and were followed for 8.5 years.[9] Several other prospective studies, using a variety of methods for assessing the TABP, also found an association between the TABP and CHD incidence.[10,11] In addition, a number of angiographic studies documented a relationship between the TABP and severity of coronary artery disease.[12-15]

A number of studies have explored the mechanisms through which Type A behavior may influence the development of CHD. One possibility is that the increased cardiovascular and neuroendocrine reactivity to stressful stimuli that characterizes the Type A individual[17,18] may promote a variety of physiologic reactions that contribute to CHD development. These include increased hemodynamic forces, such as turbulence and shear stress, and toxic effects resulting from increased levels of circulating catecholamines and cortisol.[19]

Based on the prospective and angiographic evidence linking the TABP to CHD, a panel of scientists, meeting in 1978 under the auspices of the National Heart, Lung, and Blood Institute,[16] declared the TABP to be a risk factor for CHD "over and above that imposed by age, systolic blood pressure, serum cholesterol, and smoking. . . ."

Since the panel's findings, however, research on the TABP as a risk factor for CHD has produced conflicting results. An increasing number of studies, including the prospective MRFIT study[20] and several angiographic studies,[21-23] have failed to find a link between the TABP and CHD. Most recently, a study by Ragland and Brand,[24] which reanalyzed data from 257 patients from the original WCGS who had survived a myocardial infarction, found that Type Bs were at *greater* risk for a recurrent event than were Type As. Although there are methodologic concerns with this study, it has led to a questioning of the predictive validity of the Type A concept by the scientific community. Interpretation of these conflicting results concerning the role of the TABP in CHD has focused on several possibilities, including the following:

1. Some element of the Type A pattern, or its assessment, has changed over time, so that early findings no longer generalize to populations currently under study.
2. The relationship between Type A behavior and CHD may be dependent on some third factor, such as age or risk factor status, that has varied among studies.
3. Some component or components of the TABP (for example, hostility, anger expression) are actually related to CHD, even when global Type A behavior is not.

With regard to the first possibility, the estimated prevalence of Type A behavior has been increasing, from approximately 50 percent in the WCGS to 70 percent or more in recent studies.[25] This suggests that the diagnostic criteria for determining an individual's Type A status may be changing and that certain components of the pattern more related to CHD (for example, hostility, anger) may have been emphasized in the earlier studies, leading to the finding of a positive relationship between the TABP and CHD in these studies but not in later ones.

Secondly, there is evidence that the relationship between the TABP and CHD may be dependent on the presence of other factors. For example, Williams and co-workers[26] found an interaction of Type A status and age for 2,289 angiography patients, such that the TABP was significantly associated with severity of coronary artery disease but only for patients aged 50 and younger; for individuals above age 50, a modest inverse relationship existed, which in part supports one of the findings of Ragland and Brand.[24] It appears that whereas the TABP may predict incidence of premature CHD, those patients who survive past age 50 constitute a unique group of individuals for whom the relationship between TABP and CHD may not hold.

With regard to the third possible reason for the conflicting findings in this area, a number of recent studies have focused on identifying components of the Type A pattern that may be more strongly linked to CHD than global TABP. In several of these studies, the elements of the Type A pattern most predictive of CHD were found to be hostility and mode of anger expression.[21,22,27–29] Furthermore, in a reanalysis of the data from a random sample of MRFIT participants, Dembroski and associates[30] found hostility to be more predictive of CHD incidence than a global Type A rating. Along these lines, several prospective studies have confirmed a link between a cynical, hostile personality style and cardiovascular-specific and all-cause mortality.[31,32] These findings are consistent with reactivity studies, which indicate that hostile persons are most likely to exhibit exaggerated cardiovascular and neuroendocrine responses to stressful stimuli.[33,34]

Thus, although the global Type A pattern itself appears to be less related to CHD than previously thought, the evolution of this area of research is toward a determination of those elements of the TABP that are most predictive of CHD incidence, with the goal of eventually modifying specific coronary-prone behaviors in high-risk individuals. Intervention programs in this area generally have shown that coronary-prone behaviors can be modified successfully through intensive group counseling sessions that use a combination of cognitive, affective, and behavioral techniques specifically directed toward reducing anger and hostility. Recently, in the Recurrent Coronary Prevention Project (RCPP), such behavior modification techniques were found to be protective against a recurrent coronary event (that is, MI) in a group of postinfarction patients.[35] In the future, refinement of the concept of coronary-prone behavior is expected to result in the development of interventions targeted specifically to the most pathogenic aspects of the coronary-prone behavior pattern. Such interventions would require testing through large-scale prospective studies to determine the advantages of such behavioral treatments over standard medical regimens.

INTERPERSONAL: SOCIAL SUPPORT AND CHD

Over the past two decades, evidence has accumulated linking social support to mental and physical health in general and to CHD specifically.[36–40] Investigations using a range of study populations, research methods, and social support measures consistently demonstrate an association between low levels of social support and high rates of CHD-related morbidity and mortality.[41,42] In this section, we highlight some of the epidemiologic evidence for this apparently robust phenomenon, identify limits to the available data, and suggest future agendas for research on social support and CHD. First, however, we provide a brief history and definition of social support.

DEFINING SOCIAL SUPPORT

The importance of interpersonal relationships to personal well-being has been argued by social scientists since Durkheim's[43] seminal work linking suicide rates to social isolation. However, it was not until 1974 that the physician and epidemiologist Cassel argued the importance of interpersonal relations for health maintenance. Cassel[44] hypothesized that disruptions in social relations increased susceptibility to illness. This hypothesis served as the catalyst for hundreds of studies investigating the relationship between social support and mental and physical health.[45]

Unfortunately, most early studies on social support were atheoretical and the concept rarely was explicitly defined. Thus, measures of social support have varied widely across studies, and the scientific community has had difficulty reaching agreement on a clear definition of the term.[46,47] As noted by Cohen and colleagues,[47] studies on social support use the term for a *range* of concepts that include social *network* characteristics (for example, number of friends, frequency of contact), the *functions* served by social relations (for example, emotional or tangible support), and the degree to which an individual is integrated into a community (for example, marital status, church membership, and so on). It is remarkable, in fact, that this range of definitions has yielded such similar results in linking social support to CHD.

For the purposes of this chapter, we refrain from a single definition of social support and use the distinction proposed by Cohen and Wills[48] between structural and functional support measures. Structure refers to the interconnections among social ties, whereas function refers to the *resources* provided in interpersonal relationships (for example, affection, belonging, material aid). This distinction encompasses the range of definitions of social support used in research and recognizes the possibility that different aspects of support may be plausible predictors of CHD at various stages of disease onset and progression.

EPIDEMIOLOGIC STUDIES

Epidemiologic studies linking support to CHD have used, at a minimum, a structural measure of support sometimes referred to as a social integration index, which usually includes marital status, number of close friends, participation in groups, and religious affiliation. The more recent studies have also included validated–social support *instruments* that incorporate both structural and functional components of support as well as an individual's satisfaction with support.[49] Study designs have been both prospective and cross-sectional and have included total mortality and CHD-related mortality and morbidity as outcome measures.

In general, after controlling for traditional risk factors for CHD, such as cigarette smoking, blood pressure, co-morbidity, and age, several major epidemiologic studies have confirmed that people with higher levels of social support are at lower risk for all-cause mortality than people with lower levels of support.[50–53] In all of these studies, low social support is also linked to risk for CHD mortality.

For example, in the prospective Alameda County study, participants scoring in the lowest quartile of a social network index[50] at baseline had an age-adjusted risk for all-cause mortality of 2.3 for men and 2.8 for women and had a significantly greater risk of mortality due to ischemic heart disease, specifically that which persisted even after adjusting for the standard CHD risk factors.

In the Tecumseh, Michigan Prospective Community Study,[51] marital status and some aspects of organizational involvement and leisure activity were found to be significantly related to all-cause mortality for men (after adjusting for age and CHD risk factors); however, for women, only church attendance was significantly related to all-cause mortality. Similar patterns of results were found for CHD-related mortality.

The Durham County, North Carolina study[54] found low social support to be a significant risk factor for all-cause mortality at 30-month follow-up, even when controlling for the standard CHD risk factors. Risk ratios ranged from 1.88 for the frequency of interaction dimension to 3.40 for perceptions of social support.

The Framingham Heart Disease Study[55] followed 142 female clerical workers for 8 years and found that those women with nonsupportive bosses had an increased risk of CHD (defined as MI, coronary insufficiency, angina pectoris, or CHD death). In a cross-sectional study of 3,809 Japanese-American men, aged 30 to 74 years, in San Francisco, it was found that a lack of social affiliation predicted prevalence of CHD independent of age, physical inactivity, and family history of heart attack.[56]

Several population-based studies in other countries (for example, Sweden, Finland) have obtained similar findings relating low social support and social interaction to CHD mortality.[52,57,58] A Swedish study investigating the relationship between occupational factors and CHD risk among 13,779 working men and women found an interaction between work demand, work control, and social support, such that those in high-demand, low-control, low-support occupations had an age-adjusted relative risk of 2.17 compared with those in the low-demand, high-control, and high-support occupations.[59,60]

In a study by Welin and co-workers,[57] social activity (based on participants' attendance at social and work-related activities) significantly predicted overall mortality for 1,137 Swedish men aged 50 to 60 years, even after controlling for coronary risk factors. Similarly, Orth-Gomer and Johnson[52] found that a social interaction index was significantly related to age-adjusted all-cause and cardiovascular-specific mortality for a sample of 17,433 randomly selected Swedish men and women who were followed for 6 years, after adjusting for health and socioeconomic variables. However, this relationship became nonsignificant after controlling for exercise and smoking habits.

Also, a study in North Karelia, Finland, involving a group of 13,301 men and women aged 39 to 59, found that men, but not women, who scored in the lowest quintile on a social network index had twice the overall mortality and 1.8 times the cardiovascular mortality of the highest quintile, after controlling for traditional CHD risk factors and sociodemographic factors.[58]

There is evidence also that social support is predictive of CHD mortality in people who are unhealthy at the onset of the investigation. In a prospective study of post-MI men, Ruberman and associates[53] found that men who were more socially isolated immediately following an MI had more deaths and more sudden cardiac deaths than their more socially integrated counterparts.

To summarize, both prospective and cross-sectional studies demonstrate an association between various measures of social support, all-cause mortality, and CHD-related morbidity and mortality. These relationships are strongest for white men and somewhat weaker for women and nonwhites.[36]

LIMITATIONS OF RESEARCH ON SOCIAL SUPPORT AND CHD

Although the aforementioned data are provocative, there are a number of problems in studies of social support and CHD that must be addressed. Inconsistent findings across studies may result from true population difference, variations in measures of support, and differences in outcome measures. The cross-sectional studies are plagued with a causal inference problem; that is, the questions of whether diseased people are less socially integrated or, if low social integration is a cause of disease. The prospective studies limit our ability to distinguish between individuals with pre-existing pathologic processes versus truly healthy individuals because CHD develops over a long-time course.

Despite these problems, few people would question the fact that a positive relationship exists between low levels of support and risk for CHD. As noted by Cohen and colleagues,[47] a substantial effort has has been expended since Cassel's initial hypothesis regarding support and disease susceptibility to establish this *association*. Perhaps most problematic, however, is that none of these studies addresses the factors that explain this relationship. That is, the *process or mechanisms* that account for an association between support and disease remain unknown.[40] As mentioned earlier, the mortality data tell us nothing about the relationship of support to various stages of the disease process. Furthermore, although the morbidity data[61] suggest that support is relevant to the onset of disease, these data are less consistent than the mortality data and often suffer from selection biases.[62] Studies on childhood relationships between support and disease onset are suggestive at best.[63]

All the studies on support and CHD control for risk factors for disease. This approach represents a conservative test of the hypothesized relationship.[36] That is, it is not unreasonable to suggest that support may act indirectly on disease onset by influencing the development and maintenance of risk-related behaviors (for example, diet and/or smoking). Although the literature on CHD risk factors is beyond the scope of this chapter, it should be noted that recent studies on smoking cessation and Type A behavior, for example, are consistent with a possible relationship between support and CHD risk factors.

FUTURE DIRECTIONS FOR RESEARCH ON SUPPORT AND CHD

Epidemiologic studies on support and CHD must go beyond the general social integration indices and begin to disentangle the specific components of support that account for the relationship between social support and CHD. This sophisticated approach to the issue is already evidenced in the more recent investigations.[41,61] Perhaps more importantly, however, attention needs to turn now to the mechanisms underlying this relationship. Until we have a better understanding of why and how support influences CHD, our ability to intervene effectively on this risk factor is limited.

ENVIRONMENTAL: OCCUPATIONAL STRESS AND CHD

The substantial body of evidence supporting the relationship between environmental influences and CHD incidence and mortality includes such variables as socioeconomic status (for example, education, occupation, and income) and social affiliation. Although diet, exercise, blood pressure, and smoking are acknowledged risk factors for CHD, a large portion of the variance associated with CHD remains unaccounted for, which has stimulated a broader search for additional risk factors. Demonstration of an independent effect of education and occupation on CHD-related outcomes[53,64−66] has stimulated interest in the role of occupational stress as a potential contributor to the development of CHD.

It has been proposed that certain environmental conditions may elicit acute emotional arousal, which on a repeated basis and over long periods of time may be sufficient to induce pathologic changes in the structure and function of the cardio-vascular system.[67-70] Additionally, environmental stress has been pursued as an acute precipitant of sudden death and recurrent clinical CHD, induced by exaggerated coronary vasoconstriction,[71] cardiac arrhythmias,[72,73] and wall motion abnormalities.[74,75]

The focus in behavioral medicine on the influence of environmental factors in health-relevant behaviors, including psychosocial stress, is reminiscent of an early period in public health when prevention of disease was approached largely from an environmental engineering perspective. A hallmark of that era was John Snow's removal of the handle from the Broad Street pump to prevent infection by cholera.[76] With the prospect that psychosocial stress contributes in some way to the etiology of CHD, similar emphases have been placed on determining what features of the social and physical environment act as reservoirs of toxic stimuli and influence exposure (for example, frequency and duration) and susceptibility to stress as well as to characterize the pathogenic qualities and quantities of stress.

The issue of how stressful environments may produce CHD raises the more fundamental question regarding human psychobiologic adaptation.[68,69] Folkow[69] postulates that the highly developed neocortical functions of humans provide efficient coping mechanisms to deal with a changing environment. However, humans may have limited capacities concerning quantity and quality of stimuli, and in technologically advanced societies, this threshold may be exceeded periodically. Thus, for example, demands on mental activity with little or no expenditure of physical energy may elicit the "fight-flight" response,[69,77,78] which has major relevance to cardiovascular functioning. Additionally, chronic stress may be potentiated in situations in which it is necessary to suppress physical exertion, which precludes muscle vasodilation and slows elimination of increased lipids.[69]

Occupation is thought to be a particularly important exposure in stress-related CHD because it includes long exposure periods on a daily basis and a wide variety of tasks, work procedures, and situations that may be conducive to stress, and it provides the opportunity to delineate the range of coping strategies that may be used regularly in response to stressful conditions.

Evidence from clinical studies conducted over the last two decades by Frankenhaeuser and colleagues[79-84] and others indicates that qualities of work, including time pressure, monotony, lack of controllability, and excessive noise, are among the principal determinants of occupational stress. In these studies, stress has been conceptualized as a condition of stimulus overload of the central nervous system and has been reflected on the physiologic level in cortical, autonomic, or endocrine indices of arousal and on the cognitive level in increased effort, accompanied by feelings of distress and irritation.[85] In particular, Frankenhaeuser and co-workers[86-88] manipulated various task dimensions (for example, work pace, effort, control) in a laboratory setting, demonstrating the sensitivity of epinephrine output, heart rate,[85] and systolic and diastolic blood pressure independent of heart rate response[84] to motor and mental task-related demands as the subject's performance limit is approached. These results corroborate other findings from both animal and human studies that sympathetic activation is typically increased in environmental settings that elicit emotional distress and effort.[89-92] Interestingly, there is some evidence that the lack of stimulation in task performance (underload) also increases catecholamine excretion over baseline levels, apparently in response to boredom and monotony.[80]

A key finding in the aforementioned research is that personal control over task performance (for example, self-pacing) may attenuate catecholamine and cortisol secretion rates under aversive stimulation and reduce ratings of irritation and diastolic blood pressure[84,93] and cardiac acceleration.[94] Overall, this research has dissociated *effort* from *control* of work as distinct qualities relevant to job stress: by increasing control, physiologic arousal and subjective distress associated with a given task can be substantially reduced.

On an epidemiologic level, there is reasonable evidence now to support a relationship between work and work conditions and hypertension and CHD. Measures of psychosocial components of the workplace have been developed and are beginning to provide the most well-developed focus on the linkages between chronic stress and CHD in humans.

Among the earlier investigations,[95,96] high proportions of persons with CHD worked excessively long hours for some time preceding MI. More recently, House and associates[97] concluded that work stress (for example, responsibility, pressure, quality concern, role conflict, and work load) among factory workers was positively associated with self-reported angina (WHO version of Rose Questionnaire) and systolic blood pressure independent of age, education, smoking, obesity, and work-related physical activity. Van Dijkhuizen and Reiche,[98] in a cross-sectional study among laborers employed in several companies in the Netherlands, found that self-reported high work load, poor relations with management, and job ambiguity were related to blood pressure. Increased fibrinogen levels were noted in men in the lower occupational grades examined in the Whitehall Study, suggesting an increased risk for clotting.[99]

In an effort to examine chronic stress more precisely in relation to CHD, Karasek and colleagues[100] refined the concept of work stress to include workers with high self-reported job demands and low control over work tasks. Implicit in this view is that arousal of sufficient intensity to be pathogenic will not be attained when control over work equals or exceeds demands.[101] This conceptualization of work stress has been extensively tested using Swedish national survey data and is in apparent agreement with results of Frankenhaeuser (reported previously), which suggested that the degree of control over work may represent a capacity to cope with stress in the workplace.

Karasek and colleagues[100] examined the demand-control model using self-reports of the individual on work characteristics in a longitudinal survey of CHD risk in 1,461 asymptomatic Swedish men. After six years, high-demand and low-control jobs predicted development of new self-reported symptoms of cardiovascular disease (CVD) (hypertension and clinically manifest CVD) independent of age, education, smoking, and body weight. Prevalence rose monotonically with increasing demands and decreasing work control, with incidence following a similar pattern except for the extreme levels of job strain. Alfredsson and co-workers[102] found that excessive job demands in conjunction with low levels of job control predicted future hospitalization for MI for both men and women.

In the United States, prevalence of previous MI was found to be significantly higher among men employed in high-strain (high-demand and low-control) occupations after adjusting for individual conventional risk factors.[103] LaCroix[104] found that in a subset of the Framingham cohort, men and women employed in high-strain occupations had a significantly greater risk of CHD over a 10-year period than those in low-strain occupations. Using the same method of job scoring, Karasek[105] obtained similar results using two large nationally representative United States health data bases (HES and NHANES). Employed men with jobs that were characterized by high strain had a higher prevalence of MI after accounting for age, race, education, serum cholesterol level, smoking, and systolic blood pressure.

Based on the occupational stress research, it appears that there is a relationship between occupational exposure to stress and the development of CHD. This relationship may account, in part, for the persistent differences observed in CHD mortality rates between social classes and occupations. Importantly, with the major research refinement of defining stress in terms of response to the degree of control one exerts on the environment as well as the demands of that environment on the individual, the focus has now moved beyond demographic characteristics (for example, socioeconomic status) to focus on specific aspects of how person-environment interactions may influence CHD.

Several issues need to be addressed in future studies. Important information is lacking regarding the nature and extent of the association between work-related stress and CHD, including the duration, intensity, and frequency of exposure that is necessary or sufficient for CHD. Reliable measures of blood pressure and physiologic stress indices in the work setting and ascertaining the development and progression of CHD are needed to obtain greater precision in specifying the link between occupational stress and CHD. Given the multifactorial etiologic nature of CHD, investigations should focus on the interrelationship of stress with other known risk factors for CHD in affecting abnormalities in cardiovascular structure and function (for example, heart rate and rhythm, cardiac output, blood platelet aggregation, degree and location of coronary occlusion, and so on) in healthy workers and in those with existing CHD. Finally, the work setting should be considered as a socialization influence in which peer pressure, social support, and constructive competition can be employed in the service of changing life-style behaviors in CHD risk-reducing directions.

CONCLUSIONS

In citing these examples of how psychosocial factors may impact the development of CHD, it is clear that such factors are not unitary in nature but rather multifactorial in their own right. Psychosocial factors therefore must be addressed at different levels of function, and in combination with other putative risk factors, to fully apprehend the complex architecture of the "biobehavioral" chronic disease model. Thus, one must consider age, sex, diet, exercise and smoking patterns, obesity, and family history, among other factors, as potential covariants with psychosocial factors at the individual, interpersonal, and environmental levels. Although 20 years ago such a statement would have been untestable, today's modern technology (bioinstrumentation and data acquisition and storage and analysis capabilities) provides the necessary tools to address multifactorial issues empirically at levels of extraordinary complexity. Until we *allow* ourselves to consider such multifactorial, multilevel models, however, we shall continue to be frustrated by the continuing large proportion of unexplained variance associated with the development of CHD.

REFERENCES

1. Fothergill, J: Complete collection of the medical and philosophical works. London, 1781.
2. Trousseau, A: Clinical medicine. Philadelphia, 1882.
3. Wardrop, J: Diseases of the heart. London, 1851.

4. Osler, W: Lectures on angina pectoris and allied states. Appleton, New York, 1892.

5. Friedman, M and Rosenman, RH: Type A behavior and your heart. Alfred A. Knopf, New York, 1974.

6. Rosenman, RH and Friedman, M: Neurogenic factors in pathogenesis of coronary heart disease. Med Clin N Am 58:269, 1974.

7. Friedman, M and Rosenman, RH: Association of a specific overt behavior pattern with increases in blood cholesterol, blood clotting time, incidence of arcus senilis and clinical coronary artery disease. JAMA 169:1286, 1959.

8. Rosenman, RH and Friedman, M: Association of a specific overt behavior pattern in females with blood and cardiovascular findings. Circulation 24:1173, 1961.

9. Rosenman, RH, Brand, RJ, Jenkins, CD, et al: Coronary heart disease in the Western Collaborative Group study: Final follow-up experience of 8½ years. JAMA 233:872, 1975.

10. French-Belgian Collaborative Group: Ischemic heart disease and psychological patterns: Prevalence and incidence studies, in Belgium and France. Adv Cardiol 29:25, 1982.

11. Haynes, SG, Feinleib, M, and Kannel, WB: The relationship of psychosocial factors to coronary heart disease in the Framingham Study, III: Eight-year incidence of coronary heart disease. Am J Epidemiol 111:37, 1980.

12. Blumenthal, JA, Williams, RB, Kong, Y, et al: Type A behavior pattern and coronary atherosclerosis. Circulation, 58:634, 1978.

13. Frank, KA, Heller, SS, Kornfeld, DS, et al: Type A behavior pattern and coronary angiographic findings. JAMA 240:761, 1978.

14. Friedman, M, Rosenman, RH, Strauss, R, et al: The relationship of behavior pattern to the state of the coronary vasculature: A study of 51 autopsy subjects. Am J Med 44:525, 1968.

15. Williams, RB, Haney, TL, Lee, KL, et al: Type A behavior hostility and coronary atherosclerosis: Psychosom Med 42:539, 1980.

16. Cooper, T, Detre, T, and Wiess, SM: Coronary-prone behavior and coronary heart disease: A critical review. Circulation 63:1199, 1981.

17. Contrada, RJ and Krantz, DS: Stress, reactivity and Type A behavior: Current status and future directions. Ann Behav Med 10(2):64, 1988.

18. Houston, BK: Psychological variables and cardiovascular and neuroendocrine reactivity. In Matthews, K, et al (eds): Handbook of Stress Reactivity and Cardiovascular Disease. John Wiley and Sons, New York, 1986.

19. Manuck, SB and Krantz, DS: Psychophysiologic reactivity in coronary heart disease and essential hypertension. In Matthews, K, et al (eds): Handbook of Stress Reactivity and Cardiovascular Disease. John Wiley and Sons, New York, 1986.

20. Shekelle, RB, Hulley, S, Neaton, J, et al: The MRFIT behavior pattern study: II. Type A behavior pattern and incidence of coronary heart disease. Am J Epidemiol 122:559, 1985.

21. Dembroski, TM and MacDougall, JM: Beyond global Type A: Relationships of paralinguistic attributes, hostility, and anger-in to coronary heart disease. In Field, T, McAbe, P, and Schneiderman, N: Stress and Coping. Erlbaum, Hillsdale, NJ, 1985.

22. Dembroski, TM, MacDougall, JM, Williams, RB, et al: Components to Type A, hostility and anger-in: Relationship to angiographic findings. Psychosom Med 47:219, 1985.

23. Dimsdale, JE, Hackett, TP, and Hutter, AM: Type A behavior and angiographic findings. J Psychosom Res 23:273, 1979.

24. Ragland, DR and Brand, RJ: Type A behavior and mortality from coronary heart disease. N Engl J Med 318(2):65, 1988.

25. The MRFIT Research Group: The MRFIT behavior pattern study I: Study design procedures, and reproducibility of behavior pattern judgments. J Chron Dis 32:293, 1979.

26. Williams, RB, et al: Type A behavior and angiographically documented coronary atherosclerosis in a sample of 2,289 patients. Psychosom Med 50:139, 1988.

27. Hecker, M, Chesney, MA, Black, GW, et al: Coronary-prone behaviors in the Western collaborative Group Study. Psychosom Med 50:153, 1988.

28. MacDougall, JM, Dembrowski, TM, Dimsdale, JE, et al: Components of Type A hostility, and anger-in: Further relationships to angiographic findings. Health Psychol 4:137, 1985.

29. Matthews, KA, Glass, DC, Rosenman, RH, et al: Competitive drive, pattern A, and coronary heart disease: A further analysis of some data from the Western Collaborative Group. Chron Dis 30:489, 1977.

30. Dembroski, TM: Components of hostility as predictors of sudden death and myocardial infarction in the Multiple Risk Factor Intervention Trial. Psychol Med, in press.

31. Barefoot, JC, Dahlstrom, WG, and Williams, RB: Hostility, CHD incidence and total mortality: A 25-year follow-up study of 255 physicians. Psychosom Med 43:59, 1983.
32. Shekelle, RB, Gale, M, Ostfeld, AM, et al: Hostility, risk of coronary disease, and mortality. Psychosom Med 45:219, 1983.
33. Dembroski, TM, MacDougall, JM, Shields, JL, et al: Components of the Type A coronary prone behavior pattern and cardiovascular responses to psychomotor performance challenge. J Behav Med 1:159, 1978.
34. MacDougall, JM, Dembroski, TM, and Krantz, DS: Effects of types of challenge on pressor and heart rate response in Type A and B women. Psychophysiology 18:1, 1981.
35. Friedman, M: Alteration of type A behavior and its effect on cardiac recurrences in post-myocardial infarction patients: Summary results of the Recurrent Coronary Prevention Project. Am Heart J 112(4):653, 1986.
36. Berkman, LF: The relationship of social networks and social support to morbidity and mortality. In Cohen, S and Syme, L (eds): Social Support and Health. Academic Press, New York, 1985.
37. Broadhead, WE, Kaplan, BH, James, SA, et al: The epidemiologic evidence for a relationship between social support and health. Am J Epidemiol 117:521, 1983.
38. Cohen, S and Syme, L (eds): Social Support and Health. Academic Press, New York, 1985.
39. Cohen, S: Psychosocial models of the role of social support in the etiology of physical disease. Health Psychol 7(3):269, 1988.
40. House, JS, Landis, KR, and Umberson, D: Social relationships and health. Science 241:540, 1988.
41. Orth-Gomer, K: International epidemiological evidence for a relationship between social support and cardiovascular disease. In Shumaker, SA and Czajkowski, SM (eds): Social Support and Cardiovascular Disease. Plenum Press, New York, (in press).
42. Hazuda, HP: A critical evaluation of U.S. epidemiologic evidence, including a special consideration of ethnic differences. In Shumaker, SA and Czajkowski, SM (eds): Social Support and Cardiovascular Disease. Plenum Press, New York. (In press.)
43. Durkheim, E: Suicide: A study in sociology. (Simpson, G [ed] and Spaulding, JA and Simpson, G [trans].) Glencoe: The Free Press, 1951. (Original work published 1897.)
44. Cassel, J: An epidemiological perspective of psychosocial factors in disease etiology. Am J Pub Health 64:1040, 1974.
45. Shumaker, SA and Brownell, A: Toward a theory of social support: Closing conceptual gaps. J Soc Iss 40(4):11, 1984.
46. Brownell, A and Shumaker, SA: Social support: An introduction to a complex phenomenon. J Soc Iss 40(4):1, 1984.
47. Cohen, S, Kaplan, JR, and Manuck, SB: Social support and coronary heart disease: Underlying psychologic and biologic mechanisms. In Shumaker, SA and Czajkowski, SM (eds): Social Support and Cardiovascular Disease. Plenum Press, New York. (In press.)
48. Cohen, S and Wills, TA: Stress, social support, and the buffering hypothesis. Psychol Bull 98:310, 1985.
49. Sarason, I and Sarason, B: The assessment of social support. In Shumaker, SA and Czajkowski, SM (eds): Social Support and Cardiovascular Disease. Plenum Press, New York. (In press.)
50. Berkman, LF and Syme, SL: Social networks, host resistance, and mortality: A nine-year follow-up study of Alameda County residents. Am J Epidemiol 109:186, 1979.
51. House, JS, Robbins, C and Metzner, H: The association of social relationships and activities with mortality: Prospective evidence from the Tecumseh Community Health Study. Am J Epidemiol 116:123, 1982.
52. Orth-Gomer, K and Johnson, JV: Social network interaction and mortality. J Chron Dis 40:949, 1987.
53. Ruberman, W, et al: Psychosocial influences on mortality after myocardial infarction. N Engl J Med 311:552, 1984.
54. Blazer, DG: Social support and mortality in an elderly community population. Am J Epidemiol 115:684, 1982.
55. Haynes, S and Feinleib, M: Women, work and coronary heart disease: Prospective findings from the Framingham Heart Study. Am J Pub Health 70:133, 1980.
56. Marmot, MG: Acculturation and coronary heart disease in Japanese Americans. Ph.D. Dissertation. University of California, Berkeley, CA, 1975.
57. Welin, L, et al: Prospective study of social influences on mortality. Lancet, 1:915, 1985.
58. Puska, P: The North Karelia Project. Regional Office for Europe World Health Organization, Copenhagen, 1981.

59. Orth-Gomer, K, Rosengren, A, Unden, AL, et al: Social environmental factors and cardiovascular risk in 50-year old men in Gothenburg. Paper given at the 96th Annual Meeting of the Swedish Medical Association.

60. Orth-Gomer, K, Unden, AL, and Edwards, ME: Social isolation and mortality in ischemic heart disease. Acta Med Scand.

61. Seeman, TE and Syme, SL: Social networks and coronary artery disease: A comparison of the structure and function of social relations as predictors of disease. Psychosom Med 49(4):341, 1987.

62. Cohen, S and Matthews, KA: Editorial: Social support, type A behavior and coronary artery disease. Psychosom Med 49:325, 1987.

63. Whalen, CK and Kliewer, W: Social influences on the development of cardiovascular risk during childhood and adolescence. In Shumaker, SA and Czajkowski, SM (eds): Social Support and Cardiovascular Disease. Plenum Press, New York, (in press).

64. Rose, G and Marmot, M: Social class and coronary heart disease. Br Heart J 45:13, 1981.

65. Liu, K, Lucila, B, Cedres, M, et al: Relationship of education to major risk factors and death from cardiovascular diseases and all causes. Circulation 66(6):1308, 1982.

66. Hinkle, LE, Thaler, HT, Merke, D, et al: The risk for arrhythmic death in a sample of men followed for 20 years. Am J Epidemiol 127(3):500, 1988.

67. Henry, JP and Stephens, PM: Stress, Health and the Social Environment. Springer-Verlag, New York, 1977.

68. Frankenhaeuser, M: Man in technological society: Stress, adaptation and tolerance limits. Department of Psychology Research Report # 26. University of Stockholm, Stockholm, 1974.

69. Folkow, B: Psychosocial and central nervous influences in primary hypertension. Circulation (Suppl I) 76:I-19, 1987.

70. Manuck, SB, Kaplan, JR, and Matthews, KA: Behavioral antecedents of coronary heart disease and atherosclerosis. Arteriosclerosis 6:2, 1986.

71. Mudge, GH, et al: Reflex increase in coronary vascular resistance in patients with ischemic heart disease. N Engl J Med 295:1333, 1976.

72. Verrier, RL: Mechanisms of behaviorally induced arrhythmias. Circulation (Suppl I) 76:I-48, 1987.

73. Verrier, RL and Lown, B: Experimental studies of psychophysiological factors in sudden cardiac death. Acta Med Scand (Suppl) 660:57, 1982.

74. Shepard, JT and Vanhoutte, PM: Spasm of the coronary arteries: Causes and consequences (the scientist's viewpoint). Mayo Clin Proc 60:33, 1985.

75. Rozansky, A, Bairey, N, Krantz, DS, et al: Mental stress and the induction of silent myocardial ischemia in patients with coronary disease. N Engl J Med 318:1005, 1988.

76. Snow, J: On the mode of communication of cholera, in Snow on Cholera. The Commonwealth Fund, New York, 1936.

77. Brod, J: Haemodynamic basis of acute pressor reactions and hypertension. Br Heart J 25:227, 1963.

78. Surwit, RS, Williams, R, and Shapiro, D: Behavioral approaches to cardiovascular disease. Academic Press, New York, 1982.

79. Frankenhaeuser, M and Patkai, D: Interindividual differences in catecholamine excretion during stress. Scand J Psychol 6:117, 1965.

80. Frankenhaeuser, M and Rissler, A: Catecholamine output during relaxation and anticipation. Percept Mot Skills 30:745, 1970.

81. Frankenhaeuser, M: Experimental approaches to the study of human behavior as related to neuroendocrine functions. In Levi, L (ed): Society, Stress and Disease. Oxford University Press, Oxford, 1971.

82. Frankenhaeuser, M and Gardell, B: Overload and underload in working life: Outline of a multidisciplinary approach. J Human Stress 2(3):35, 1976.

83. Lundberg, U and Frankenhaeuser, M: Pituitary-adrenal and sympathetic-adrenal correlates of distress and effort. J Psychosom Res 24:125, 1980.

84. Bohlin, G, Eliasson, K, Hjemdahl, P, et al: Pace variation and control of work as related to cardiovascular, neuroendocrine, and subjective responses. Biol Psychol 23:247, 1986.

85. Frankenhaeuser, M and Johansson, G: Task demand as reflected in catecholamine excretion and heart rate. J Hum Stress 2(3):15, 1976.

86. Frankenhaeuser, M: Behavior and circulating catecholamines. Brain Res 31:142, 1971.

87. Frankenhaeuser, M: Experimental approaches to the study of catecholamines and emotion. In Levi, L (ed): Emotions: Their Parameters and Measurement. Raven Press, New York, 1975.

88. Johansson, G and Frankenhaeuser, M: Temporal factors in sympatho-adrenomedullary activity following acute behavioral activation. Biol Psychol 1:63, 1973.
89. Akerstedt, T, Gillberg, M, Hjemdahl, P, et al: Comparison of urinary and plasma catecholamine responses to mental stress. Acta Physiol Scand 117:19, 1983.
90. Henry, JP: Coronary heart disease and arousal of the adrenal cortical axis. In Dembroski, TM, Schmidt, TH, and Blumchen, G (eds): Biobehavioral Bases of Coronary Heart Disease. S. Karger, Basel, 1983.
91. Atterhog, JH and Hjemdahl, P: Sympathoadrenal and cardiovascular responses to mental stress, isometric handgrip, and cold pressor test in asymptomatic young men with primary T-wave abnormalities in the electrocardiogram. Br Heart J 46:311, 1981.
92. Ward, MM, Mefford, IN, Parker, SD, et al: Epinephrine and norepinephrine responses in continuously collected human plasma to a series of stressors. Psychosom Med 45:471, 1983.
93. Frankenhaeuser, M: The psychoendocrine response to challenge. In Dembroski, TM, Schmidt, TH, and Blumchen, G (eds): Biobehavioral Bases of Coronary Heart Disease. S. Karger, Basel, 1983.
94. Elliott, R, Bankart, B, and Light, T: Differences in the motivational significance of heart rate and palmar conductance: Two tests of a hypothesis. J Pers Soc Psychol 14:166, 1970.
95. Russek, HL and Zohman, BL: Relative significance of heredity, diet and occupational stress in coronary heart disease of young adults. Am J Science 235:266, 1958.
96. Buell, P and Breslow, L: Mortality from coronary heart disease in California men who work long hours. J Chron Dis 11(6):615, 1960.
97. House, JS, et al: Occupational stress and health among factory workers. J Health Soc Behav 20:139, 1979.
98. Van Dijkhuizen, N and Reiche, H: Psychosocial stress in industry: A heartache for middle management? Psychother Psychosom 34:124, 1980.
99. Markowe, HL, Marmot, MG, Shipley, M, et al: Fibrinogen: A possible link between social class and coronary heart disease. Br Med J 291:1312, 1985.
100. Karasek, R, Baker, D, Marxer, F, et al: Job decision latitude, job demands, and cardiovascular diseases: A prospective study of Swedish men. Am J Pub Health 71:694, 1981.
101. Johnson, JV: The impact of workplace social support job demands and work control upon cardiovascular disease in Sweden. Department of Psychology Report No. 1, University of Stockholm, Stockholm, 1986.
102. Alfredsson, L, Karasek, R, and Theorell, T: Myocardial infarction risk and psychosocial work environment characteristics: An analysis of the male Swedish work force. Soc Sci Med 16:463, 1985.
103. Karasek, R, Triantis, K, and Chaudhry, S: Coworker and supervisor support as moderators of associations between task characteristics and mental strain. J Occup Behav 3:181, 1982.
104. LaCroix, A and Haynes, S: Gender differences in the health effects of workplace roles. In Barnett, RC, Biener, L, and Baruch, G (eds): Gender and Stress. Free Press, New York, 1987.
105. Karasek, R, Theorell, T, Schwartz, J, et al: Job characteristics in relation to the prevalence of myocardial infarction in the US Health Examination Survey (HES) and the Health and Nutrition Examination Survey (HANES). Am J Pub Health 78:910, 1988.

CHAPTER 10

Nutritional Treatment of Hyperlipidemia and Obesity

Morton H. Maxwell, M.D.
David Heber, M.D., Ph.D.

A number of recent events, including the publication of the Lipid Research Clinics Coronary Primary Prevention Trial in 1984,[1] the awarding of the Nobel Prize in 1985 to Brown and Goldstein for their work on the receptor-mediated control of cholesterol synthesis,[2] and the availability for clinical use in 1987 of a new class of cholesterol synthesis inhibitors[3] have increased the awareness of patients and their doctors to the problem of controlling blood lipid levels.

One of the commonest secondary causes of hyperlipidemia is excess body fat or obesity.[4,5] Obesity is an independent risk factor for coronary heart disease (CHD) when body weight is greater than 130 percent of ideal levels. However, elevations of blood lipids, including cholesterol, can occur with much smaller amounts of excess fat. Attention directed at the achievement of ideal or desirable body weight is a cornerstone of the dietary treatment of hyperlipidemia.[6]

There are many other factors in the diet, including total fat content, total calories, fiber, and amounts of specific classes of fat, such as polyunsaturated fat, that affect blood lipids. When nutritional counseling is directed at developing new food choices that maximize those elements promoting lower lipid levels, heightened awareness of food choices often leads to modest weight changes even in patients who do not have obvious obesity.

In this chapter, the general recommendations for dietary treatment of hypercholesterolemia outlined by the National Cholesterol Education Program (NCEP) of the National Heart, Lung, and Blood Institute (NHLBI)[7] are reviewed and the role of dietary fiber is specifically discussed in detail. Additionally, the available evidence on the beneficial effects of weight loss on serum cholesterol levels is reviewed.

NUTRITIONAL TREATMENT OF HYPERLIPIDEMIA

The nutritional management of patients with hyperlipidemia has been outlined carefully as the NCEP Step 1 and Step 2 diets by the NHLBI (Table 10-1).

Table 10–1. National Cholesterol Education Program
Diets for Treatment of Hypercholesterolemia

Nutrient	Step 1 Diet	Step 2 Diet
Total fat	Less than 30%	Less than 30%
Total calories	To achieve and maintain desirable weight	
Saturated fat	Less than 10%	Less than 7%
Polyunsaturated fat	Up to 10%	Up to 10%
Monounsaturated fat	10–15%	10–15%
Carbohydrates	50–60%	50–60%
Protein	10–20%	10–20%
Cholesterol	<300 mg/day	<200 mg/day

This program emphasizes the use of dietary change rather than drugs whenever possible to lower cholesterol levels. The diagnosis of hypercholesterolemia and the recommendation of the Step 1 diet are the responsibility of the primary physician counseling the patient. For those patients who do not respond to simple diet guidelines after a 6-month period, referral to a registered dietitian for instruction in the Step 2 diet or further education and counseling in implementing the Step 1 diet is indicated. It must be emphasized that dietary adherence can be accomplished only with appropriate follow-up, and, when this is done, serum lipids can be lowered to desirable levels in the majority of patients.

CLASSIFICATIONS OF HYPERLIPIDEMIA

For the purpose of the dietary treatment of hyperlipidemias, one can classify hyperlipidemias simply into the following three types: (1) elevated cholesterol with normal triglyceride, (2) elevated cholesterol and triglyceride, and (3) elevated triglyceride with normal cholesterol. Only the first two types of hyperlipidemia are considered risk factors for CHD based on elevated serum cholesterol levels.

All types of hyperlipidemia are influenced by genetic and environmental factors. In the past, hyperlipidemias have been classified as primary (genetic) or secondary (environmental or due to an associated condition). Obesity is the most common environmental factor, but other common conditions include diabetes mellitus; hypothyroidism; nephrotic syndrome; obstructive liver disease; and use of certain drugs, including progestins and anabolic androgens. The recognition and treatment of these conditions is an important aspect of the clinical evaluation of hyperlipidemia, which should be done prior to recommending dietary therapy.

In addition to the aforementioned broad classifications, the degree of elevation in serum cholesterol can be used to subdivide patients according to their risk of developing CHD. Individuals with blood levels >240 mg/dl (corresponding to low-density lipoprotein (LDL) cholesterol level >160 mg/dl) are classified as high risk. Individuals with blood cholesterol levels between 200 mg/dl and 240 mg/dl (corresponding to LDL cholesterol levels between 130 mg/dl and 160 mg/dl) are classified as borderline high cholesterol. Individuals with cholesterol levels below 200 mg/dl are classified as having desirable blood cholesterol levels. The rationale for this graded classification is based on the observations of CHD risk in 361,662 men ages 35 to 57 over an average follow-up of 6 years in the Multiple Risk Factor Intervention Trial.[8] This large-scale study demonstrated a continuous increase in

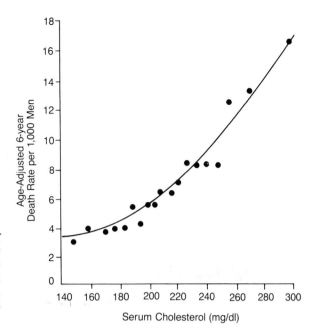

Figure 10-1. Relationship of serum cholesterol to coronary heart disease death rate in 361,662 men 35–57 years of age during an average follow-up of six years. Each point represents the median value for 5% of the population.[8]

the risk for CHD death in men with blood cholesterol levels greater than 180 mg/dl (Fig. 10–1). Although the slope of the line defining increased risk with increased blood cholesterol rises more steeply above 240 mg/dl, from a public health point of view many more individuals with CHD in the United States have blood cholesterol levels within the borderline range.[7]

Not all experts agree with the consensus recommendations of the NCEP regarding intervention in individuals with borderline high cholesterol (200 to 239 mg/dl). Studies of patients with coronary artery disease have revealed significant subpopulations with normal cholesterol levels but abnormalities of apoprotein B composition.[9] The large variation in LDL cholesterol levels observed in populations consuming similar diets cannot be accounted for by diet but seems to be genetically determined. The incidence of familial hyperlipidemias is so low that they cannot account for this large variation. Recently, commonly occurring polymorphisms of apoprotein E have been associated with hypercholesterolemia and have been estimated to account for about 7 percent of the observed variation in cholesterol levels of populations consuming similar diets.[10] It is likely that in the future many polymorphisms of the apoprotein B-100 molecule, which is made up of 4536 amino acids, will be found to account for some of the large variation in cholesterol levels in subpopulations. Forty-three polymorphisms of apo B-100 have been identified to date, including some associated with increased serum LDL cholesterol levels. Recently, a variation of the apo B-100 gene not affecting the coding region of the gene has been associated with increased cholesterol levels.[11]

The majority of individuals with hypercholesterolemia have multifactorial hypercholesterolemia. The term *multifactorial* is used to denote the polygenic inheritance of this trait and the fact that its expression is affected by environmental factors such as diet.[12] Despite our current lack of understanding of multifactorial hypercholesterolemia, it has been estimated that in three fourths of patients with cholesterol levels above 240 mg/dl, serum cholesterol can be lowered to a desirable range with dietary modifications alone.

The NCEP recommends institution of dietary therapy in all individuals with cholesterol levels above 240 mg/dl. In individuals with borderline cholesterol (200 to 239 mg/dl), dietary intervention is recommended only under two circumstances: first, if they have specific CHD defined by history of a prior myocardial infarction or active anginal symptoms, or second, if they have two of the following risk factors:

1. Male gender
2. Family history of premature CHD
3. Cigarette smoking
4. Hypertension
5. Low high-density lipoprotein (HDL) cholesterol (<35 mg/dl)
6. Diabetes mellitus
7. Definite cerebrovascular accident or peripheral vascular disease
8. Severe obesity (>30 percent above ideal weight)

ELEMENTS OF THE DIET AFFECTING CHOLESTEROL

The recommended foods are listed in Table 10–2 according to food group. The recommendations are simple and can be implemented by the general population without impairing the nutritional value of the diet. There are four major elements of the diet that can affect the level of serum cholesterol to varying degrees in different individuals.

Total Fat and Calories

First, total fat and calories are directly related to serum cholesterol by their effects on increasing body fat. Increased body fat in susceptible individuals affects insulin action and metabolism and results in increased very low-density lipoprotein (VLDL) synthesis in the liver, leading to elevated serum cholesterol and triglycerides.[5]

Dietary Fat Quality

Second, dietary fat quality can affect serum cholesterol. If total fat and calories are kept constant but the type of fat is varied from saturated fats (largely derived from meats, dairy products, and selected vegetable sources) to polyunsaturated fats (largely derived from vegetable sources), serum cholesterol levels will decrease.[13] Monounsaturated fats derived from olive oil or avocados have no effect on LDL cholesterol levels but have been shown to increase HDL cholesterol in some studies.[14] A special group of polyunsaturated fats derived from cold-water fish, the so-called n–3 fatty acids have been shown to decrease triglyceride levels in most studies and to decrease cholesterol slightly in some individuals with increased VLDL cholesterol levels.[15] However, although the fish oils have potentially important anti-inflammatory and antithrombotic effects, which operate by different mechanisms, they have no beneficial effects on LDL cholesterol levels.[16]

Dietary Cholesterol

Third, dietary cholesterol, separate from the effects of dietary fats, has been said to affect serum cholesterol levels markedly. In population studies, there often

Table 10–2. Food Choices in the Step 1 Diet

<table>
<tr><td colspan="2" align="center">Fish, Fowl, and Meats</td></tr>
<tr><td>Choose</td><td>Decrease</td></tr>
<tr><td>Fish, poultry with no skin</td><td>Fatty meats, cold cuts</td></tr>
<tr><td>Lean cuts of meat, shellfish</td><td>Organ meats, bacon, roe</td></tr>
<tr><td colspan="2" align="center">Dairy Products</td></tr>
<tr><td>Choose</td><td>Decrease</td></tr>
<tr><td>Skim or 1% milk</td><td>Whole milk</td></tr>
<tr><td>Nonfat or low-fat yogurt</td><td>Evaporated, condensed, 2% milk, nondairy creamers</td></tr>
<tr><td>Low-fat cottage cheese</td><td>Whipped toppings</td></tr>
<tr><td>Low-fat cheeses (2–6 gm/oz)</td><td>Sour cream, cream cheese</td></tr>
<tr><td>Sherbet, sorbet</td><td>Ice cream</td></tr>
<tr><td colspan="2" align="center">Eggs</td></tr>
<tr><td>Choose</td><td>Decrease</td></tr>
<tr><td>Egg whites (2 whites for 1 egg)</td><td>Egg yolks</td></tr>
<tr><td>Cholesterol-free egg substitutes</td><td></td></tr>
<tr><td colspan="2" align="center">Fruits and Vegetables</td></tr>
<tr><td>Choose</td><td>Decrease</td></tr>
<tr><td>Fresh, frozen, canned, dried fruits and vegetables</td><td>Creamed vegetables or sauces as topping</td></tr>
<tr><td colspan="2" align="center">Breads and Cereals</td></tr>
<tr><td>Choose</td><td>Decrease</td></tr>
<tr><td>Homemade baked goods using oils sparingly</td><td>Commercial baked goods</td></tr>
<tr><td></td><td>Pies, cookies, doughnuts</td></tr>
<tr><td></td><td>Crackers, croissants</td></tr>
<tr><td>Rice, pasta</td><td>Egg noodles</td></tr>
<tr><td>Whole-grain breads and cereals</td><td>Breads in which eggs are a major ingredient</td></tr>
<tr><td colspan="2" align="center">Fats and Oils</td></tr>
<tr><td>Choose</td><td>Decrease</td></tr>
<tr><td>Baking cocoa</td><td>Chocolate</td></tr>
<tr><td>Unsaturated oils</td><td>Butter, coconut, bacon fat</td></tr>
<tr><td>Margarine or shortening</td><td></td></tr>
<tr><td>Diet margarine</td><td></td></tr>
<tr><td>Mayonnaise made with unsaturated oils</td><td>Dressings made with egg yolk</td></tr>
<tr><td>Low-fat dressings</td><td></td></tr>
<tr><td>Seeds and nuts</td><td>Coconut</td></tr>
</table>

appear to be direct statistical correlations between dietary cholesterol intake and observed levels of serum cholesterol.[17] These observations are likely to be attributable to increased dietary fat intake because in most countries dietary cholesterol is usually eaten in proportion to sources of saturated fat in the diet. In fact, the most concentrated sources of cholesterol in the diet are eggs and organ meats. The majority of studies in which the intake of these concentrated sources is increased without increasing dietary fat intake significantly have demonstrated little effect on serum cholesterol.[18,19]

Dietary cholesterol is taken up from the gut, where it is absorbed from micelles made up of bile acids and other emulsifying components. Together with chylomicron remnants, this dietary cholesterol then enters hepatocytes, where it can inhibit synthesis both of cholesterol and of LDL receptors. Because the clearance of LDL cholesterol from the bloodstream depends on the activity of the hepatic LDL receptors, down-regulation of these receptors will tend to elevate serum cholesterol. On the other hand, when intracellular cholesterol is depleted, the receptors are up-regulated within several hours both in cultured cells and in the liver in vivo.[20] The extent of down-regulation of the hepatic LDL receptors by dietary cholesterol then depends on the ability of the hepatocyte to excrete intracellular cholesterol into the enterohepatic circulation as bile acids.

There are at least five ways in which the body can adapt to increased dietary cholesterol to maintain serum cholesterol constant. First, it is possible to increase bile acid synthesis and excretion, as discussed previously. Second, it is possible to decrease intracellular cholesterol synthesis. This was recently documented in a clinical study of cholesterol homeostasis by McNamara and associates,[21] in which 52 of 75 healthy volunteers maintained normal blood cholesterol levels when dietary cholesterol was increased from 250 mg/day to 800 mg/day. Sixty-one percent of these individuals decreased sterol synthesis in monocytes by greater than 15 percent. Third, it is possible to decrease the fractional absorption of cholesterol from the gut. In the aforementioned study, both compensators and noncompensators decreased their fractional absorption of cholesterol in response to increased dietary cholesterol. Fourth, it is possible to increase excretion of cholesterol as fecal neutral steroids.[22] Finally, it is possible to expand extrahepatic tissue stores of cholesterol.[23]

The issue of heterogeneity of cholesterol homeostasis in individuals is an exciting area for investigation. The differences between individuals in their ability to compensate for a dietary cholesterol load are poorly understood. Whether the noncompensator is also genetically the same individual predisposed to CHD has not been determined. Historically there has been a great deal of controversy on the issue of whether eggs and organ meats can elevate cholesterol.[21] It is now clear that this question can only be answered in individuals by studying them to determine whether they are compensators or noncompensators. From a public health point of view, the current consensus is that decreasing egg and organ meat consumption will help a significant subgroup of the population in the United States without harming the majority.[7]

Dietary Fiber

The Step 1 diet specifies changes in total fat, calories, types of fat, and cholesterol but does not specifically recommend changes in dietary fiber intake. From a practical standpoint, inasmuch as the diet recommends increasing intake of fruits and vegetables, it will result in increased fiber intake. Nonetheless, it should be recognized that dietary fiber is a major determinant of serum cholesterol levels in man.

Dietary fibers are plant substances that are resistant to digestion and include both nonstarch polysaccharides and lignin. They can be divided into two broad classes: soluble fiber and insoluble fiber.[24]

Soluble fibers are soluble in water and are generally digestible. They include gums, pectins, mucilages, and hemicelluloses. These fibers tend to lower cholesterol when their intake is increased.

Insoluble fibers, on the other hand, are not digestible and do not lower cholesterol levels. These fibers include cellulose, lignin, and some hemicellulose. They benefit bowel function by shortening intestinal transit time, and are used in the treatment of irritable bowel syndrome and constipation. These fibers are those found primarily in bran cereals, and they increase stool bulk by virtue of the remaining residue of undigested fibers.

The soluble fibers, by contrast, are fermented in the large bowel and increase stool bulk by an increase in bacterial mass. Increased intake of these soluble fibers from such sources as oat bran, corn bran, apples, and beans will tend to decrease cholesterol levels from 5 to 15 percent. The long-term safety and effectiveness of fiber supplements such as guar, Metamucil, and konjak are not proven, but represent potential for increasing fiber intake as an adjunct to dietary changes.

OBESITY AND HYPERCHOLESTEROLEMIA

When the aforementioned changes have been instituted in free-living adults, a significant amount of weight loss usually has been observed. As total fat is decreased, the nutrient density of foods decreases, and the same amount of food yields fewer calories per bite. Whether weight loss per se or the decrease in saturated fat and cholesterol intake results in a decrease in serum cholesterol has been debated.[26] It is clear from several large studies that decreases in serum cholesterol accompany weight loss achieved through the use of formula diets or very low calorie diets. Anderson and co-workers[27] measured serum cholesterol biweekly in 85 obese subjects participating in a very low-calorie diet program in which only 520 calories per day were allowed. Serum cholesterol values decreased rapidly, reaching a nadir at 4 to 6 weeks and increasing toward control values as weight loss continued. The reason for the increase in cholesterol values as weight loss progressed is not well understood. It has been proposed that cholesterol is mobilized from adipose stores, but this has not been proved.

The long-term effects of weight loss in a massively obese population also have been documented. Funfar and colleagues[28] studied 88 obese individuals at 1 to 5 years after joining a weight-reduction program. At baseline, significant correlations were found between total body fat (body mass index) and serum cholesterol as well as between upper body fat (waist-to-hip ratio) and serum cholesterol. At follow-up, serum cholesterol, triglyceride, and LDL cholesterol all decreased significantly. There was no significant change in HDL cholesterol. Although there was no correlation between the change in body weight or total body fat with the decrease in serum cholesterol, there was a statistically significant correlation between serum cholesterol changes and the change in upper body fat measured by a decrease in waist to hip ratio. It appears that weight loss via formula diets has enduring effects on serum cholesterol and that these effects may be due to changes in fat distribution.

These data obtained on obese patients have implications for the nonobese individual with increased upper body fat and elevated or borderline serum cholesterol. Such individuals have been called "metabolically obese," inasmuch as the loss of only 10 or 20 pounds can result in dramatic and sustained changes in serum cholesterol levels.[29] The separate effects of weight loss and dietary composition in the mildly or obviously overweight patient are of little practical significance because these two problems would be addressed clinically in any case. Obesity is recognized both as an independent risk factor for CHD and as a secondary cause of hypercholesterolemia. Weight loss in the obese individual is indicated as part of the initial management of hyperlipidemia, and once desired weight is achieved, the Step 1 diet can be instituted as a maintenance regimen for the optimization of serum lipids and body weight.

REFERENCES

1. Lipid Research Clinics Program: The Lipid Research Clinics Coronary Primary Prevention Trial results: I. Reduction in incidence of coronary heart disease. JAMA 251:351, 1984.

2. Brown, MS and Goldstein, JL: Lipoprotein receptors in the liver: Control signals for plasma cholesterol traffic. J Clin Invest 72:743, 1983.

3. Illingworth, DR and Sexton, GJ: Hypocholesterolemic effects of mevinolin in patients with heterozygous hypercholesterolemia. J Clin Invest 74:1194, 1984.

4. Egusa, G, Beltz, WF, and Grundy, SM: Influence of obesity on the metabolism of apolipoprotein B in humans. J Clin Invest 76:596, 1985.

5. Kesaniemi, YA and Grundy, SM: Increased low density lipoprotein production associated with obesity. Arteriosclerosis 3:170, 1983.

6. Lowering blood cholesterol to prevent heart disease. Consensus Conference. JAMA 253:2080, 1985.

7. Report of the Expert Panel on Detection, Evaluation, and Treatment of High Blood Cholesterol in Adults. NIH Publication No. 88-2925, 1988.

8. Multiple Risk Factor Intervention Trial Group: Risk factor changes in morbidity results. JAMA 248:1465, 1982.

9. Sniderman, A, Shapiro, S, and Marpole, D: Association of coronary arteriosclerosis with hyperapobetalipoproteinemia (increased protein but normal cholesterol levels in human plasma low density lipoprotein). Proc Nat Acad Sci USA 77:604, 1980.

10. Davignon, J, Gregg, RE, and Sing, CF: Apolipoprotein E polymorphism and atherosclerosis. Arteriosclerosis 7:526a, 1988.

11. Talmud, PJ, et al: Apolipoprotein B gene variants are involved in the determination of serum cholesterol levels: A study in normo- and hyperlipidemic individuals. Atherosclerosis 67:81, 1987.

12. Muench, KH: Genetic Medicine. Elsevier, New York, 1988.

13. Mattson, FH and Grundy, SM: Comparison of saturated, monounsaturated, and polyunsaturated fatty acids on plasma lipids and lipoproteins. J Lipid Res 26:194, 1985.

14. Grundy, SM: Comparison of monounsaturated fatty acids and carbohydrates for plasma cholesterol lowering. N Engl J Med 314:745, 1986.

15. Phillipson, RE, Rothrock, DW, and Connor, WE: Reduction of plasma lipids, lipoproteins, and apoproteins by dietary fish oils in patients with hypertriglyceridemia. N Engl J Med 312:1210, 1985.

16. Schechtman, G and Kissebah, AH: Effect of marine lipid concentrate dose on plasma lipoproteins in hypertriglyceridemic individuals. Clin Res 370A, 1987.

17. Keys, A, Anderson, JT, and Grande, F: Serum cholesterol responses to changes in the diet: II. The effect of cholesterol in the diet. Metabolism 14:759, 1965.

18. Slater, G, et al: Plasma cholesterol and triglycerides in men with added eggs in the diet. Nutr Rep Int 14:249, 1976.

20. Goldstein, JL and Brown, MS: The low density lipoprotein pathway and its relation to atherosclerosis. Ann Rev Biochem 46:897, 1977.

21. McNamara, DJ, et al: Heterogeneity of cholesterol homeostasis in man. J Clin Invest 79:1729, 1987.

22. Grundy, SM, Ahrens, EH, and Davignon, J: The interaction of cholesterol absorption and synthesis in man. J Lipid Res 10:304, 1969.

23. Quintao, ECR, Brummer, S, and Stechhahn, K: Tissue storage and control of cholesterol metabolism in man on high cholesterol diets. Atherosclerosis 26:297, 1977.

24. Prosky, L: Analysis of total dietary fiber: The collaborative study. In Vahouny, GV, and Kritchevsky, D (eds): Dietary Fiber. Plenum, New York, 1985.

25. Jenkins, DJA, et al: Effect of processing on digestibility and the blood glucose response: A study of lentils. Am J Clin Nutr 36:1093, 1982.

26. Wolf, RN and Grundy, SM: Influence of weight reduction on plasma lipoproteins in obese patients. Arteriosclerosis 3:160, 1983.

27. Anderson, JW, et al: Serum lipid responses of obese men and women to very low calorie diets. Am J Clin Nutr 47:763(abstr.#22), 1988.

28. Funfar, J, Heshka, S, and Heymsfield, SB: Long-term effects of weight reduction on serum lipids. Am J Clin Nutr 47:763(abstr.#23), 1988.

29. Olefsky, J, Reaven, GM, and Farquhar, JW: Effects of weight reduction on obesity: Studies of lipid and carbohydrate metabolism in normal and hyperlipoproteinemic subjects. J Clin Invest 53:64, 1974.

CHAPTER 11

Treatment of Lipoprotein Disorders

W. Virgil Brown, M.D.
Wm. James Howard, M.D.

After recent detailed review of the evidence that lowering blood cholesterol will lead to a reduction in the incidence of coronary heart disease (CHD), the National Cholesterol Education Program (NCEP) has issued detailed guidelines for classification and treatment of *borderline high* and *high blood cholesterol*.[1] The basis for this system of classification and treatment is built not only on epidemiologic correlations[2,3] and the analysis of clinical trial data[4-7] but also is supported by extensive animal studies[8] as well as the growing knowledge of lipoprotein and cellular physiology.[9] Although all the questions have not been answered about the etiology of arteriosclerosis, it has become clear that the plasma levels of low-density lipoproteins (LDL) have a close and causal relationship.[2,3] It is also well demonstrated that LDL levels can be changed by diet and pharmacologic therapy and that the correlate of this change is a proportional change in the rate of heart attack and sudden death.[4,5,7] It is for this reason that the NCEP has used LDL cholesterol as the major parameter for defining risk related to cholesterol levels and as the major target for treatment.

There are several other risk factors for coronary artery disease that have been repeatedly documented by long-term community-based studies[1-3] (Table 11–1). These risk factors amplify the effects of LDL cholesterol and heighten the potential value of reducing LDL. As defined by the NCEP guidelines, these risk factors deserve careful evaluation and treatment as separate issues, and, when two or more are present, the recommendation is to set lower targets for goal levels of LDL cholesterol.

Having all the scientific data and these new guidelines helps significantly in developing an approach to managing elevated cholesterol in medical practice, but many practical issues remain. The first issue is to come to psychologic grips with the fact that the majority of adults seen each day in the physician's office will have borderline high or high blood cholesterol by the new definitions.[10] Thus, the systematic determination of blood cholesterol should become a routine part of every practice. The NCEP recommends that every adult in the United States should have a test to measure his or her cholesterol level. Those individuals with cholesterol levels

Table 11–1. Risk Factors for Coronary Artery Disease Other Than LDL-Cholesterol

Male gender
Family history of premature coronary artery disease
Cigarette smoking
Hypertension
Glucose intolerance/diabetes mellitus
Low HDL cholesterol (<35 mg/dl)
History of other atherosclerotic vascular diseases
Significant obesity ($>30\%$ overweight)

LDL = Low-density lipoprotein.
HDL = High-density lipoprotein.

above the desirable level of 200 mg/dl will want to have this measurement confirmed and then undergo further evaluation to determine their risk for coronary artery disease. The great majority of patients with cholesterol levels above the desirable range will not need medicinal management but will administer their own therapy through life-style and dietary changes. However, this does not diminish the physician's role in identifying the problem, in providing effective counseling to induce appropriate life-style changes, in assisting the patient to remain compliant to his or her new habits, and in confirming the success of those habits in the reduction of blood cholesterol. A patient's personal physician is the most trusted source of health information, and the physician's strong endorsement of healthy living styles can be a major inducement to the patient's beginning a desirable behavior pattern.

Finally, there are a variety of drugs that can effectively lower LDL cholesterol when used in an artful manner.[11,12] These need to be carefully selected to fit the individual patient's needs. Fortunately, the clinical trials have given us both long-term and short-term information to guide our choice of drugs for the specific problem at hand. Using this information, the NCEP has made recommendations concerning the choice of the most appropriate drugs for particular lipid abnormalities[1,11,12] (Table 11–2).

Table 11–2. Drug Therapy for Lipid Disorders

Drugs for Hypercholesterolemia
Cholestyramine, colestipol
Nicotinic acid
Lovastatin
Probucol
Drugs for Combined Hypercholesterolemia and Hypertriglyceridemia
Nicotinic acid
Gemfibrozil
Lovastatin
Drugs for Hypertriglyceridemia
Nicotinic acid
Gemfibrozil

Table 11–3. Classification Based on
LDL-Cholesterol

Desirable LDL-cholesterol	<130 mg/dl
Borderline high-risk LDL-cholesterol	130–159 mg/dl
High-risk LDL-cholesterol	≥ 160 mg/dl

CLASSIFICATION

Because the relationship between LDL cholesterol and the risk of cardiovascular disease (CVD) is continuous and positive over virtually the entire range of LDL cholesterol values found in Western humans,[2,3] choosing any particular values for classification of cardiovascular risk is arbitrary. In looking to populations that are low in their rate of coronary disease (that is, 10 to 20 percent of the current United States rate), average LDL cholesterol values are approximately 100 mg/dl.[13,14] Although such values might be considered "ideal," in its attempt to establish practical and achievable goals, the NCEP wisely chose a somewhat higher LDL cholesterol value of 130 mg/dl and designated those individuals with values below this level as having "desirable" LDL cholesterol. Reductions from 130 to 100 mg/dl might produce some additional risk reduction. Although achieving this goal would indeed be ideal, the benefit for many Americans may well not be worth the cost. At the LDL level currently determined as desirable, emphasis is placed more productively on identifying and treating other cardiovascular risk factors, such as cigarette smoking and obesity, rather than on the further reduction of cholesterol. Even at these levels, however, prudent dietary change to reduce the intake of saturated fat, cholesterol, and sodium can be advised.[15]

At a level of 160 mg/dl for LDL cholesterol, a middle-aged man's risk of dying from CHD is approximately doubled when compared with an LDL cholesterol of 130 mg/dl.[1-3] The NCEP recommended that we classify those individuals with LDL cholesterol values greater than 130 mg/dl but less than 160 mg/dl as being in a *borderline high risk* category. These individuals need counseling from their physician and monitoring to document that the LDL cholesterol has been reduced by life-style changes, particularly dietary change. Above 160 mg/dl the term *high-risk* LDL cholesterol is recommended. These individuals need dietary therapy, more frequent monitoring, and, in some cases, drugs may be indicated.

At 190 mg/dl and above, the coronary risk for a middle-aged man is four to five times greater than that for individuals with LDL cholesterol below 130 mg/dl.[1-3] These individuals may be designated as having a *very high risk* LDL cholesterol, and if the values remain above 190 mg/dl after an adequate trial of dietary therapy, some form of pharmacologic management would be indicated in virtually all adults. The definition of the terms used to classify LDL cholesterol is given in Table 11–3. It is strongly recommended that we physicians and health professionals use this terminology so that we can be speaking a common language with our patients about the importance of controlling LDL cholesterol.

INITIAL EVALUATION

It is appropriate to use the total plasma cholesterol in the initial evaluation of the patient. It is neither cost-effective nor practical to measure lipoprotein levels initially for three major reasons:

Table 11–4. Classification Based on
Total Cholesterol

Desirable total cholesterol	<200 mg/dl
Borderline high total cholesterol	200–239 mg/dl
High total cholesterol	≥240 mg/dl

1. Added expense of two- to threefold
2. Necessity of fasting for 12 to 14 hours
3. Lack of possibility for immediate feedback information

In addition, the total plasma cholesterol can now be accurately measured in the physician's office using a table-top analyzer.[16] This can be done at any time without the necessity of fasting and provides an additional value in the record, which the physician can use to judge biologic fluctuations within the patient. The following scheme is suggested by the NCEP to use total plasma cholesterol as a guide to further action. In concordance with the definitions for *desirable, borderline high risk,* and *high risk* LDL cholesterol values, the corresponding total plasma cholesterol levels found in the average individual with the specified LDL cholesterol values are given in Table 11–4. Thus, an individual with a total plasma cholesterol value under 200 mg/dl would be referred to as having "desirable blood cholesterol." From 200 to 239 mg/dl, the designation should be "borderline high cholesterol," and at 240 mg/dl or greater, the patient should be designated as having a "high blood cholesterol." Because LDL cholesterol and not total plasma cholesterol is used specifically to classify risk status, the term *risk* was omitted from the designations for total plasma cholesterol. For example, the total cholesterol may be elevated in the presence of a desirable LDL cholesterol due to an unusually high HDL cholesterol. In this situation, the patient's coronary risk is actually decreased. Therefore, the total plasma cholesterol should be used as a guide to determine whether further risk evaluation is necessary through the measurement of lipoprotein levels.

It is worth noting that the use of one of several desktop analyzers for the measurement of total plasma cholesterol may prove very useful in the classification and monitoring of patients. These analyzers, if properly cared for and with the use of proper standardization and quality control procedures, can provide both accurate and precise values.[16] In fact, with the new enzymatic methods used in virtually all such analyzers, accuracy may actually exceed that of some large clinical chemistry laboratories that continue to use older methodology that may overestimate the total plasma cholesterol by 10 to 15 percent.[17] A clear tipoff to this point is the use by some laboratories of a value of 300 to 310 mg/dl as the 95th percentile. With more accurate methods, the 95th percentile value in the general population is closer to 265 mg/dl.[1,10] Having grown accustomed to these artifactually high values, many physicians are uncomfortable with the new NCEP guidelines inasmuch as they appear to foster marked over-diagnosis of *borderline high* or *high* blood cholesterol.

FOLLOW-UP

For individuals with *desirable* blood cholesterol, the value should be repeated at the time of the next complete physical examination, or at the latest within 5 years.

Table 11–5. Lipoprotein Analysis

Confirm elevated total cholesterol
12-hour fast
Measure total cholesterol, HDL cholesterol, and triglycerides
Estimate LDL cholesterol by Friedewald formula

LDL cholesterol = total cholesterol
HDL cholesterol
Triglycerides/5

For those with *borderline high* blood cholesterol (200 to 239 mg/dl), the patient should be given a brief discussion of appropriate dietary changes (see below) and the total plasma cholesterol repeated 4 to 8 weeks later. If found within the desirable range (less than 200 mg/dl), a subsequent measurement 6 months to 1 year later should be made to document continued adherence to the dietary change. For those individuals with borderline high blood cholesterol and the presence of arteriosclerosis or the presence of two major risk factors, a full lipoprotein analysis should be made on a fasting blood sample (Table 11–5). Subsequent management should be based on the LDL cholesterol value.

If *high* blood cholesterol is present on the initial screen (greater than 240 mg/dl), the lipoprotein analysis should be performed within 1 to 8 weeks. If the LDL cholesterol is 160 mg/dl or greater, dietary therapy should be instituted and a repeat lipoprotein measurement made 4 to 8 weeks later. If the LDL cholesterol has not fallen below 160 mg/dl, further dietary modification should be made and a subsequent lipoprotein analysis scheduled (4 to 8 weeks later). Repeated measurement of total plasma cholesterol, lipoprotein values, or both is important because of both laboratory error, which should be less than 3 percent,[16] and biologic variation, which will average 6 to 7 percent.[18] Thus, a 10 percent variation from visit to visit can be expected with no apparent therapeutic intervention. Therefore, it is recommended that two or more measurements be made before any major therapeutic decision, such as beginning drug therapy, is undertaken.

DIETARY THERAPY

The goal of dietary therapy is to reduce the LDL cholesterol to less than 130 mg/dl or the surrogate total plasma cholesterol to less than 200 mg/dl in every adult in the United States. In those individuals with CHD or with two major risk factors (Table 11–1), dietary therapy should be initiated when the LDL cholesterol is 130 mg/dl or greater. A systematic treatment program and monitoring schedule should be put into place in order to help the patient achieve these goals. For individuals without either coronary disease or two major risk factors, a more conservative approach can be taken. In such individuals, an LDL cholesterol of 160 mg/dl (total plasma cholesterol 240 mg/dl) is acceptable but certainly far from ideal.

CHANGING THE DIET

In Western humans, the major dietary changes that have been documented to reduce the total plasma cholesterol and LDL cholesterol are:

1. Reduction in dietary saturated fat
2. Reduction in dietary cholesterol
3. Reduction in excess body fat

In making these dietary changes, it is always valuable to remember that maintaining a wide variety of foods in the diet is the best method of assuring nutritional adequacy in terms of vitamins, minerals, essential amino acids, and calories. Therefore, very few foods, if any, should be completely eliminated, and the emphasis should be on reducing the quantity of certain food groups while increasing the amount of others.

Reducing the saturated fat content of the diet remains the intervention with the most likely efficacy in reducing LDL cholesterol.[15] Americans are currently eating 13 to 15 percent of their calories as saturated fat. This can easily be reduced by one-third, to less than 10 percent of calories, while maintaining a palatable diet. This in fact is the recommendation of both the American Heart Association and the NCEP (Table 11–6). When the Step 1 dietary recommendation does not achieve the aforementioned goals, moving on to Step 2 requires the further reduction of saturated fat to approximately 7 percent of calories.[1] This is a bit more difficult. At a saturated fat level of 7 percent of total calories, it is possible to have an appealing and varied diet, but detailed instructions are required and consultation with a registered dietician is necessary. Discussing caloric percentages is of little direct use to the patient. It is thus recommended that changes in eating patterns be discussed as outlined in Table 11–7.

Reducing dietary cholesterol from the current intake of about 400 to 500 mg per day to less than 300 mg per day is recommended in the Step 1 diet. A further reduction to less than 200 mg per day is an important change in the Step 2 diet. It should be kept in mind that no dietary cholesterol is required for normal growth and development or for health in adult life. Vegetarians eat virtually no cholesterol as a consequence of avoiding animal products. Current evidence indicates that they have much less vascular disease with few, if any, ill health consequences.[19,20] The importance of dietary cholesterol may go well beyond its impact on the fasting levels of LDL cholesterol inasmuch as several thorough studies of the relationship between dietary composition and subsequent CHD have shown the intake of dietary cholesterol to be an independent risk factor even after correcting for its effects on blood lipid levels.[21,22] A list of practical steps to be taken in order to achieve a significant reduction in dietary cholesterol is given in Table 11–8.

The third important issue is reduction in excess body fat mass. Obesity, and particularly truncal obesity, is a major risk factor for CHD.[23] This risk is only partly explained by the increased incidence of elevated blood cholesterol, lower high-density lipoprotein (HDL) cholesterol, and a higher incidence of elevated blood pres-

Table 11–6. Dietary Therapy of Elevated
LDL-Cholesterol*

Nutrient	Step 1 Diet	Step 2 Diet
Total fat	<30% of total calories	<30% of total calories
Saturated fat	<10% of total calories	<7% of total calories
Polyunsaturated fat	Up to 10% of total calories	Up to 10% of total calories
Monounsaturated fat	10–15% of total calories	10–15% of total calories
Carbohydrate	50–60% of total calories	50–60% of total calories
Protein	10–20% of total calories	10–20% of total calories
Cholesterol	<300 mg/day	<200 mg/day

*Percent total calories to achieve and maintain desirable body weight.

Table 11–7. Recommended Changes in Eating Patterns to Reduce Dietary Saturated Fat

1. Choose lean cuts of meat, trim visible fat, and cook so that the fat drains away
2. Decrease the frequency of and reduce the size of meat portions
3. Decrease the consumption of red meats
4. Remove the skin from poultry
5. Use low-fat milk and dairy products
6. Avoid baked goods made with butter, whole milk, and other saturated fats such as palm oil and coconut oil
7. Substitute vegetable-oil margarine for butter
8. Decrease the consumption of egg yolks
9. Avoid foods containing coconut and palm oils—read labels
10. Substitute fish for meats

sure. Losing this excess fat has been shown to improve these measurable and related risk factors. From an epidemiologic perception, the major cause for excess body weight in Western humans is the lack of exercise rather than high caloric consumption.[24] Of course the final issue is the balance between the two. In many patients, increasing regular exercise is often a more successful recommendation. Sustaining a long-term weight loss purely by caloric restriction is one of the more difficult dietary issues for even the most expert specialist in metabolic disease. An appropriately planned exercise regimen may have added benefit in improving the collateral coronary circulation, and in the younger patient may result in larger lumenal diameter of the coronary arteries.[25]

Monounsaturated and Polyunsaturated Fats

Some of the interest in the use of monounsaturated and polyunsaturated fats as a dietary substitute for saturated fats has been engendered by various clinical trials over time.[15] It now seems evident that the degree to which LDL cholesterol is reduced is most clearly a result of removing saturated fat, and that either monounsaturates or polyunsaturates are good substitutes for this purpose. All fats are, however, a rich source of calories; for that reason an attempt to keep the total fat intake below 30 percent of calories is recommended by both the American Heart Association and the NCEP. Furthermore, we have very little long-term data on populations that have consumed more than 10 percent of their calories from polyunsaturated fats of vegetable origin, and therefore a recommended upper limit at 10 percent is offered in these diet plans. This would allow an increase of 30 to 40 percent above the current average intake for Americans (currently about 6 to 7 percent of calories). Monounsaturates have been consumed by large populations at levels approaching 20 percent of calories with no adverse effects. Therefore, there

Table 11–8. Recommended Changes in Eating Patterns to Reduce Dietary Cholesterol

1. Limit or eliminate intake of egg yolks
2. Avoid baked goods made with egg yolks
3. Limit intake of liver and organ meats
4. Decrease the frequency of meat and shellfish and limit cooked portion sizes to 3 ounces
5. Use low-fat milk and dairy products

Table 11–9. Comparison of Dietary Fats

Fats and Oils	Total Fat (g/tbs)	Fatty Acids			Cholesterol (mg/tbs)
		Sat	Mono (g/tbs)	Poly	
Olive oil	13.5	1.8	9.9	1.1	0
Rapeseed (canola)	13.6	0.9	7.6	4.5	0
Safflower oil	13.6	1.2	1.6	10.1	0
Sunflower oil	13.6	1.4	2.7	8.9	0
Corn oil	13.6	1.7	3.3	8.0	0
Soybean oil	13.6	2.0	3.2	7.9	0
Peanut oil	13.5	2.3	6.2	4.3	0
Palm oil	13.6	6.7	5.0	1.3	0
Palm kernel oil	13.6	11.1	1.5	0.2	0
Coconut oil	13.6	11.8	0.8	0.2	0
Vegetable shortening	12.8	3.2	5.7	3.3	0
Lard	12.8	5.0	5.8	1.4	12
Butter	11.4	7.1	3.3	0.4	31

SOURCE: U.S. Department of Agriculture, Human Nutrition Information Service, HNIS/PT-101.

seems to be no rationale for a similar restriction of monounsaturated fats. Vegetable oils rich in monounsaturated and polyunsaturated fats are given in Table 11–9.

Fish and Fish Oils

Data from the Zutphen study,[22] the Ireland-Boston Diet Heart Study,[26] and the Western Electric Study[21] indicate that individuals who eat fish two to three times per week have significantly less heart disease than similar individuals who avoid fish completely in these communities. This does not appear to be due to differences in plasma cholesterol levels or difference in the saturated fat intake. Thus, there may be positive results from the regular consumption of fish. One explanation has been the high content of polyunsaturated fats of the so called Omega-3 variety.[27] Ocean fish and shellfish contain these Omega-3 fatty acids in high concentrations. The Omega-3 fatty acids, including eicosapentaenoic and docosahexaenoic fatty acids, are known to suppress the synthesis of triglycerides when given in large quantities to humans and animals. They also markedly change the synthesis of certain prostaglandins, including thromboxane, thereby affecting platelet aggregation.[29] However, they do not lower LDL cholesterol or specifically raise HDL cholesterol and are, therefore, not recommended as treatment of an elevated cholesterol level. The long-term impact of fish oil on arteriosclerosis in humans is yet to be determined. At the moment, the recommendation that fish be consumed two or three times per week is soundly based in the epidemiologic literature; however, the rationale for the use of fish oil extract is not yet adequately developed, and there is no rationale for attempting to lower LDL cholesterol with these preparations.

Fiber

There is now considerable evidence that the consumption of foods high in water-soluble fiber may lower total plasma and LDL cholesterol.[30] Foods high in these fibers include legumes (beans and peas), oats, corn, and certain fruits. One of the most concentrated forms is psyllium seed, used in over-the-counter preparations as stool softeners. One preparation (Metamucil) has been reported to produce a significant reduction in LDL cholesterol when taken regularly.[31] Foods containing primarily cellulose and other insoluble fiber have little direct impact on plasma cholesterol levels. The mechanism of the effect of soluble fiber on cholesterol reduction is not understood. Studies to date have failed to confirm the proposed mechanism of binding to intestinal bile acids, and further studies are needed.[32] In recommending high-fiber foods, it should be kept in mind that in general they are low-cholesterol, low-saturated-fat substances that make excellent dietary substitutes. The direct impact of soluble fiber may add a small increment in the LDL reduction, but in general, it is impractical to expect more than a 3 to 5 percent reduction by the addition of such foods.[33]

In summary, it is most important to reduce the consumption of saturated fats by decreasing the intake of certain dairy products, reducing the frequency and portion-size of meat consumption, and virtually eliminating egg yolks and organ meats. Whether or not foods high in mono, poly, or Omega-3 fatty acids are consumed is of much less importance. Foods high in soluble fiber provide vitamins and minerals and are excellent in many ways, but their direct impact on cholesterol reduction probably will be undetectable in the individual.

ACHIEVING DIETARY COMPLIANCE

Many physicians do not advocate dietary intervention for their own personal reasons. In spite of the adequate scientific evidence demonstrating that a change in saturated fat and cholesterol intake will markedly reduce LDL cholesterol, the experience with the individual patient in practice may seem quite the contrary. There are several factors that may explain this observation. For the short term, the problem is usually not patient compliance. Most individuals will readily adopt a diet low in saturated fat and cholesterol, particularly if they are properly motivated by their physician. Increasingly, the "problem" of lack of responsiveness relates to the fact that most individuals already know the necessary dietary changes, and when appearing with a disorder such as CHD, dietary changes may already have been made. Thus, the initial dietary treatment should involve dietary assessment. The majority of patients with known vascular disease already may have adopted a diet that is similar to the Step 1 diet, and the appropriate dietary intervention should involve closing any loopholes found on dietary assessment and proceeding to the Step 2 regimen. If the patient is already on an optimum diet when first seen, three important issues must be kept in mind:

1. Avoid suggesting that dietary composition is not important simply because you fail to see further reduction in LDL cholesterol after dietary instruction. This may result in the patient resuming previous habits that led to much higher plasma cholesterol levels and contributed to the coronary disease.
2. Emphasize the importance of continued reduced saturated fat and cholesterol in the diet because, as coronary symptoms stabilize or disappear with nutritional therapy, the patient's commitment to dietary adherence often diminishes.

3. Evaluation of the diet for unwarranted restrictions that reduce the palatability of the diet and the use of a broad spectrum of healthful foods may lead to increased compliance. Adding a small portion of lean beef on occasion or pointing out that margarine contains no cholesterol and very little "bad saturated fat" may improve long-term dietary compliance markedly.

DRUG TREATMENT

In most cases, patients should be allowed to develop new dietary patterns and life-style changes for at least 6 months before considering drug treatment for elevated LDL cholesterol. Only in a few cases, in which the LDL cholesterol is very high (greater than 220 mg/dl) or desired dietary modifications are assessed to be fully implemented, should the physician consider more immediate drug therapy. Even in these instances, several LDL cholesterol values over a period of 6 to 12 weeks are needed to document the baseline against which pharmacologic therapeutic efficacy will be judged. Before beginning drug therapy, secondary forms of hyperlipidemia should be ruled out. The presence of diabetes mellitus, hypothyroidism, hepatic diseases, and nephrotic syndrome or other renal diseases should be assessed with appropriate blood tests.

With the use of a hypolipidemic agent, several important issues are worthy of consideration, including the following:

1. Is this drug likely to produce a significant reduction in LDL cholesterol without adversely affecting other lipoprotein levels?
2. Has this drug been shown to reduce the risk for CHD in long-term clinical trials?
3. Are long-term, serious complications possible with its use?
4. What are the common side effects, and how do they fit with the patient's clinical findings?
5. Is ease of administration an issue with this particular patient?
6. Is the mechanism of action understood?
7. Is there burdensome cost?

Each of the commonly used lipid-lowering agents is discussed in light of these important questions.

ESTABLISHING GOALS FOR TREATMENT

All patients with very high LDL cholesterol (greater than 190 mg/dl) should be considered candidates for drug treatment following a prolonged and well-documented attempt to alter diet and other important life-style parameters. In general, 6 months of therapy using nonpharmacologic means should be considered a minimal time for most patients. For individuals without CHD and without two major risk factors, a minimal goal of reduction of LDL cholesterol to less than 160 mg/dl is recommended. Increments in the dose of a medication is appropriate step-by-step until this goal is achieved. For individuals with CHD or with two major risk factors, the persistence of LDL cholesterol above 160 mg/dl following prolonged dietary change should also be considered appropriate for drug treatment. In such individuals, the goal of reducing the LDL below 130 mg/dl is suggested by the NCEP. As further data are gathered with ongoing clinical trials, a clear rationale for even greater reductions in LDL cholesterol in such high-risk patients may be documented.

Because most interventions (diet or drug) require 4 to 6 weeks before they fully impact on lipoprotein levels, it is sensible to evaluate and consider therapeutic adjustments at 4- to 8-week intervals. With many cholesterol-lowering agents, side effects, ease of administration, and, certainly, cost are dose related. Thus, it is logical to begin with a low dose and to adjust the dose upward at intervals of at least 4 weeks, assessing for side effects and efficacy in LDL reduction. Maintaining the patient on the lowest effective dose of medication is most likely to achieve the long-term adherence necessary for prevention of CHD. In some cases in which side effects are transient, such as the flushing episodes with niacin or the constipation with the bile acid sequestrants, a higher dose may be tolerated only after a period of adjustment to lower doses. On the other hand, failing to move forward to the dose level required for the desired efficacy may deny the patient the full benefits of drug treatment that have been documented in previous clinical trials.[4-6]

BILE ACID SEQUESTRANTS

Cholestyramine (Questran or Cholybar) and colestipol (Colestid) are long-chain polymers containing strong positively charged ionic groups. These nonabsorbable anionic exchange resins act in the intestinal tract. Questran and Colestid are provided as insoluble powders that must be suspended in a liquid and taken orally, usually twice daily. They are provided in bulk cans or in individual foil-wrapped doses. The standard dose of Questran provides 4 gm of cholestyramine, whereas that of Colestid provides 5 gm of colestipol. These doses are equivalent in reducing LDL cholesterol. Cholybar provides a dose of 4 gm of cholestyramine in a gum-based bar sweetened by fructose. The usual dose ranges are:

Cholestyramine—4 to 12 gm twice daily
Colestipol—5 to 15 gm twice daily.

Expected Efficacy

At full therapeutic doses (cholestyramine, 12 gm twice daily and colestipol, 15 gm twice daily), reduction of LDL cholesterol of approximately 25 percent and elevation of HDL cholesterol of 5 to 10 percent may be achieved.[2,34] However, triglycerides often increase by 20 to 100 percent.

Clinical Efficacy

Questran was used in the Lipid Research Clinic Coronary Primary Prevention Trial (LRC CPPT) with demonstrated efficacy in the prevention of CHD.[5] Colestid was used in the Cholesterol Lowering Atherosclerosis Study (CLAS),[35] in which a significant reduction in the rate of development of angiographically demonstrable coronary artery lesions occurred.

Side Effects

At full dosage of both cholestyramine and colestipol, constipation has been reported in 10 to 20 percent of patients, and gastric distress, nausea, vomiting, and diarrhea have been reported in 1 to 3 percent of patients.[11] Negatively charged drugs will absorb to these medications and should be taken at least 1 hour before or 4 hours after the dose of the bile acid sequestrants. Triglyceride levels may be doubled or tripled in hypertriglyceridemic patients; therefore, individuals with triglycerides in excess of 250 mg/dl should not be treated with bile acid sequestrants as the primary hypolipidemic agent.[36] Transient elevations of triglycerides in normal individuals usually disappear after 8 to 12 weeks of treatment.

Contraindications

Triglycerides in excess of 250 mg/dl and severe anal-rectal disorders that might be aggravated by constipation are contraindications to the use of a bile acid sequestrant.

Mechanisms of Action

As anionic exchange resins, cholestyramine and colestipol bind bile acids in the intestines, preventing their reabsorption and thereby increasing their loss in the stool. The liver responds to the lack of bile acid reabsorption by increasing the conversion of intrahepatic cholesterol to bile acid and by increasing the number of cell surface receptors for LDL. The net effect is an increased clearance of LDL from the plasma and a reduction in LDL cholesterol levels.

Clinical Use

The side effects commonly experienced with the bile acid sequestrants can be avoided by the appropriate initial usage of these medications. The starting dose of 4 gm of cholestyramine or 5 gm of colestipol twice daily should be given with a vehicle that is pleasing to the palate. These agents can be mixed in a variety of juices, water, yogurt or placed in oatmeal or cereal. The fluid content of the diet should also be increased, and resulting constipation may be reduced by adding a soluble fiber preparation such as one of the psyllium-containing products. At the end of 4 to 6 weeks on this initial dose, lipoproteins should be measured and the dose increased if the goal LDL cholesterol levels have not been achieved. With time, most of the bothersome side effects dissipate as the gastrointestinal tract adjusts to the medication. Total daily doses of 24 gm for cholestyramine or 30 gm for colestipol are usually effective. Higher doses of 32 gm or 40 gm respectively have been used in occasional patients.

Nicotinic Acid (Niacin)

Nicotinic acid is required as a coenzyme in intermediary metabolism at a dose level of less than 20 mg per day. When given at much higher dosages (500 mg to 3 gm three times daily), this agent has profound lipid-lowering effects.[11] Nicotinic acid reduces the LDL cholesterol by 15 to 40 percent at the upper dosage levels. It also reduces very low-density lipoprotein (VLDL) triglycerides by 40 to 50 percent and raises HDL cholesterol by 10 to 30 percent. It is supplied by a variety of manufacturers in various dosage forms, including long-acting preparations. In general, the most effective and least expensive form of this medication is the ordinary nicotinic acid tablet. It should be pointed out that *nicotinamide* is frequently purchased by patients as an over-the-counter medication instead of nicotinic acid; although well-tolerated, nicotinamide has no lipid-lowering effect.

Mechanisms of Action

Nicotinic acid transiently suppresses the release of free fatty acids from adipose tissues, but its major effect appears to occur in the liver, where there is a reduction in VLDL synthesis with a concomitant reduction in plasma triglycerides and LDL cholesterol.[37] The biochemistry of its action in the liver to reduce VLDL synthesis is not fully understood. The mechanism by which HDL is increased is also without biochemical explanation.

Side Effects

The most common side effect of nicotinic acid is cutaneous flushing occurring 15 minutes to 2 hours after a dose, with a frequency of over 90 percent in patients begun at dose levels above 250 mg. Other skin reactions include pruritus and, rarely, acanthosis nigracans. Some patients experience nausea, abdominal discomfort, and diarrhea on this medication. Inflammatory disorders of the intestinal tract may be exacerbated, including peptic ulcer disease, regional enteritis, and ulcerative colitis. Headaches and hypotension sometimes occur. Toxic amblyopia apparently due to macular edema is a very rare side effect. The metabolic side effects of nicotinic acid include hyperuricemia and glucose intolerance. However, many diabetics tolerate the medication without necessitating a change in their specific antidiabetic therapy. At dosages greater than 3 gm per day, 1 to 5 percent of patients will show liver dysfunction with elevations of the transaminases and alkaline phosphatase levels. These abnormalities of liver function are rapidly reversible after discontinuing treatment. Liver function tests, uric acid, and blood glucose levels should be monitored during the initiation of treatment and for 2 to 3 months after establishing the effective dose regimens. Increased frequency of cardiac arrhythmias has been reported in patients with coronary artery disease.

Contraindications

Contraindications to the use of nicotinic acid are:

1. Severe inflammatory disorders of the gastrointestinal tract
2. Known cardiac arrhythmias
3. Hyperuricemia
4. Pre-existing liver disease.

Clinical Use

Many of the side effects of nicotinic acid can be avoided by beginning with a low dose and slowly titrating the dose until therapuetic levels are achieved. For example, an initial dose of 100 mg administered three times daily immediately after meals is a reasonable regimen for initiating therapy. The unpleasant cutaneous flushing may be avoided by administering aspirin (325 mg) or Ibuprofen (200 mg) beginning the evening before the first dose and continuing twice daily until the final dosage regimen is established. The nicotinic acid dose may then be doubled at 3 to 7 day intervals. When the dose exceeds 400 mg three times a day, the 250 mg or 500 mg tablet is more convenient, and after the patient has taken a dose of 500 mg three times daily for 4 to 6 weeks, lipoproteins should be measured and glucose, liver function, and uric acid levels should be evaluated. If all are in order, further reduction in LDL cholesterol may be achieved by increasing the nicotinic acid in increments of 0.5 gm after each meal at monthly intervals. The lipoprotein, blood glucose, liver functions, and uric acid levels should continue to be monitored at each visit.

Clinical Efficacy

In the Coronary Drug Project, treatment with nicotinic acid resulted in a significant reduction in new myocardial infarctions; and, after 15 years of monitoring, a significant reduction in both cardiovascular mortality and total mortality was observed in the nicotinic acid–treated group as compared with the placebo-treated group.[38] Nicotinic acid was also used in the CLAS in conjunction with colestipol.[35] In the latter study, a significant reduction was observed in the rate of progression of vascular lesions in the native coronary arteries and in bypass grafts of patients who had undergone coronary artery bypass surgery. There was even a suggestion that some lesions regressed after two years of aggressive cholesterol lowering.

FIBRIC ACID DERIVATIVES

Clofibrate (Atromid-S) and gemfibrozil (Lopid) are the only fibric acid preparations available in the United States at present. Fenofibrate and bezafibrate are currently in clinical trials in the United States and have been used in Europe and other parts of the world for several years. Clofibrate is supplied as a 500 mg capsule and gemfibrozil as a 300 mg capsule. The usual dose is two capsules twice daily with both medications. The newer fibric acid derivatives are effective at a lower dose level.

Mechanisms of Action

The fibric acid derivatives increase lipoprotein lipase activity with a resulting increase in VLDL triglyceride clearance. In patients with normal triglycerides and elevated LDL cholesterol, an increase in LDL clearance is also observed. Animal studies suggest that this reduction in LDL cholesterol may be the result of decreased hepatic cholesterol synthesis.[40] The mechanism responsible for increasing HDL cholesterol levels is not known. The fibrates also increase biliary cholesterol output while diminishing the output of bile acids, resulting in a more lithogenic bile.

Side Effects

Both gemfibrozil and clofibrate are well tolerated, although they both produce occasional nausea and abdominal discomfort, and 1 to 3 percent of patients describe breast tenderness and decreased libido with clofibrate. In the World Health Organization (WHO) Study[41] as well as the Coronary Drug Project,[4] a significant increase in the incidence of cholelithiasis was observed in patients treated with clofibrate, and, in the WHO study, a significantly higher mortality rate from noncardiac causes was observed in the clofibrate-treated group when compared with control subjects receiving placebo. This increased mortality was attributable to complications resulting from the cholelithiasis and subsequent cholecystectomy as well as a variety of other causes, including an increase in malignant neoplasms. On subsequent follow-up, the increment in noncardiac deaths did not persist in the clofibrate group after discontinuing therapy. Increased cancer rates were not observed in the Coronary Drug Project. This may have been a statistical artifact. The more recent Helsinki Heart Study using gemfibrozil found no statistically significant increase in gallstone disease and no change in cancer death rates. The only statistically significant observation was an increase in abdominal discomfort. An increase in hepatic transaminase enzymes and a relatively uncommon myositis-like syndrome have been reported with both fibric acid derivatives, although the latter appears to be more common with clofibrate.[42] Clofibrate and perhaps gemfibrozil potentiate the activity of the coumarin anticoagulants, and the combined use of these agents requires very careful monitoring.

Clinical Efficacy

Both clofibrate and gemfibrozil are very effective in reducing elevated VLDL triglyceride levels by as much as 30 to 50 percent.[39] In patients with normal triglyceride levels and an elevated LDL cholesterol, a 10 to 20 percent reduction in LDL may be seen. In hypertriglyceridemic patients, the LDL response to these drugs is variable. In more severe cases of hypertriglyceridemia, LDL may actually rise moderately. There is a consistent increase in HDL cholesterol of approximately 10 to 20 percent.

In the WHO Study, new myocardial infarctions were significantly reduced; however, the overall death rate in the clofibrate-treated group was accentuated.[41] In the more recent Helsinki Heart Study, an average decline of 9 percent in LDL and an increase in HDL of approximately 9 percent was associated with a 34 percent reduction in myocardial infarctions and sudden deaths.[6]

Clinical Use

Because the fibric acid derivatives are much less effective in reducing LDL cholesterol than the bile acid-binding resins, nicotinic acid, or the HMG Co-A reductase inhibitors discussed here, they should be reserved as second-line agents for treating patients with pure hypercholesterolemia. In patients with both elevated VLDL triglyceride and LDL cholesterol, they are effective in controlling the triglyceride level and may also reduce LDL cholesterol. Combination therapy beginning with gemfibrozil and later adding a bile acid-binding resin, if necessary, provides effective treatment for elevations of both LDL and VLDL. In the rare syndrome of dysbetalipoproteinemia, either gemfibrozil or clofibrate is effective therapy when used alone.[11]

HMG CO-A REDUCTASE INHIBITORS

Lovastatin (Mevacor) is the most recently released new drug for reducing plasma cholesterol levels. Two additional drugs, simvastatin and pravastatin, are currently in phase 3 clinical trials and may be available in the near future after Food and Drug Administration (FDA) review of their safety and efficacy. Lovastatin is supplied as a 20 mg scored tablet. The usual dose is 10 to 40 mg as a single dose in the evening. Maximum dosage levels are 40 mg twice daily.

Mechanisms of Action

This group of agents acts by competitive inhibition of the enzyme HMG Co-A reductase. The major effect appears to be in the liver, with a small reduction in hepatic cholesterol synthesis that results in an increase in the cell-surface receptors for LDL.[44] This in turn causes an increase in the clearance of LDL particles from the plasma with a reduction in the plasma level of LDL cholesterol.

Side Effects

Liver dysfunction occurs in a mild form in 3 to 5 percent of patients, usually within the first 3 months.[43] A more severe liver dysfunction, with a rise in transaminase levels of more than three times normal, has been reported in approximately 2 percent of patients and requires the discontinuation of the medication. Muscle tenderness with a rise in creatine phosphokinase (CPK) has been reported in approximately 1 in 200 patients. A number of cases have been reported in patients receiving immunosuppressive drugs, such as cyclosporin, in whom the incidence of this muscle disorder approaches 30 percent.[45] There is also a higher incidence of myositis in patients who are receiving combination therapy with fibric acid derivatives and perhaps nicotinic acid. Rarely, rhabdomyolysis has occurred in this group of patients, with accompanying acute renal failure. Patients showing significant CPK elevations should discontinue lovastatin immediately. Beagle dogs receiving HMG Co-A reductase inhibitors in very high doses have developed subcapsular cataracts, and therefore very careful monitoring of lenticular changes are required during treatment with these agents. To date, several hundred patients have been so monitored for 3 to 5 years without evidence of drug-related lenticular disease.[46]

Combination Therapy

In patients with severe elevations of LDL cholesterol, the combination of a bile acid sequestrant and an HMG Co-A reductase inhibitor has given mean reductions in LDL of 55 to 65 percent.[47] It appears that increasing the elimination of cholesterol via binding bile acids while simultaneously inhibiting the synthesis of new cholesterol can markedly potentiate the hepatic removal of LDL from the plasma space with at least an additive effect by the two drugs.

Clinical Efficacy

Lovastatin produces a reduction in LDL cholesterol that is dose related with approximately a 25 percent reduction at 20 mg daily, a 35 percent reduction at 40 mg, and over 40 percent reduction at 40 mg twice daily.[43] Some patients are very sensitive, with a dramatic response at 10 mg (½ tablet) daily, whereas others show no detectable reduction in LDL cholesterol at this dosage level. There is often a modest reduction in VLDL triglyceride of 10 to 20 percent, and the HDL levels tend to increase by 5 to 10 percent.

To date, no trials of HMG Co-A reductase inhibitors in the prevention of CHD have been completed. In the absence of prolonged randomized controlled trials, the long-term safety (that is, greater than 5 years) remains undetermined, and in the absence of this information, conservative recommendations are warranted for the use of the HMG Co-A reductase inhibitors.

PROBUCOL (LORELCO)

Probucol, a lipophilic drug with modest cholesterol-lowering potential, has been available for a number of years. A recent resurgence of interest in this agent has resulted from the demonstration that probucol is a potent antioxidant and may have actions, in addition to lowering cholesterol, which in animal studies retard the development of atherosclerosis. This medication is supplied as 500 mg capsules. The usual dose is one capsule twice daily.

Lipoprotein Effects

LDL reductions of 8 to 15 percent are seen with probucol, but its cholesterol-lowering effect is highly variable from patient to patient.[11] A reduction in HDL of 10 to 30 percent is observed routinely with this drug. Although the mechanism of this effect on HDL is not fully explained, it appears to be due primarily to a reduction in the cholesterol content of HDL particles with a lesser effect on the apolipoprotein content. Of some interest is the observation that LDL cholesterol reduction is achieved in patients with familial homozygous hypercholesterolemia, a disorder in which no LDL receptors may be functioning.[48] In such patients, tendon xanthomata have been noted to regress. It is fascinating that the degree to which xanthomata regress in familial hypercholesterolemia has been correlated with the degree to which HDL cholesterol is reduced.[49] This drug is of research interest because it is incorporated into LDL particles after oral consumption and in this location prevents oxidation of the lipoprotein lipid. One current hypothesis relates LDL levels to the generation of lipid-laden macrophages, or foam cells, in the arterial wall with the formation of a fatty streak, the initial lesion of atherosclerosis. This mechanism proposes that the oxidation of the lipids in the LDL particle accentuates the uptake and storage of cholesterol by these cells.[50] LDL-containing probucol is markedly resistant to oxidation, and animals studied using probucol have been shown to develop fewer arterial lesions at the same total plasma LDL level.[51] Additional human studies are needed to determine any potential clinical efficacy of probucol as a lipid antioxidant agent.

Side Effects

Mild diarrhea with accompanying flatulence, abdominal discomfort, and nausea occurs in approximately 5 percent of patients. Other less frequent complaints include hyperhidrosis, fetid sweat, and angioneurotic edema. The drug rarely produces a prolongation of the QT interval on the electrocardiogram. This effect has been observed in dogs and nonhuman primates, and ventricular arrhythmias have been reported in these animals.

PATIENT ADHERENCE TO THE THERAPEUTIC REGIMEN

Successful prevention of CHD by reducing LDL cholesterol requires a very long-term view of therapy. In the clinical trials that have been successful in preventing myocardial infarction and sudden death, very little evidence of therapeutic benefit was evident until 3 or more years of treatment.[5,6] After that point, the benefits of treatment became increasingly evident, and, in the Coronary Drug Project, therapeutic benefits continued for 10 to 15 years with a resulting significant decline in total mortality.[38] Over many months, the artful physician can develop an effective course of therapy that fits the patient's specific needs and that will result in long-term adherence. There are several important steps in building this therapeutic program. The physician must let the patient know that he is very serious about the significance of the patient's risk factors and about the importance of altering them. However, he must simultaneously impart an enthusiastic, positive attitude about the possibility of effective treatment and risk reduction. He also must be willing to listen to the patient, who frequently will describe acceptable and unacceptable approaches to therapy. Attempting to force unacceptable therapy on a patient without resolving the issue of why that particular therapeutic approach is unacceptable is doomed to failure.

Enlisting the patient as a more-than-equal participant in this therapeutic venture is essential. Teaching the patient to understand and interpret the numbers that describe the LDL cholesterol, the HDL cholesterol, and other risk factors helps impart the lesson of his or her own responsibility for reducing risk. Helping the patient to understand that his or her treatment regimen is personal and must be developed through trial and testing can blunt the negative impact and loss of confidence that can result when the first therapeutic regimen fails to achieve therapeutic goals. For similar reasons, it is useful to describe the more important side effects of medication on several occasions and to encourage communication from the patient (by telephone, for instance) when questions arise, rather than discontinuing the medication immediately.

The patient who is educated and apppears motivated while in the physician's office may be totally disheartened if he or she returns home to a family that lacks similar education and understanding. Thus, it is particularly important that the spouse and other members of the household participate in dietary instruction and understand as much as possible about the nature of the patient's individual risk parameters. Understanding how and why the medication is to be used may result in a husband or a wife whose motivation actually exceeds that of the patient and provides that necessary support during the initial weeks when good habits are being formed. In studies of compliance, one of the most important predictors is spousal involvement.[52] Furthermore, clarifying the goal of therapy and providing regular systematic monitoring so that the patient can understand the impact of each therapeutic step can be very beneficial to long-term success. Finally, educating the office staff to be aware of each patient's important dietary and drug-related issues can add to the support group that has a positive impact on the patient's experience and builds confidence in the validity of a combined effort. LDL cholesterol reduction can be achieved in the long-term in the great majority of patients, and a significant reduction of morbidity and death should result.

REFERENCES

1. Cholesterol Adult Treatment Panel Report: Report of the National Cholesterol Education Program Expert Panel on Detection, Evaluation, and Treatment of High Blood Cholesterol in Adults. Arch Intern Med 148:36, 1988.
2. Castelli, WP, Garrison, RJ, Wilson, PWF, et al: The Framingham Study: Incidence of coronary heart disease and lipoprotein cholesterol levels. JAMA 256:2835, 1986.
3. Stamler, J, Wentworth, D, and Neaton, JD, for the MRFIT Research Group: Is relationship between serum cholesterol and risk of premature death from coronary heart disease continuous and graded? JAMA 256:2823, 1986.
4. The Coronary Drug Project Research Group: Clofibrate and niacin in coronary heart disease. JAMA 231:360, 1975.
5. Lipid Research Clinics Program: The Lipid Research Clinics Coronary Primary Prevention Trial results: Reduction in the incidence of coronary heart disease. JAMA 251:351, 1984.
6. Helsinki Heart Study: Primary-prevention trial with gemfibrozil in middle-aged men and dyslipidemia. N Engl J Med 317:1237, 1987.
7. Lipid Research Clinics Program: The Lipid Research Clinics Coronary Primary Prevention Trial results: The relationship of reduction in incidence of coronary heart disease to cholesterol lowering. JAMA 251:365, 1984.
8. Stehbens, WE: An appraisal of cholesterol feeding in experimental atherogenesis. Progr Cardiovasc Dis 29:107, 1986.

9. Grundy, SM: Cholesterol and coronary heart disease. JAMA 256:2849, 1986.

10. Consensus Development Conference: Lowering blood cholesterol to prevent heart disease. JAMA 253:2080, 1985.

11. Illingworth, DR: Lipid-lowering drugs: An overview of indications and optimum therapeutic use. Drugs 33:259, 1987.

12. Howard, WJ and Brown, WV: Pharmacologic therapy of hypercholesterolemia. Curr Opin Cardiol 3:525, 1988.

13. Supplement Number 1: Coronary heart disease in seven countries. Circulation 41:I-1, 1970.

14. Kato, H, Tillotson, J, Nichaman, MZ, et al: Epidemiologic studies of coronary heart disease and stroke in Japanese men living in Japan, Hawaii, and California: Serum lipids and diet. Am J Epidemiol 97:372, 1973.

15. Grundy, SM, et al: Rationale of the diet-heart statement of the American Heart Association. Circulation 65(4):839A, 1982.

16. Burke, JJ II and Fischer, PM: A clinician's guide to the office measurement of cholesterol. JAMA 259:3444, 1988.

17. Blank, DW, Hoeg, JM, Kroll, MH, et al: The method of determination must be considered in interpreting blood cholesterol levels. JAMA 256:2867, 1986.

18. Jacobs, D and Barrett-Conner, E: Re-test reliability of plasma cholesterol and triglycerides: The Lipid Research Clinics Prevalence Study. Am J Epidemiol 116:878, 1982.

19. Taylor, CB, Allen, ES, Mikkelson, B, et al: Serum cholesterol levels of Seventh-Day Adventists. Par Arter 3:175, 1976.

20. Wynder, EL and Lemon, FR: Cancer, coronary artery disease and smoking: A preliminary report on differences in incidences between Seventh-Day Adventists and others. Calif Med 89:267, 1958.

21. Shekelle, RB, Shyock, AM, Paul, O, et al: Diet, serum cholesterol and death from coronary heart disease: The Western Electric Study. N Engl J Med 304:65, 1981.

22. Kromhout, D, Bosschieter, EB, and DeLezenne Coulander, C: The inverse relation between fish consumption and 20-year mortality from coronary heart disease. N Engl J Med 312:1205, 1985.

23. Bjorntorp, P, Smith, U, and Lonnroth, P: Health implications of regional obesity. Acta Med Scand Symposium Series No. 4.

24. Ravussin, E, et al: Reduced rate of energy expenditure as a risk factor for body-weight gain. N Engl J Med 318:467, 1988.

25. Kramsch, DM, Aspen, AJ, Abramowitz, BM, et al: Reduction of coronary atherosclerosis by moderate conditioning exercise in monkeys on an atherogenic diet. N Engl J Med 305:1483, 1981.

26. Kushi, LH, Lew, RA, Stare, EJ, et al: Diet and 20-year mortality from coronary heart disease: The Ireland-Boston Diet-Heart Study. N Engl J Med 312:811, 1985.

27. Von Schacky, C: Prophylaxis of atherosclerosis with marine omega-3 fatty acids. Ann Intern Med 107:890, 1987.

28. Phillipson, BE, Rothrock, DW, Connor, WE, et al: Reduction of plasma lipids, lipoproteins, and apoproteins by dietary fish oils in patients with hypertriglyceridemia. N Engl J Med 312:1210, 1985.

29. Von Schacky, C, Fischer, S, and Weber, PC: Long-term effects of dietary omega-3 fatty acids upon plasma and cellular lipids, platelet function, and eicosanoid formation in man. J Clin Invest 76:1626, 1985.

30. Keys, A, Grande, F, and Anderson, JT: Fiber and pectin in the diet and serum cholesterol concentration in man. Proc Soc Exp Biol Med 105:555, 1961.

31. Anderson, JW, Zettwoch, N, Feldman, T, et al: Cholesterol-lowering effects of psyllium hydrophilic mucilloid for hypercholesterolemic men. Arch Intern Med 148:292, 1988.

32. Le, NA: Unpublished material,.

33. VanHorn, LV, et al: Serum lipid response to oat product intake with a fat-modified diet. J Am Diet Assoc 86:759, 1986.

34. Gordon, DJ, Knoke, J, Probstfield, JL, et al, for the Lipid Research Clinics Program: High-density lipoprotein cholesterol and coronary heart disease in hypercholesterolemic men: The Lipid Research Clinics coronary primary prevention trial. Circulation 6:1217, 1986.

35. Blankenhorn, DH, Nessim, SA, Johnson, RL, et al: Beneficial effects of combined colestipol niacin therapy on coronary atherosclerosis and coronary venous bypass grafts. JAMA 257:3233, 1987.

36. Crouse, JR III: Hypertriglyceridemia: A contraindication to the use of bile acid binding resins. Am J Med 83:243, 1987.

37. Grundy, SM, Mok, HYI, Zack, L, et al: The influence of nicotinic acid on metabolism of cholesterol and triglycerides in man. J Lipid Res 22:24, 1981.

38. Canner, PL, Berge, KG, Wenger, NK, et al, for the Coronary Drug Project Research Group: Fifteen year mortality in coronary drug project patients: Long-term benefit with niacin. JACC 8:1245, 1986.

39. Grundy, SM and Vega, GL: Fibric acids: Effects on lipids and lipoprotein metabolism. Am J Med 83:9, 1987.
40. Vega, GI and Grundy, SM: Gemfibrozil therapy in primary hypertriglyceridemia associated with coronary heart disease: Effects on metabolism of low density lipoproteins. JAMA 253:2398, 1985.
41. World Health Organization (WHO): Cooperative trial on primary prevention of ischemic heart disease using clofibrate to lower serum cholesterol. Lancet 2:379, 1980.
42. Blane, GF: Comparative toxicity and safety profile of fenofibrate and other fibric acid derivatives. Am J Med 83:26, 1987.
43. Hoeg, JM and Brewer, HB Jr: 3-Hydroxy-3-methylglutaryl-coenzyme A reductase inhibitors in the treatment of hypercholesterolemia. JAMA 258:3532, 1987.
44. Brown, MS and Goldstein, JL: A receptor-mediated pathway for cholesterol homeostasis. Science 232:34, 1986.
45. Tobert, JA: Rhabdomyolysis in patients receiving lovastatin after cardiac transplantation (reply to Letter to the Editor). N Engl J Med 318:48, 1988.
46. Hunninghake, DB, Miller, VT, Palmer, RH, et al: Lovastatin Study Group II: (Letter to the editor). Inhibitors of cholesterol synthesis and cataracts. JAMA 257:1598, 1987.
47. Malloy, MJ, Kane, JP, Kunitake, ST, et al: Complementarity of colestipol, niacin and lovastatin in treatment of severe familial hypercholesterolemia. Ann Intern Med 107:616, 1987.
48. Bilheimer, DW: Lipoprotein fractions and receptors: A role for probucol? Am J Cardiol 57:7H, 1986.
49. Yamamoto, A, Matsuzawa, Y, Yokoyama, S, et al: Effects of probucol on xanthomata regression in familial hypercholesterolemia. Am J Cardiol 57:29H, 1986.
50. Carew, TE, Schwenke, DC, and Steinberg, D: Antiatherogenic effect of probucol unrelated to its hypocholesterolemic effect: Evidence that antioxidants in vivo can selectively inhibit low density lipoprotein degradation in macrophage-rich fatty streaks and slow the progression of atherosclerosis in the Watanabe heritable hyperlipidemic rabbit. Proc Natl Acad Sci 84:7725, 1987.
51. Kita, T, Nagana, Y, Yokode, M, et al: Probucol prevents the progression of atherosclerosis in Watanabe heritable hyperlipidemic rabbit: An animal model for familial hypercholesterolemia. Proc Natl Acad Sci 84:5928, 1987.
52. Haynes, RB: A critical review of the "determinants" of patient compliance with therapeutic regimens. In Sacket, DL and Haynes, RB: Compliance with Therapeutic Regimens. The Johns Hopkins University Press, Baltimore, 1976.

CHAPTER 12

The Role of Exercise in the Primary and Secondary Prevention of Coronary Atherosclerotic Heart Disease

Henry B. Sadlo, M.D.
Nanette K. Wenger, M.D.

As the levels of health information and health consciousness have increased both among the general public and among cardiac patients, the populations of most industrialized nations have continued to assume a more active role in health enhancement and disease prevention. The morbidity and mortality from coronary atherosclerotic heart disease have decreased progressively and significantly in the United States during the past 20 years; coronary mortality has decreased faster than that from any other cause except stroke. This development has contributed substantially to the recent increase of more than two years in life expectancy for both men and women in the United States.[1] Primary and secondary preventive efforts have played an important role and can be further expected to impact favorably on coronary morbidity and mortality. Primary prevention refers to the modification of coronary risk factors prior to clinical evidence of disease. Secondary prevention involves measures that are designed to decrease the progression of clinically apparent coronary atherosclerosis, attempting to prevent recurrent myocardial infarction or sudden cardiac death.[2]

The relationship of habitual physical activity levels to the development of coronary atherosclerosis was highlighted in the 1950s by the pioneering work of Morris,[3] who described a lowered incidence of coronary events associated with an increase in occupational physical activity levels. To date, there is no unequivocal proof of this "exercise hypothesis"[4] for the primary prevention of coronary disease; only suggestive data are available regarding secondary prevention.[5] Despite the considerable and continuing debate about the contributions of exercise to reducing coronary risk, many, if not most, physicians consider that exercise (or physical activity) plays an important role in the prevention of coronary atherosclerosis and also recommend physical activity as a component of long-term management for coronary patients.[6] The American Heart Association Council on Cardiovascular Disease in the Young[7] has emphasized the importance of shaping ideas and habits of proper exercise beginning in childhood, citing the potential for instituting coronary risk modification at an early age.

This chapter reviews (1) the development of the concept of exercise/activity in the primary and secondary prevention of coronary atherosclerosis, (2) the analysis of exercise as a single coronary risk variable, (3) the effects of exercise on other coronary risk factors, and (4) the pivotal studies of exercise in the primary and secondary prevention of coronary atherosclerosis.

THE EXERCISE/CORONARY ATHEROSCLEROTIC HEART DISEASE RELATIONSHIP

Benefits of exercise in preserving one's health have been cited since ancient times. Cicero, in about 100 BC, commented that, "exercise and temperance can preserve something of our strength in old age."[8] Maimonides, a twelfth-century scholar and physician, recommended daily exercise and wrote in the Mishneh Torah that "anyone who sits around idle and takes no exercise will be subject to physical discomforts and failing strength."[8] The specific focus on the potential impact of exercise in the primary prevention of coronary atherosclerosis initially gained recognition in the 1950s with the British study of Morris and associates,[3] which suggested that the habitual activity level of an individual might favorably affect the development of coronary atherosclerosis.

During the subsequent four decades, physical activity has increasingly been considered a component of primary and secondary prevention. Based on a compilation of data on the extent of exercise in United States and Canadian populations in 1985, Stephens and associates[9] concluded that "approximately 20 percent exercise with an intensity and frequency generally recommended for cardiovascular benefit. An additional 40 percent are active at a more moderate level or less frequently, perhaps sufficient to receive some health benefits," and "at least 40 percent may be considered completely sedentary." A Gallup poll of daily leisure physical activity over the past three decades published in the Los Angeles Times Syndicate in 1984 suggested a 246 percent increase in leisure activity. When asked, "Aside from any work you do at home or at the job, do you do anything regularly, that is, on a daily basis, that helps keep you physically fit?" 24 percent answered positively in 1961, 47 percent in 1977, and 59 percent in 1984.[10] If the "exercise hypothesis" for the prevention of coronary atherosclerosis is true, whereas some United States and Canadian residents may have increased their habitual physical activity, a larger percentage of the population remains sedentary, with potential for improvement in future decades.

In 1987, the European Atherosclerosis Society Study Group concluded that although "proof of a causal role of exercise in reducing the risk of coronary heart disease is incomplete . . . the Study Group regards the evidence of a favorable effect as being sufficient to justify the recommendation of regular, frequent, appropriate aerobic exercise as part of a healthy life-style"[11] for primary prevention. Local authorities and central government were urged to become involved by "providing suitable facilities widely," for example, by providing bicycle paths, allowing adults to use school sports facilities, and developing "forest pathways and other rural facilities."[11]

Prior to the 1950s, most cardiologists advocated protracted bed rest for patients after myocardial infarction and further recommended that "when he becomes ambulatory, return to activities should be gradual and in most cases it will be desirable to urge that he should permanently diminish his activities to some extent."[12] In contemporary secondary prevention, early ambulation is routine following myocardial infarction, coronary artery bypass surgery, and percutaneous transluminal coronary angioplasty; most physicians recommend physical activity for patients following an uncomplicated myocardial infarction[13] and other coronary events.

EXERCISE AS A SINGLE CORONARY RISK VARIABLE

It is difficult to analyze the effect of exercise as a single variable in the prevention of coronary atherosclerosis.[14] Most men and women who are motivated to exercise also make health-related modifications in other aspects of daily living, such as improved dietary choices (lower cholesterol, lower saturated fat foods), weight control, and cessation of cigarette smoking. Thus, it is virtually impossible to find a study of the effect of exercise on coronary morbidity and mortality in which exercise has been the only variable modified in comparison with a control group.

Over the years, this problem has led to difficulty in scientifically establishing the role of exercise in the prevention of coronary morbidity and mortality. Designing a unifactorial trial of the effect of exercise on coronary morbidity and mortality—that is, attempting to alter only the exercise level between the study and control groups—would be unethical today, given the probable important role of cessation of cigarette smoking, control of hypertension, and modification of lipid profiles in the prevention of coronary atherosclerotic heart disease. Thus, whereas multifactorial trials are more appropriate, they decrease the ability to isolate exercise as a relevant factor in the reduction of coronary morbidity and mortality.

Because coronary atherosclerosis develops over many years, studies of exercise and its effect(s) on the primary prevention of coronary atherosclerosis would have to be carried out over decades before the appearance of sufficient clinical manifestations of coronary disease to enable statistically significant differences to be detected.

INFLUENCE OF EXERCISE ON OTHER CORONARY RISK FACTORS

In examining the effect(s) of exercise on the primary and secondary prevention of coronary atherosclerosis, it is appropriate to review the effects of exercise on each of the accepted major risk factors for the development of coronary atherosclerosis. Exercise has a favorable effect, directly or indirectly, on hyperlipidemia, hypertension, tobacco use, and diabetes mellitus. There are also significant beneficial effects of exercise on less well-proven risk factors for coronary atherosclerosis: coagulation factors, obesity, and psychologic profiles. The effect of exercise on each will be examined serially.

EXERCISE, LIPIDS, AND LIPOPROTEIN PROFILES

The Adult Treatment Panel of the United States National Cholesterol Education Program[15] recommends as desirable a blood cholesterol level below 200 mg/

dl and a low-density lipoprotein cholesterol (LDL-C) level below 130 mg/dl. A review of the chronic effects of physical activity on total cholesterol level concluded that the "relationship between physically active vocations and cholesterol concentration has not yet been resolved."[16] However, exercise appears to alter the lipoprotein subfractions of cholesterol. In some studies, high-density lipoprotein cholesterol (HDL-C) levels were substantially higher in endurance-trained athletes. However, a short-term (9 week) study of the effect of moderate exercise on HDL-C in healthy sedentary, nonsmoking, nonobese men did not show significant changes.[17] The effect of exercise on plasma LDL-C is small and variable. Exercise decreases triglyceride levels, owing primarily to enhanced triglyceride removal by skeletal muscle.[18] However, the role of triglycerides in the development of coronary atherosclerosis is not as well established as are decreased HDL-C and increased LDL-C levels.

Although moderate exercise appears to favorably alter the HDL-C/LDL-C ratio, further long-term studies are required to define with certainty the effect of exercise on lipoprotein profiles and its resultant influence on the primary and secondary prevention of coronary atherosclerosis.

A recent prospective, controlled study of overweight sedentary men by Wood and associates[61] demonstrated that losses in body fat, over a one-year period, regardless of whether achieved by dieting or by exercise, resulted in similar and significant increases in HDL-C when compared with the control group. Total cholesterol and LDL-C levels were not significantly changed.

EXERCISE AND HYPERTENSION

For some years, exercise has been recommended as one of the nonpharmacologic measures that can reduce elevated blood pressure levels. A recent review of the role of exercise in lowering blood pressure in persons with essential hypertension concluded that exercise training could produce an approximately 10 mm Hg reduction in systolic and diastolic blood pressures in these individuals.[19] The exact mechanism that produces this effect is unknown; changes in cardiac output or total peripheral resistance, or a combination of the two, could effect the beneficial blood pressure lowering. This and other reviews of the effects of exercise on hypertension have led both the IV U.S. Joint National Committee[20] and the World Health Organization[21] to recommend physical activity as an aid to the control of hypertension. Exercise-induced reductions in systolic and diastolic blood pressures should play a small but important role in retarding the atherosclerotic process.

EXERCISE AND SMOKING HABITS

Cigarette smoking is well established as a major risk factor for coronary atherosclerotic heart disease. One might postulate that individuals in an active exercise regimen would be more motivated than those in a control population to decrease or stop cigarette smoking; this is not necessarily so. Secondary prevention studies reported by Palatsi,[22] Kentala,[23] and Wilhelmsen[24] have shown no significant difference between the percentage of cigarette smokers in the exercise compared with the control group. Marra and associates[25] reported that, after 8 to 9 weeks of exercise, 22 percent of the exercise group continued to smoke as compared with 31.2 percent of the control group, which was not a statistically significant difference.

Although the percentage of smokers decreases following an initial episode of myocardial infarction, exercise programs do not appear to provide additional motivation for individuals to stop smoking cigarettes. In 9 years of follow-up after myocardial infarction, Roman and colleagues[26] showed that cigarette smoking decreased significantly in both the cardiac exercise rehabilitation and the control groups.

EXERCISE AND DIABETES MELLITUS

Regular exercise has a number of beneficial effects in patients with controlled diabetes mellitus; these benefits include enhanced insulin sensitivity, improved glucose tolerance, and lower plasma insulin levels.[27] Although these effects are important to a diabetic patient for control of the diabetes and potential slowing of its secondary complications, the effect and magnitude of exercise-improved diabetic control on atherogenesis has not been defined.

EXERCISE AND COAGULATION FACTORS

A recent review of the acute effects of exercise showed a number of alterations in blood coagulation factors. These alterations included a decrease in whole blood clotting time, an increase in plasma viscosity, an increase in factor VIII procoagulant activity, and increases in the platelet count, platelet aggregation, and production of beta-thromboglobulin and platelet factor IV in some patients.[28] These changes might lead one to infer that, from a coagulation standpoint, exercise is deleterious to individuals with coronary atherosclerosis. However, exercise also acutely increases fibrinolysis and endothelial prostacyclin, a vasodilator and an inhibitor of platelet aggregation, to produce a more balanced system.[28] As the role of coagulation factors, including endothelial factors, is further explored, a clearer picture of exercise-related coagulation changes may emerge, as may their ultimate effect on coronary morbidity and mortality.

EXERCISE AND OBESITY

The link between coronary atherosclerosis and obesity is less well-defined than that of the previously cited risk factors. The effect of obesity on atherogenesis cannot be evaluated independently, in that weight reduction is associated with a reduction in blood pressure levels and blood glucose levels and an increase in HDL-C levels. Thus, weight reduction in an obese individual may aid indirectly in prevention of coronary morbidity and mortality owing to its beneficial effect on hypertension and HDL cholesterol.

EXERCISE AND PSYCHOLOGIC WELL-BEING

There has been considerable controversy during the past few decades as to whether personality profiles influence the development of coronary atherosclerotic heart disease. Studies have examined differences in cardiovascular morbidity and mortality in persons with a Type A or *stress* behavior compared with those having Type B or less-stressed behavior profiles.

Although this debate continues, most agree that regular exercise of at least moderate intensity is associated with a reduction in symptoms of tension and may have an antidepressant effect.[29] Over time, the effect of exercise on the psychologic profile of an individual may influence the occurrence of coronary events; however, present data are only suggestive and further studies are needed.

EXERCISE AND THE PRIMARY PREVENTION OF CORONARY HEART DISEASE

During the past 4 decades, evidence has been mounting favoring the *exercise hypothesis* in the primary prevention of morbidity and mortality from coronary atherosclerotic heart disease. Several reviews have examined a variety of prospective and retrospective studies.[4,30–32] Of the 12 coronary incidence studies charted in a review by Oberman,[33] 8 revealed a positive correlation between physical inactivity and coronary atherosclerotic heart disease. Powell and associates[32] at the Centers for Disease Control examined 43 studies and provided a comprehensive assessment of the quality of each; they concluded that an inverse relationship between activity and coronary atherosclerotic heart disease "is consistently observed, especially in the better designed studies." They also considered the relative risk of inactivity "to be similar in magnitude to that of hypertension, hypercholesterolemia, and smoking" and recommended that "public policy that encourages regular physical activity should be pursued." The following section reviews several of these studies that merit special consideration.

A 1952 English study of the *exercise hypothesis* by Logan and Glasg[34] noted that coronary deaths were most common in professional men and least common in unskilled workers. In 1953, Morris and associates[3] published their comparison of coronary heart disease events among London transport workers, focusing on the differences between the more physically active conductors on the double-deck buses and the less active bus drivers. Both more fatal myocardial infarctions and more episodes of sudden death occurred among the more sedentary drivers. This study has been challenged subsequently in that the drivers tended to be more overweight even at hiring, had higher blood pressures, and higher blood cholesterol levels. Nevertheless, this landmark study stimulated interest in the relationship between a group's physical activity level and coronary atherosclerosis.

A large number of diverse populations were subsequently analyzed in separate studies: Los Angeles civil servants,[35] United States railroad workers,[36] North Dakota residents,[37] residents of rural Italy,[38] East and West Finland residents,[39] Israeli kibbutzim residents,[40] and Evans County, Georgia residents,[41] to name a few that illustrate this diversity. Most earlier studies focused more on the measurement of coronary events than on the measurement of physical activity and thus were somewhat less than convincing. Powell and associates[32] rated the quality of the physical activity measures in 20 early studies as unsatisfactory in 13, satisfactory in 6, and good in only one (San Francisco longshoremen[42]). Thus, variations in activity measurement in the earlier studies compounded the difficulty of comparing one study with another. Despite these weaknesses, most early studies demonstrated an increased relative risk of coronary heart disease in the less active groups. This stimulated the organization of prospective studies with more detailed and scientific analyses of physical activity levels.

The San Francisco longshoremen study of Brand and associates,[42] in which nearly 4000 longshoremen were followed for 22 years, was one of the earliest prospective studies to define physical activity measurements in metabolic terms (kcal per min). After adjusting for factors such as age, race, systolic blood pressure, smoking, body mass index, glucose intolerance, and electrocardiographic status, men with a high work activity (7 kcal per min above basal metabolic level) had about half the rate of fatal heart attack of men in the lowest work activity category (1 kcal per min). Despite some minor weaknesses, this study provided further support for the exercise hypothesis and offered a "prudent basis for the possible protective effect against coronary heart disease of physical exercise by a healthy individual."[42]

The Framingham Heart Study contributed further data about exercise and coronary atherosclerosis. In a cohort study published in 1979, Kannel and Sorlie[43] reported that both overall mortality and mortality from cardiovascular and ischemic heart disease in men were inversely related to their level of physical activity. Daily activity was tabulated by assigning a 1.0 weight factor to basal activity (sleep, rest) up to a 5.0 weight factor for heavy activity; this approach enabled the summation of a total daily activity score for each individual. A person who slept or was at rest for an entire day, for example, received a score of 24. The age-adjusted death rate of men aged 35 to 64, free of cardiovascular disease, revealed an incidence rate of cardiovascular death of 8.5 percent in the group with the lowest (24 to 29) physical activity index, compared with a 5 percent incidence in the group with the highest physical activity index (38 to 83). The incidence rates of ischemic heart disease deaths were 6 and 4 percent, respectively, for the lowest and highest physical activity groups. Despite the subjective measurement of physical activity based on recall, Powell and associates[32] rated the quality of the measure of physical activity, of the coronary heart disease (CHD) measure, and of the epidemiologic methods as good for all three categories. This study was one of only 2 among 16 cohort studies reviewed that received "good" ratings in all three categories. The other study that merited a high-quality rating, an evaluation of 8155 male Puerto Rican residents, also demonstrated an increase in cardiovascular morbidity and mortality as physical activity decreased ($p < 0.05$).[44]

Further support to the exercise hypothesis for primary prevention was provided by Paffenbarger and associates in 1978 in a cohort study of 19,936 Harvard alumni.[45] Questionnaires were mailed to the Harvard alumni who had entered Harvard between 1916 and 1950. Those free of apparent heart attack were followed for the study endpoints of heart attack, death from any cause, age 75, or until the end of the observation period (1972); follow-up ranged from 6 to 10 years. Activity, analyzed by questionnaire, involved the number of flights of stairs climbed daily, the number of city blocks or equivalent walked each day, and the amount of time (weekly) of participation in light and strenuous sports. A physical activity index, measured in kcal per week, was derived from these data. A sharp reduction in both nonfatal and fatal heart attack rates occurred up to an activity level of 2000 to 2999 kcal per week; beyond this level of activity, no further significant change was apparent. Thus, the less active group (<2000 kcal per week) was at a 64 percent increased risk of heart attack when compared with the more active group (2000+ kcal per week). Importantly, previous strenuous activity (for example, varsity athletics during college years) did not confer a lower risk. Ex-varsity athletes retained their lower risk status only if they sustained high physical activity indexes as alumni. This argues against "self selection," a concept discussed as a prime weakness of some of the earlier population studies; that is, a more coronary-prone person might select a less active job. Paffenbarger and associates[45] concluded that the "risk of heart attack is increased if physical activity is reduced below favorable levels, and risk is lowered if adequate exercise is maintained."

A more recent primary prevention study, the Multiple Risk Factor Intervention Trial (MRFIT), evaluated the contribution of several factors, including physical activity, to the reduction in CHD mortality among 12,138 middle-aged men.[46] Study subjects were divided into three categories based on the amount of their leisure-time physical activity. Total mean leisure-time physical activity measured 15.2 minutes per day in the low-activity group, compared with 47.4 minutes per day in the moderate-activity group and 133.6 minutes per day in the high-activity group. There was a significant ($p < 0.01$) reduction in fatal coronary events between the low-activity and moderate-activity groups but not between the moderate-activity and high-activity groups. The age-adjusted risk ratios for coronary death were 1.00, 0.63, and 0.64, respectively for the low, moderate, and high leisure-time physical activity groups. Fewer differences were evident in fatal/nonfatal myocardial infarction among the three groups (1.00/low, 0.88/moderate, and 0.81/high). The overall conclusion was that, "leisure-time physical activity has a modest inverse relation to coronary heart disease and overall mortality in middle-aged men at high risk for coronary heart disease."[46]

The Lipid Research Clinics Mortality Follow-up Study enabled Ekelund and associates[62] to examine physical fitness as a predictor of cardiovascular mortality in asymptomatic North American men. Treadmill exercise testing, using a modified Bruce protocol, was used to measure cardiovascular fitness. A healthy group, patients without evidence of cardiovascular disease, was divided into quartiles depending on their peak heart rate after at least 1 minute of stage II of the exercise test. The rate of coronary and cardiovascular death over a mean of 8.5 years of follow-up revealed a substantial increase in each quartile as the cardiovascular fitness decreased. The conclusion was that "a lower level of physical fitness is associated with a higher risk of death from coronary heart disease and cardiovascular disease in clinically healthy men, independent of conventional coronary risk factors."

The recent U.S. Railroad Study[65] showed that leisure-time physical activity, particularly in occupationally sedentary men, protected against death from CHD and decreased all-cause mortality.

Not all studies support the exercise hypothesis. Paul[47] considers the evidence that exercise prevents coronary artery disease inconclusive and reviews the data that failed to demonstrate a protective effect of exercise. Studies by Rosenman,[48] Elmfeldt,[49] and Paul[50] and their colleagues did not show significant differences in coronary heart disease between the active and less active groups. Four of 12 recent coronary incidence studies also revealed no relationship between physical inactivity and CHD.[33]

Nonetheless, the majority of studies demonstrate a favorable effect of exercise on the primary prevention of CHD. Thus, many leaders in preventive medicine and cardiovascular epidemiology recommend exercise, in addition to avoidance of cigarette smoking, control of blood pressure, and control of serum cholesterol levels, for the primary prevention of CHD.

EXERCISE AND THE SECONDARY PREVENTION OF CHD

The benefit of exercise in the secondary prevention of CHD is a more recent concept. The historical perspective, as discussed by Wenger,[51] notes the change in ideas about physical activity following myocardial infarction. In the early 1900s, immobilization and protracted bed rest was the rule; in the 1940s, the Levine "chair treatment of coronary thrombosis" allowed the patient to sit in a chair for 1 to 2 hours daily beginning on the first day after infarction; currently, structured early ambulation regimens are routine for many patients recovering from myocardial infarction.

Beginning in the 1970s, reports of prospective randomized studies examined the potential benefits of posthospital exercise in patients with CHD. Siegel and associates[52] reviewed pooled data from nine randomized controlled trials of exercise in survivors of myocardial infarction. A statistically significant reduction in mortality was evident among the exercisers, although compliance with the recommended exercise was generally poor. Only 13 to 60 percent of patients in the different studies attended more than 70 percent of the exercise sessions, and a number of the "control" patients participated in regular exercise. Another review of pooled data regarding exercise rehabilitation following myocardial infarction also revealed a statistically significant reduction in cardiovascular death in the intervention groups (9.9 percent in the rehabilitation groups versus 12.6 percent in the control groups).[53] Several of the larger exercise trials are described subsequently.

The United States National Exercise and Heart Disease Project[54] was a multicenter, randomized clinical trial of the effects of 3 years of prescribed supervised exercise on 651 survivors of myocardial infarction. The cumulative 3 year mortality rate, 7.3 percent for the control group and 4.6 percent for the exercise group, did not show a statistically significant difference. Nor did the rate of recurrent myocardial infarction, 7.0 percent in the control group and 5.3 in the exercise group, differ significantly. The weaknesses of this study include the small numbers of patients enrolled, the short time period of follow-up (3 years), and the late enrollment of patients (over 40 percent entered the study 12 months or longer after their initial infarction). Also, it is noteworthy that 23 percent of the exercise group patients were not exercising after 2 years, whereas 31 percent of the control patients alleged that they exercised regularly.

The Ontario (Canada) Exercise–Heart Collaborative Study[55] involved a similar number of patients recovered from myocardial infarction who were randomized to a *low-intensity* or a *high-intensity* exercise group. Note that there was no true control population. All patients received a preliminary exercise test to document the heart rate and its relation to oxygen uptake. The low-intensity exercise group met once weekly for "relaxation and supervised recreational activities such as volleyball, bowling, or swimming;" the patient's heart rate was checked to ensure that it did not exceed the heart rate observed at 50 percent of that individual's estimated maximal oxygen uptake. The high-intensity group exercised four times each week by walking or jogging at a pace that raised the heart rate to a level corresponding to 65 to 85 percent of the individual's estimated maximal oxygen uptake. The study analyzed only the endpoint of re-infarction and found no statistically significant differences between the two groups. Again, the dropout rate was high, 45.4 percent, although similar in both groups. There was no evidence of increased risk from high-intensity exercise.

Studies of cardiac rehabilitation/physical training after myocardial infarction from Italy,[25] Chile,[26] and Sweden[24] also were unable to demonstrate statistically significant differences between the control and exercise groups. The Italian study[25] showed a trend for the exercising group to be more symptom-free (44 versus 30 percent) and to have a lower rate of re-infarction (6.1 versus 11.2 percent); however, the numbers were small. The study from Chile[26] also showed a trend toward reduced mortality rate and a statistically significant reduction in angina frequency in the exercise group compared with the control group. The Swedish study[24] showed a decrease in 4-year total mortality in the exercising group, but this finding did not reach statistical significance.

More recently, Blumenthal and colleagues[63] enrolled 45 patients with a recent myocardial infarction (median 8 weeks) in either a low- or high-intensity training group. During 3 months, the low-intensity group exercised three times weekly for 30 to 45 minutes at an intensity level less than 45 percent of their maximal oxygen consumption rate. The high-intensity group exercised at similar intervals but gradually increased the exercise intensity from 50 percent to 75 percent of their maximal oxygen consumption rate. Both groups demonstrated statistically similar improvements in mean maximal oxygen consumption rates, an 11 percent increase in the high-intensity versus a 14 percent increase in the low-intensity group; and both groups experienced significant increases in HDL-C. The authors concluded that comparable cardiorespiratory improvement occurred with low-intensity and high-intensity exercise during the initial 3 months of exercise training following acute myocardial infarction.

Although individual studies of exercise in the secondary prevention of CHD have been unable to demonstrate a statistically significant reduction in coronary morbidity and mortality, possibly because of the small number of patients and the short duration of the studies, pooled data suggest benefit.[5,52,53] Despite the potential risks of exercise in patients known to have coronary disease these secondary prevention trials demonstrated that supervised exercise was reasonably safe and could reduce anginal symptoms and provide other noncardiac benefits, including improvement in the patient's psychologic profile. Exercise training also may demonstrate to the patient the amount of physical activity that can be safely performed without concern of sudden death or re-infarction. In summary, as suggested by Furberg,[5] although "trials of adequate size are needed to determine with certainty the preventive value of physical exercise," its contemporary clinical application is widespread.

POTENTIAL EXERCISE RISKS AND EXERCISE CONTRAINDICATIONS IN PATIENTS WITH CORONARY ARTERY DISEASE

The potential risks of exercise training for secondary prevention include an increase in angina pectoris, myocardial infarction, arrhythmias, and sudden cardiac death as well as musculoskeletal problems (mostly sprains but occasionally more complex orthopedic injuries). Absolute contraindications to exercise training for coronary patients include uncontrolled arrhythmias, uncontrolled hypertension, uncontrolled congestive heart failure, unstable angina pectoris, and the initial days following acute myocardial infarction. Numerous cardiac and noncardiac relative contraindications should be evaluated on an individual basis by a physician familiar with the patient. In a 1978 multicenter review of cardiovascular complications during exercise training of cardiac patients, Haskell[56] reported data for 13,570 patients in 30 North American centers, for a total of 1,629,634 patient-hours of supervised exercise. There were 50 cardiac arrests, of which 8 were fatal, and 7 myocardial infarctions, 2 fatal. A more recent review by Van Camp and Petersen[57] collected data from 167 rehabilitation programs involving 51,303 exercising patients; a total of 21 cardiac arrests occurred (3 fatal), and 8 episodes of nonfatal myocardial infarction. This represents one cardiac arrest for every 111,996 patient-hours of exercise and one myocardial infarction for every 293,990 patient-hours. Neither the size of the exercise group nor the presence or extent of ECG monitoring made any statistically significant difference. These data support the reasonable safety of exercise training for appropriately selected coronary patients. Another study evaluated home versus supervised group exercise training in low-risk patients following myocardial infarction;[58] improvement in functional capacity was similar in both groups at 26 weeks, and there were no training-related complications in either group. Because not all coronary patients can or choose to participate in a structured and supervised cardiac exercise program, the safety and efficacy of unsupervised home exercise for low-risk coronary patients is encouraging.

SUMMARY: EXERCISE RECOMMENDATIONS

Exercise is recommended increasingly by physicians as a component of the primary and secondary prevention of CHD. At present, the evidence appears adequate to recommend exercise training, although studies with larger numbers of patients for longer time periods are necessary to document benefit unequivocally. It is unlikely that exercise as an isolated intervention will ever be evaluated by a major study.

An important but unanswered question is the amount of exercise required for cardiovascular benefit. For primary prevention, the American Heart Association[59] recommends "repetitive, large muscle dynamic exercise for extended periods of time. The intensity of the exercise should increase the heart rate to more than 60 percent of the individual's work intensity. The exercise should be maintained for at least 30 minutes and be performed at least three times weekly."

Åstrand's[60] recommendations for maintaining physical fitness are similar. He advises daily physical activity to total at least 60 minutes of moving, walking, climbing stairs, and so on, in any combination (i.e., 1 minute 60 times a day or 12 minutes 5 times a day) for a total of approximately 1.2 MJ or 300 kcal per week. In addition, he advises intense exercise such as brisk walking, jogging, aerobic dancing, swimming, cycling, or cross-country skiing to total 30 minutes two or three times weekly; this level of activity entails 3 MJ or 750 kcal per week. This combination should help maintain physical fitness and aid in the primary prevention of CHD. Individuals over 35 years of age or those with a family history of premature coronary atherosclerosis or other medical problems should check with a physician prior to beginning an exercise program.

For secondary prevention, the exercise intensity should be individualized for each patient, prescribed by a physician, and based on the results of recent exercise testing. Traditionally, it is recommended that patients with coronary disease exercise to 70 to 85 percent of the highest heart rate safely achieved at exercise testing. This regimen includes a period of stretching or warm-up exercise, followed by higher-intensity exercise to achieve the target heart rate range for about 30 minutes two to three times weekly, followed by a cool-down period. Many middle-aged or older patients find longer exercise sessions (for example, 45 to 60 minutes) at a lesser intensity (that is, a 60 to 75 percent heart rate range) more enjoyable; similar training benefit appears to be attained in this manner, with an increased likelihood of patient adherence and potential lessened risk in an unsupervised setting.

It appears likely that the morbidity and mortality of CHD will continue to decline during the next decade and that exercise training will contribute to this favorable trend.

Guidelines for exercise implementation for individuals both with and without ischemic heart disease are presented by Haskell;[64] examples of exercise prescriptions are provided, with a discussion of some of the pitfalls of exercise programs and methods to avoid them.

ACKNOWLEDGMENT

The authors acknowledge with gratitude the technical assistance of Mrs. Denise Fennell in the preparation of this manuscript.

REFERENCES

1. Levy, RI and Moskowitz, J: Cardiovascular research: Decades of progress, a decade of promise. Science 217:121, 1982.
2. Wenger, NK and Schlant, RC: Prevention of coronary atherosclerosis. In Hurst, JW (ed): The Heart, ed 6. McGraw-Hill Book Company, New York, 1986.
3. Morris, JN, Heady, JA, Raffle, PAB, et al: Coronary heart disease and physical activity of work. Lancet 2:1053, 1953.
4. Eichner, ER: Exercise and heart disease: Epidemiology of the "exercise hypothesis." Am J Med 75:1008, 1983.
5. Furberg, CD: Secondary prevention trials after acute myocardial infarction. Am J Cardiol 60:28A, 1987.
6. Wenger, NK, Hellerstein, HK, Blackburn, H, et al: Physician practice in the management of patients with uncomplicated myocardial infarction—changes in the past decade. Circulation 65:421, 1982.
7. Riopel, DA, Boerth, RC, Coates, TJ, et al: Coronary risk factor modification in children: Exercise. A Statement for Physicians by the Committee on Atherosclerosis and Hypertension in Childhood of the Council on Cardiovascular Disease in the Young, American Heart Association. Circulation 74:1189A, 1986.
8. Wynder, EL: The Book of Health. The American Health Foundation. Franklin Watts, New York, 1981.
9. Stephens, T, Jacobs, DR, and White, CC: A descriptive epidemiology of leisure-time physical activity. Pub Health Rep 100:147, 1985.
10. The Gallup Poll: Six of 10 adults exercise daily. Los Angeles Times Syndicate, Los Angeles, May 1984.
11. Study Group, European Atherosclerosis Society: Strategies for the prevention of coronary heart disease: A policy statement of the European Atherosclerosis Society. Eur Heart J 8:77, 1987.
12. Levine, SA: Clinical Heart Disease, ed 2. WB Saunders, Philadelphia, 1940.
13. Wenger, NK: Rehabilitation of the coronary patient: Status 1986. Prog Cardiovasc Dis 29:181, 1986.
14. Stamler, J: Review of primary prevention trials of coronary heart disease. Acta Med Scand (Suppl)701:100, 1985.
15. The Expert Panel: Report of the National Cholesterol Education Program Expert Panel on detection, evaluation and treatment of high blood cholesterol in adults. Arch Intern Med 148:36, 1988.
16. Goldberg, L and Elliot, DL: The effect of physical activity on lipid and lipoprotein levels. In Goldberg, L and Elliot, DL (eds): Symposium on Medical Aspects of Exercise. Med Clin North Am 69:1, 1985.
17. Raz, I, Rosenblit, H, and Kark, J: Effect of moderate exercise on serum lipids in young men with low high density lipoprotein cholesterol. Arteriosclerosis 8:245, 1988.
18. Sady, SP, Cullinane, EM, Saritelli, A, et al: Elevated high-density lipoprotein cholesterol in endurance athletes is related to enhanced plasma triglyceride clearance. Metabolism 37:568, 1988.
19. Hagberg, JM and Seals, DR: Exercise training and hypertension. Acta Med Scand (Suppl)711:131, 1986.

20. IV Joint National Committee: The 1988 Report of the Joint National Committee on Detection, Evaluation, and Treatment of High Blood Pressure. Arch Intern Med 148:1023, 1988.
21. Guidelines for treatment of mild hypertension: Memorandum from a WHO/ISH meeting. Hypertension 5:394, 1983.
22. Palatsi, I: Feasibility of physical training after myocardial infarction and its effect on return to work, morbidity and mortality. Acta Med Scand (Suppl)599:1, 1976.
23. Kentala, E: Physical fitness and feasibility of physical rehabilitation after myocardial infarction in men of working age. Ann Clin Res (Suppl 9)4:1, 1972.
24. Wilhelmsen, L, Sanne, H, Elmfeldt, D, et al: A controlled trial of physical training after myocardial infarction. Effects on risk factors, nonfatal reinfarction and death. Prev Med 4:491, 1975.
25. Marra, S, Paolillo, V, Spadaccini, F, et al: Long-term follow-up after a controlled randomized post-myocardial infarction rehabilitation programme: Effects on morbidity and mortality. Eur Heart J 6:656, 1985.
26. Román, O, Guitierrez, M, Luksic, I, et al: Cardiac rehabilitation after acute myocardial infarction. Cardiology 70:223, 1983.
27. Schneider, SH, Vitug, A, and Ruderman, N: Atherosclerosis and physical activity. Diabetes/Metabolism Rev 1:513, 1986.
28. Colwell, JA: Effects of exercise on platelet function, coagulation, and fibrinolysis. Diabetes/Metabolism Rev 1:501, 1986.
29. Dishman, RK: Medical psychology in exercise and sport, In Goldberg, L and Elliott, DL (eds): Symposium on medical aspects of exercise. Med Clin North Am 69:123, 1985.
30. Oberman, A: Exercise and the primary prevention of cardiovascular disease. Am J Cardiol 55:10D, 1985.
31. Leon, AS: Physical activity levels and coronary heart disease: Analysis of epidemiologic and supporting studies. In Goldberg, L and Elliot, DL (eds): Symposium on medical aspects of exercise. Med Clin North Am 69:3, 1985.
32. Powell, KE, Thompson, PD, Caspersen, CJ, et al: Physical activity and the incidence of coronary heart disease. Ann Rev Public Health 8:253, 1987.
33. Oberman, A: The role of exercise in preventing coronary heart disease. In Rapaport, E (ed): Current Controversies in Cardiovascular Disease. WB Saunders Company, Philadelphia, 1980.
34. Logan, WPD and Glasg, MD: Mortality and coronary and myocardial disease in different social classes. Lancet 1:758, 1952.
35. Chapman, JM, Goerke, LS, Dixon, W, et al: The clinical status of a population group in Los Angeles under observation for two to three years. Am J Pub Health 47:33, 1957.
36. Taylor, HL, et al: Five year follow-up of employees of selected U.S. railroad companies. Circulation 41 (Suppl)1:20,1970.
37. Zukel, WJ, et al: A short-term community study of the epidemiology of coronary heart disease. Am J Pub Health 49:1630, 1959.
38. Fidanza, F, et al: Five year experience in rural Italy. Circulation (Suppl 1)41:63, 1970.
39. Punsar, S and Karvonen, MJ: Physical activity and coronary heart disease in populations from East and West Finland. Adv Cardiol 18:196, 1976.
40. Brunner, D, et al: Physical activity at work and the incidence of myocardial infarction, angina pectoris, and death due to ischemic heart disease: An epidemiological study in Israeli collective settlements (kibbutzim). J Chronic Dis 27:217, 1974.
41. Cassel, J, et al: Occupation and physical activity and coronary heart disease. Arch Intern Med 128:920, 1971.
42. Brand, RJ, et al: Work activity and fatal heart attack studied by multiple logistic risk analysis. Am J Epidemiol 110:52, 1979.
43. Kannel, WB and Sorlie, P: Some health benefits of physical activity: The Framingham Study. Arch Intern Med 139:857, 1979.
44. Garcia-Palmieri, MR, Costas, R, Jr, Cruz-Vidal, M, et al: Increased physical activity: A protective factor against heart attacks in Puerto Rico. Am J Cardiol 50:749, 1982.
45. Paffenbarger, RS, Wing, AL, and Hyde, RT: Physical activity as an index of heart attack risk in college alumni. Am J Epidemiol 108:161, 1978.
46. Leon, AS, Connet, J, Jacobs, DR, et al: Leisure-time physical activity levels and risk of coronary heart disease and death: The Multiple Risk Factor Intervention Trial. JAMA 258:2388, 1987.
47. Paul, O: Exercise and the prevention of coronary artery disease: The evidence is inconclusive. In Rapaport, E (ed): Current Controversies in Cardiovascular Disease. WB Saunders Company, Philadelphia, 1980.

48. Rosenman, RH, Brand, RJ, Jenkins, CD, et al: Coronary heart disease in the Western Collaborative Group Study: Final follow-up experience of 8½ years. JAMA 233:875, 1975.
49. Elmfeldt, D, Wilhemsson, C; Vedin, A, et al: Characteristics of representative male survivors of myocardial infarction compared with representative population samples. Acta Med Scand 199:387, 1976.
50. Paul, O: Physical activity and coronary heart disease. Am J Cardiol 23:303, 1969.
51. Wenger, NK: Early ambulation after myocardial infarction: Rationale, program components, and results. In Wenger, NK and Hellerstein, HK (eds): Rehabilitation of the Coronary Patient. 2nd ed. John Wiley, New York, 1984.
52. Siegel, D, Grady, D, Browner, WS, et al: Risk factor modification after myocardial infarction. Ann Intern Med 109:213, 1988.
53. Oldridge, NB, Guyatt, GH, Fischer, ME, et al: Cardiac rehabilitation after myocardial infarction: Combined experience of randomized clinical trials. JAMA 260:945, 1988.
54. Shaw, LW: Effects of a prescribed supervised exercise program on mortality and cardiovascular morbidity in patients after a myocardial infarction: The National Exercise and Heart Disease Project. Am J Cardiol 48:39, 1981.
55. Rechnitzer, PA, Cunningham, DA, Andrew, GM, et al: Relation of exercise to the recurrence rate of myocardial infarction in men: Ontario Exercise–Heart Collaborative Study. Am J Cardiol 51:65, 1983.
56. Haskell, WL: Cardiovascular complications during exercise training of cardiac patients. Circulation 57:920, 1978.
57. Van Camp, SP and Peterson, RA: Cardiovascular complications of outpatient cardiac rehabilitation programs. JAMA 256:1160, 1986.
58. Miller, NH, Haskell, WL, Berra, K, et al: Home versus group exercise training for increasing functional capacity after myocardial infarction. Circulation 70:645, 1984.
59. American Heart Association: Statement on Exercise. Circulation 64:1327A, 1981.
60. Åstrand, P: Why exercise? An evolutionary approach. Acta Med Scand (Suppl)711:241, 1986.
61. Wood, PD, Stefanick, ML, Dreon, DM, et al: Changes in plasma lipids and lipoproteins in overweight men during weight loss through dieting as compared with exercise. N Engl J Med 319:1173, 1988.
62. Ekelund, L-G, Haskell, WL, Johnson, JJ, et al: Physical fitness as a predictor of cardiovascular mortality in asymptomatic North American men: The Lipid Research Clinics Mortality Followup Study. N Engl J Med 319:1379, 1988.
63. Blumenthal, JA, Rejeski, WJ, Walsh-Riddle, M, et al: Comparison of high- and low-intensity exercise training early after acute myocardial infarction. Am J Cardiol 61:26, 1988.
64. Haskell, WL: Elements and evaluation of physical activity in the prevention and management of ischemic heart disease. J Am Coll Cardiol 12:1091, 1988.
65. Slattery, MC, Jacobs, DR, Jr, and Nichaman, MZ: Leisure-time physical activity and coronary heart disease death. The U.S. Railroad Study. Circulation 79:304, 1989.

CHAPTER 13

Supervised and Unsupervised Exercise for the General Population and Patients with Known Cardiac Disease

Jerome D. Cohen, M.D.
Mark D. Wittry, M.D.

Cardiovascular disease is by far the number one cause of death in the United States despite the fact that over the past two decades deaths have diminished. Acute myocardial infarction occurs in approximately 1.5 million people per year, and one third of all cases are fatal.[1,2] An alteration of cardiac risk factors therefore can have a potentially large impact. Unfortunately, some cardiac risk factors cannot be modified (that is, advancing age, male sex, and a family history of coronary artery disease), whereas others may be altered only at potentially great cost (for example, pharmacologic treatment of hypertension). A sedentary life-style is the most prevalent of the cardiac risk factors and given the potential that exercise can have on disease progression, from a public health perspective, increasing physical activity is the most beneficial alteration that Americans can make.[3]

In addition to the benefits of exercise training on cardiovascular fitness per se, increased physical activity may have beneficial effects on several other risk factors. Although there are potential risks, in the great majority of people the benefits outweigh the risks. In this chapter, the potential benefits and complications of routine exercise are discussed as they pertain to both the general population and to individuals with known heart disease. Guidelines for initial screening of individuals wishing to participate in regular exercise are discussed as well as recommendations for structuring both supervised and unsupervised exercise aimed at improving cardiovascular conditioning.

BENEFITS OF EXERCISE

CARDIOVASCULAR EFFECTS

The cardiovascular effects of physical conditioning have been well studied. Blood pressure response during exercise and as a result of conditioning may vary dependent on the age of the subject. In young, normal subjects, systolic blood pressure increases during exercise while diastolic pressure remains unchanged.[4] In the absence of weight loss, little or no change occurs in resting blood pressure after a physical training program, although some studies have suggested that resting systolic and diastolic blood pressures may be lowered an average of 10 mm Hg dependent on activity level.[5-8] For older individuals and those with hypertension, this response differs. During acute exercise, the peak systolic blood pressure and pressure-rate products will rise higher compared with younger individuals, indicating a decrease in arterial compliance.[9] Improvement in exercise capacity usually results in a lowering of systolic, diastolic, and mean arterial blood pressures. Several studies have suggested a decrease in cardiac events for hypertensive individuals who routinely exercise compared with hypertensive sedentary individuals.[10]

Routine exercise will lower heart rate response to exercise.[11] The reasons are most likely due to alterations in stroke volume, a resetting of carotid baroreceptors, or both. A downgrading of the autonomic nervous system may result in lower circulating catecholamine levels, with a resultant decrease in resting pulse rate.[12]

An increase in stroke volume occurs in response to acute exercise, with a resultant increase in cardiac output at peak exercise.[13] Repetitive exercise results in a persistent increase in stroke volume, probably via both central (cardiac) and peripheral adaptations.[14] The increased stroke volume largely accounts for the improved maximal cardiac output regularly observed from training. Oxygen and nutrient delivery are augmented, allowing muscles to convert from oxidative to anaerobic metabolism (anaerobic threshold) at a higher level of exertion. This adaptation is readily documented by an increased maximal oxygen consumption (VO_2max),[15] which is reflected in an increased endurance and in more efficient heart rate responses to submaximal workloads.

Although blood pressure and pulse-rate responsiveness may be lowered and cardiac output and anaerobic threshold improved, the major benefit of exercise may be a reduction in cardiovascular morbidity and mortality. Many studies have established the role of physical inactivity as a cardiac risk factor, and they show a trend toward lower cardiac risk in individuals who are physically active.[16-18]

Kannel and Sorlie[19] reviewed the risk of cardiovascular disease due to physical inactivity in the Framingham population. When multivariate analysis was performed, increased physical activity had a separate, protective effect for both men and women. The relative risk of physical inactivity for all cardiovascular disease increased with advancing age; it was 1.1 for individuals between the ages of 35 and 44 and 1.3 in older age groups.

In a study by Morris and colleagues,[20] the incidence of first clinical cardiac events was twice as common in sedentary male civil servants as compared with those who performed vigorous exercise during leisure time (activities included swimming, jogging, and cycling). The degree of disparity was even more marked for overall fatality, with a threefold reduction (1.5 percent versus 5.0 percent).

Analysis of the Multiple Risk Factor Intervention Trial also has documented the role of physical exercise in lowering the risk of first cardiac events.[21] During 7 years of follow-up, moderate physical activity was associated with 37 percent fewer fatal cardiac events when compared with low levels of leisure activity. Similar benefits also were observed for men with high levels of physical leisure-time activity. These results were statistically significant even after adjustment for other factors, and they were observed in both the special intervention and usual care groups. Similar reductions in mortality and overall event rates have been reported by several other workers as well.[22–24]

Among individuals who have survived a myocardial infarction, data suggest that routine exercise is also of benefit. The National Exercise and Heart Disease Project demonstrated a 48 percent reduction in mortality,[25] and although not statistically significant owing to the small sample, the results are comparable with other studies. No change in the incidence of nonfatal events has been detected, suggesting that the benefits of exercise may be related to mechanisms that influence the acute event, including a reduction in ischemia, ventricular fibrillation threshold, and platelet effects.

BLOOD LIPID EFFECTS

In the absence of weight loss, total serum cholesterol is unaffected by routine exercise. However, high-density lipoprotein cholesterol (HDL-C) usually increases directly with the frequency and intensity of exercise,[26] and very low-density lipoprotein cholesterol (VLDL-C) decreases with a concomitant reduction in serum triglycerides.[27–30] These changes occur after several months of exercise and disappear when exercise is discontinued. Wood and associates[31] have examined these relationships and have quantified the change in each that can be expected for a specific level of exercise. Although these changes are potentially beneficial with respect to the risk of coronary artery disease, it is uncertain whether these effects are related to physiologic changes resulting from exercise. It is common to find accompanying changes in diet composition and body weight, each of which may contribute to favorable changes in blood lipid profiles, including a reduction in LDL-C.

EFFECTS ON BODY WEIGHT AND COMPOSITION

Many studies have documented the benefits of increasing physical activity on weight loss. In three separate studies, when dietary intake was controlled, a routine exercise regimen resulted in an average weight loss of 6.7 kg.[32–35] Among obese individuals, weight loss has definite cardiovascular benefits. Peripheral arterial resistance is usually decreased, and aerobic exercise capacity is increased. Favorable changes in blood lipids, carbohydrate metabolism, and uric acid production have all been well documented.

Physical inactivity at an extreme can cause disuse atrophy with loss of muscle mass. There is a change in body composition with an increase in body fat among those who are sedentary. With routine physical training, weight loss that occurs is due primarily to a decrease in percent body fat, and lean body mass loss is minimized as well.[36] This is why at least modest exercise should be part of every weight loss program.

CHANGES IN CARBOHYDRATE METABOLISM

In normal individuals, there is no change in serum glucose levels during exercise, despite a reduction in serum insulin levels. Similar responses are found with submaximal exercise in diabetic patients. With progressively higher-intensity exertion, differences in the response of well-controlled diabetics can be seen compared with those poorly controlled.[37] Acute exercise results in a progressive lowering of serum glucose in controlled diabetics.[38] There is the potential for hypoglycemia, which should be guarded against. In uncontrolled diabetics, the serum glucose level usually remains constantly high.

Of more importance is the response to chronic exercise. Insulin-dependent diabetics appear to have a slower clearance of exogenous insulin, with a resultant lowering of insulin requirements.[39,40] Noninsulin-dependent diabetics demonstrate a lowering of serum glucose levels, with both an increase in insulin receptors and endogenous insulin production.[41] Although these changes can facilitate the management of the diabetic patient, close supervision is necessary, and there is the need to maintain the exercise regimen because the effects are lost within 2 weeks of inactivity.

PSYCHOLOGIC EFFECTS

Vigorous routine exercise consistently has been associated with a reduction in anxiety and the physiologic manifestations of stress.[42] Individuals who exercise generally improve their self-esteem. Self-confidence and cognition may also be improved.[43] An improvement in IQ may occur in mentally retarded individuals.[44] Exercise can help the depressed or schizophrenic patient, but maintaining motivation is often a problem.[45]

POTENTIAL COMPLICATIONS OF VIGOROUS EXERCISE

Like other types of intervention, exercise has potential complications, but most are minor. However, serious complications, including death, can occur. These untoward results can be minimized if proper precautions are taken.

ORTHOPEDIC PRECAUTIONS

The joints of the lower extremities are prone to trauma from even low-intensity physical exertion. Trained athletes are able to minimize these occurences by applied kinesiology and gradual buildup in training routines. Nevertheless, even well-trained athletes encounter minor orthopedic injuries such as sprained ankles, stress fractures, and tendinitis.[46-48]

The average person usually begins to exercise at a level of intensity that is too high and with too little knowledge of the proper precautions, techniques, and risks and without warm-up and cool-down periods. The so-called *weekend warrior* is thereby at higher risk for injury, which may result in cessation of exercise. Fortunately, the majority of such injuries are minor and temporary. With proper instruction one can resume exercise.

CARDIOVASCULAR PRECAUTIONS

Siscovick and colleagues[49] have demonstrated that any vigorous exercise, regardless of the level of prior training, transiently increases the risk of sudden cardiac death. This is despite the fact that, when not exercising, persons who engage in habitual exercise have a lower risk of sudden death than their sedentary counterparts. During low-intensity exercise by apparently normal men, the relative risk for sudden cardiac death is 56 times higher than during sedentary activity. The absolute risk, however, is still quite low, occurring in one per 19,000 men who exercise. In individuals who routinely perform high levels of physical activity, the risk of sudden death during exercise is still increased, but only five times higher than when not exercising.

A review of deaths among joggers in Rhode Island by Thompson and colleagues[50] also established a low fatality rate of one death per 7260 joggers per year. Importantly, of 11 deaths during jogging that were cardiac in nature, 8 had documentation of either prior myocardial infarction or angina. The incidence of exercise-related fatality appeared to be seven times the estimated death rate of the nonexercising general population and was higher in older age groups.

Acute myocardial infarction has been reported among exercisers in the general population, but the majority of these individuals had antecedent cardiac symptoms, making this complication very unlikely in the truly asymptomatic individual. In a study of individuals with known coronary artery disease who performed regular exercise, Haskell[51] estimated the fatality rate at one-per-thousand with a case ratio of one death per 116,402 patient hours of participation. Eight of these deaths were due to sudden cardiac death, with two cases each of acute myocardial infarction, pulmonary edema, and pulmonary embolism. The incidence of cardiac complications and death appeared to be lower when there was supervised exercise with continuous electrocardiographic monitoring for patients with coronary artery disease who participated in supervised cardiac rehabilitation. Although these individuals had electrocardiographic monitoring, the overall incidence of nonfatal cardiac arrest was 10 times higher than in the normal population, occurring roughly once in every 2500 patients. The case ratio per hour of exercise was low, with an average of one case of cardiac arrest occurring for every 34,000 hours of supervised exercise. Nonfatal acute myocardial infarction was even rarer, with only seven cases occurring for 1.6 million hours of physical activity. Rare instances of pulmonary embolism and acute pulmonary edema have also been reported.

EVALUATION PRIOR TO BEGINNING AN EXERCISE PROGRAM

Previous studies of "normal" individuals who have died during exercise have found that in the majority of cases, antecedent cardiac symptoms were reported by family members.[52] All individuals should undergo a complete history analysis and physical examination before participating in an exercise program or competitive athletics (Table 13–1). Routine questioning can uncover symptoms of cardiac disease in the apparently healthy adult, and a thorough physical examination might reveal significant abnormalities.

Screening for cardiac risk factors should be performed routinely. Sex, age, resting blood pressure, smoking history, and family history of coronary artery disease are obtained by the history and physical examination. Serum glucose and total cholesterol should be performed along with a blood count and urinalysis. If the total cholesterol is elevated (>200 mg per dl), HDL-C and triglyceride levels should be obtained after a 12-hour fast. A resting 12 lead electrocardiogram (ECG) also is recommended.

Table 13–1. Screening Regimen for Pre-exercise Evaluation in
Apparently Healthy Adults

Complete medical history
Detailed physical examination
Total cholesterol level
Serum fasting/random glucose level
Urinalysis
Total blood count
Lipid profile (HDL-cholesterol and triglycerides)*
12 lead resting electrocardiogram†
Graded exercise test†

*If total cholesterol >200 mg/dl
†Optional if <35 years of age

Further evaluation depends on the patient's status as follows: (1) Men and women under 35 years of age and women between the ages of 35 and 45 who are apparently healthy; (2) apparently healthy men between 35 and 45 years of age; and (3) men and women over the age of 45 or persons of any age with known cardiac disease or two or more cardiac risk factors.

1. Patients who are less than 35 years of age may be cleared for exercise without further evaluation if all of the aforementioned screening is normal. The 12 lead ECG is useful as a baseline for future reference. A graded exercise test is not routinely recommended. In a population with a low prevalence of coronary disease, a positive graded exercise test is more likely to be a false-positive and of limited value as a diagnostic tool when used routinely. It can be useful for determining an individual's exercise capacity when an individual exercise prescription is indicated.

2. The prevalence of coronary disease is high enough in men over the age of 35 years to recommend routine graded exercise testing if any cardiac risk factor is present. The percentage of false-positive tests is relatively low, with approximately 70 percent sensitivity for the detection of coronary artery disease.[53] In addition, if the individual reaches stage IV of the Bruce protocol, the chances of a cardiac event are less than 1 percent.[54] In asymptomatic women in this age group, exercise testing should be performed if two cardiac risk factors are present. However, there still is a high incidence of false-positive results, and the concurrent use of radionuclide isotopes ([201]thallium perfusion imaging or [99m]technetium radionuclide angiography) can improve the diagnostic accuracy.[55,56]

3. For all patients over the age of 45 and for those of any age with either suspected cardiac symptoms or known cardiac disease, graded exercise testing is clearly indicated. The prevalence of coronary disease is high enough to offset the additional cost in this population. A chest x-ray and pulmonary function tests also may be of value if there is a history of smoking or environmental exposures. If any screening test is abnormal, appropriate follow-up is recommended prior to clearing the individual for an exercise program. Table 13–2 summarizes the recommendations for use of routine graded exercise testing in the evaluation of patients prior to initiating an exercise program.

Table 13–2. Recommendations for Graded Exercise
Testing in Pre-exercise Evaluation

Health Status	Age		
	≤ 34 Years	35–44 Years	≥ 45 Years
Apparently healthy	−	−	+
≥ 1 cardiac risk factors	−	+	+
Known cardiac disease	+	+	+

− = Graded exercise test not routinely recommended.
+ = Graded exercise test routinely recommended.

EXERCISE PRESCRIPTION

After an individual has passed a pre-exercise evaluation, an appropriate exercise program can be recommended or prescribed.[57] The individual may already have a specific program in mind or may rely on the physician for an exercise prescription. All exercise programs should be thoroughly reviewed with the patient so that expectations are appropriate and the risk of cardiac and orthopedic complications can be minimized. Every exercise program should include a warm-up period, a period of aerobic training, and a cool-down phase (Table 13–3).

The overall goal of exercise is to improve cardiovascular conditioning. The optimal frequency to achieve this goal is three to five sessions per week.[58] Although some individuals will show a modest gain in cardiovascular fitness when exercising twice a week, there will be little decrease in weight or percent body fat. If exercise is performed more than five times per week, additional gains in cardiovascular and musculoskeletal fitness are limited, and there is an increased risk of orthopedic injuries.

The use of heart rate to monitor intensity during all phases of an exercise session is important in patients with known heart disease or risk factors and in those over 35 years of age. A target heart rate for each individual is determined, as discussed below, and his or her response is followed to determine both the adequacy of exercise and the potential for overexertion. Exercising to a modifiable target heart rate allows for changes in exercise capacity as cardiovascular fitness improves and allows for consistency of the exercise regimen in a changing environment and for constant intensity levels during different exercise regimens.

Table 13–3. Components of an Aerobic Training Session

Warm-Up Period (5–10 Minutes)
    General—light stretching and cardiovascular preparation
    Specific—preparation of muscles for the type of exercise to be performed

Aerobic Phase (15–45 Minutes)
    Continuous exercise to maintain pre-determined target heart rate

Cool-Down Period (5–60 Minutes)
    Gradual decrease in cardiovascular demand
    Stretching and flexibility exercises
    Heart rate should return to resting level

Unsupervised exercise can be performed safely in the apparently healthy individual who has passed the initial evaluation. The risk for cardiac complications is extremely low. These individuals, like all who are starting an exercise program, need information about proper training because improper exercise techniques predispose to musculoskeletal injuries. The following recommendations should be given with individual modifications as required.

WARM-UP

Exercise sessions should begin with a warm-up period to prepare the body for the more vigorous phase that will follow. The warm-up period is designed to increase muscle temperature and 2,3 diphosphoglycerate levels, resulting in increased release of oxygen from hemoglobin with the potential for a higher metabolic rate.[4] The increase in muscle temperature also allows for more rapid recruitment of the myofibrils during the aerobic phase. In addition, vasodilation of the arterial bed occurs, augmenting oxygen and nutrient delivery and promoting lactate removal.[59]

A generalized warm-up increases the temperature and perfusion of all muscle groups. The warm-up should not work muscles to their extreme limits of use. It should consist of well-controlled activity designed to raise the heart rate to within approximately 20 beats per minute of the target rate. This allows adequate time for the cardiovascular system to adapt to the increased demands during the high intensity phase. Similarly, these warm-up exercises should not force joints into their extreme ranges of motion; they are not intended to improve flexibility or increase muscle bulk. Light stretching and range of motion exercises are all that is recommended when the muscles are cold.

Although a general warm-up involves all of the major muscle groups and joints, a specific warm-up phase concentrates on the specific muscle groups to be used during the aerobic phase. Again, the aim is to prepare the muscles for the high-intensity phase and should not overwork them to the point that fatigue sets in early.

The duration of the warm-up period will vary and should be guided by heart rate response and activation of sweating. The onset of perspiration is a good sign that the autoregulatory systems are activated and the body is prepared for a higher intensity workload in the aerobic phase. The heart rate should be within 20 beats per minute of the target heart rate.

AEROBIC PHASE OF EXERCISE

The intensity of exercise performed during the aerobic phase is the most critical variable that the physician should monitor and regulate. Exercising at too high an intensity may lead to serious complications. This is seen more often in over-achievers and can be predicted by a personality-screening questionnaire.[60] The aim of the exercise program is to induce a cardiovascular training effect without producing metabolic demands that cannot be met by the heart. This level is objectively determined by the patient's VO$_2$max. Optimal training intensity for aerobic exercise is usually considered to be between 60 and 80 percent of VO$_2$max but may be less than 50 percent in some individuals. Except for elite, competitive athletes, aerobic training at a level of 90 percent VO$_2$max or higher is not recommended because the incidence of musculoskeletal injuries and cardiovascular complications

(S-T segment depression, ventricular dysrhythmias, myocardial infarction, and sudden cardiac death) are increased,[61,62] and the value of such high-intensity training is limited. Although laboratory determination of VO_2max may be helpful in some individuals (for example, patients with chronic obstructive pulmonary disease (COPD) or congestive heart failure), an estimation is usually sufficient for exercise prescriptions.

VO_2max can be estimated if the individual has undergone a graded exercise test. Readily available tables provide data for conversion to VO_2max from the total duration of exercise and the peak exercise level for both men and women.[63] A target heart rate for aerobic exercise can be determined by identifying a heart rate that places the patient at 60 to 80 percent VO_2max. A much simpler method, suggested by the American Heart Association,[64] is to have the individual exercise to 70 to 85 percent of their *age-predicted maximal heart rate.** At this level of intensity, the patient should still be able to talk in short sentences. If he or she is unable to do so, the level of exercise is too high regardless of the heart rate.

The aerobic phase should last for 15 to 45 minutes. Longer periods are associated with an increased incidence of musculoskeletal injuries, and shorter periods do not allow adequate time for cardiovascular training to occur. However, a deconditioned individual initially may be unable to exercise for 15 minutes and may have to progressively increase each exercise session over several weeks or months until sustained aerobic exercise can be performed.

The types of exercise recommended include activities that provide rhythmic exercise to the large muscle groups. Activities associated with maximal cardiovascular conditioning are those that allow a sustained intensity and give a relatively constant heart rate. These include walking, jogging, running, cross-country skiing, swimming, cycling, and aerobic dance. It is most important that individuals choose activities that appeal to them. Activities that an individual does not like will not be pursued for any length of time, and the goal is for a long-term conditioning effect. Sports such as basketball, squash, tennis, and soccer do not have the constancy of the level of exercise and are less consistent in producing cardiovascular training. Isometric exercise, such as free-weight training, should be avoided since there is no cardiovascular training effect, whereas there are profound effects on blood pressure and myocardial oxygen demand.

COOL-DOWN

The cool-down phase should immediately follow the high-intensity phase. It allows the body to recover gradually from strenuous exercise. The activity performed should be at a lower intensity level than that attained in the aerobic phase and should gradually decrease in intensity. This maintains venous return to the heart, decreasing the potential for orthostasis or presyncope. It also induces recruitment of slow-twitch myofibrils that enhance lactate removal through its oxidative utilization.[65,66] The gradual decrease in demands on the cardiovascular system allows the heart time to adapt while dissipating heat by vasodilation of the integument. Maximal stretching and flexibility exercises should be performed during the cool-down period when the muscles are still warm. Cool-down should last at least

---

*Age-predicted heart rate (beats per minute) = 220 − age (in years).

5 minutes, and, depending on the individual's level of fitness and environmental conditions, may take up to an hour. Ideally, heart rate should return to the baseline resting level by the end of the cool-down phase.

Special Considerations for Cardiac Patients

The optimal levels of aerobic training are the same for patients with known coronary artery disease as they are for the general population. However, a more gradual buildup in duration and intensity of exercise is necessary to minimize cardiovascular complications. A graded treadmill test is most important. Exercise intensity should be kept initially to 60 to 80 percent of the heart rate at which ischemia occurred during exercise testing (ischemic threshold). This level will be sufficient to initiate cardiovascular training and can be increased under physician supervision if the patient desires and if the degree of aerobic training is not satisfactory. While self-monitored, unsupervised aerobic exercise may be performed in this population after appropriate evaluation and individual recommendations are given, re-evaluations should be performed at least annually to assess the ischemic threshold and to ascertain that the patient is exercising within this limitation. If the patient develops new cardiac symptoms or has a change in symptoms, the training regimen should be interrupted and repeat exercise testing should be performed prior to continuing the training program.

The patient with recent myocardial infarction presents a unique training situation during the early convalescent period. Because the majority of recurrent cardiac events take place within the first 3 months,[67] supervised exercise with heart rate monitoring is recommended during this time. A graded exercise test is necessary to determine the patient's ischemic threshold and whether there is exercise-induced left ventricular dysfunction. Initial levels of exercise are kept to 40 to 70 percent of the heart rate at which ischemia, left ventricular dysfunction, or both occur, or 40 to 70 percent of the patient's maximal predicted heart rate (VO_2max), whichever is lower. If the patient has documented ischemia during the graded exercise test, electrocardiographic monitoring during exercise is recommended to minimize the chances of developing either silent ischemia, ventricular dysrhythmias, or both. Exercise programs that use this approach have a low incidence of cardiac complications.[51]

As the patient's aerobic capacity improves, the intensity level of exercise can be increased, with a target heart rate similar to the normal population (70 to 85 percent of the age-predicted maximal heart rate). It should be emphasized that individuals taking beta-blockers (or some calcium-channel antagonists) have lower heart rate responses compared with their VO_2max. It is essential to monitor these patients closely and to avoid overexertion. A maximal target heart rate of 120 beats per minute is recommended. If available, the direct measurement of VO_2max is preferred in these patients and those with COPD or congestive heart failure and is recommended for both the initial pre-exercise screening and periodic follow-up.

Once the patient with recent myocardial infarction is beyond the 3-month convalescent period, the risk of recurrent cardiac events is lower and similar to patients with known cardiac disease who have not had a recent myocardial infarction. Unsupervised exercise then can be initiated after a repeat graded exercise test is performed to reassess the ischemic threshold and VO_2max. Repeat graded exercise testing should be performed at least annually to redefine the ischemic threshold or uncover patient symptoms or other problems.

CONCLUSION

Aerobic exercise can be performed safely in most individuals, including those with known heart disease. The benefits of exercise include improved cardiovascular fitness (increaed VO$_2$max), a potential for lowering blood pressure and body weight, improved glucose tolerance, higher HDL-C levels, and an improved psychologic profile. With routine pre-exercise evaluation, the risks of exercise can be minimized for both normal and cardiac patients. A detailed exercise regimen should be prescribed, particularly for high-risk patients and those with known heart disease. Reevaluation of the cardiac patient's status should be performed at regular intervals. If these guidelines are followed, the benefits of exercise can be achieved and enjoyed with minimal risk.

REFERENCES

1. American Heart Association: Sudden Coronary Death Outside the Hospital, Monograph 74 (proceedings). American Heart Association, Dallas, 1974.
2. Goldstein, S: Sudden Death and Coronary Heart Disease. Futura Publishing Co, Inc, New York, 1974.
3. Caspersen, CJ, Christenson, GM, and Pollard, RA: Status of the 1990 physical fitness and exercise objectives—evidence from NHIS 1985. Public Health Rep 101:587, 1986.
4. Scheuer, J and Tipton, CM: Cardiovascular adaptations to physical training. Ann Rev Physiol 39:221, 1977.
5. Hagberg, JM and Seals, DR: Exercise training and hypertension. Acta Med Scand (Suppl) 711:131, 1986.
6. deVries, HA: Physiological effects of an exercise training regimen upon men aged 52 to 88. J Gerontol 25:325, 1970.
7. Kiyonaga, A, Arakawa, K, Tanaka, H, et al: Blood pressure and hormonal responses to aerobic exercise. Hypertension 7:125, 1985.
8. Wilmore, JH, Royce, J, Girandola, RN, et al: Physiological alterations resulting from a 10-week program of jogging. Med Sci Sports Exerc 2:7, 1970.
9. Cade, R, Mars, D, Wagemaker, H, et al: Effect of aerobic training on patients with systemic arterial hypertension. Am J Med 77:785, 1984.
10. Seals, DR and Hagberg, JM: The effect of exercise training on human hypertension: A review. Med Sci Sports Exerc 16:207, 1984.
11. Foster, C: Central circulatory adaptations to exercise training in health and disease. Clin Sports Med 5:589, 1986.
12. Hagberg, JM, Goldring, D, Heath, GW, et al: Effect of exercise training on plasma catecholamines and hemodynamics of adolescent hypertensives during rest, submaximal exercise, and orthostatic stress. Clin Physiol 4:117, 1984.
13. Higginbotham, MB: Cardiac performance during submaximal and maximal exercise in healthy persons. Heart Failure 3:68, 1988.
14. Wilmore, JH: Training for Sport and Activity, ed 2. Boston, Allyn, and Bacon, Inc, Boston, 1982.
15. Leff, AR (ed): Cardiopulmonary Exercise Testing. Grune and Stratton, Orlando, 1986.
16. Erikssen, J: Physical fitness and coronary heart disease morbidity and mortality. Acta Med Scand (Suppl) 711:189, 1986.
17. Wilhelmsen, L, Sanne, H, Elmfeldt, D, et al: A controlled trial of physical training after myocardial infarction. Prevent Med 4:491, 1975.
18. Powell, KE, et al: Physical activity and the incidence of coronary heart disease. Ann Rev Pub Health 8:253, 1987.
19. Kannel, WB and Sorlie, P: Some health benefits of physical activity. Arch Intern Med 139:857, 1979.
20. Morris, JN, Pollard, R, Everitt, MG, et al: Vigorous exercise in leisure-time: Protection against coronary heart disease. Lancet 2:1207, 1980.
21. Leon, AS, Connett, J, Jacobs, DR, Jr, et al: Leisure-time physical activity levels and risk of coronary heart disease and death. The Multiple Risk Factor Intervention Trial. JAMA 258:2388, 1987.

22. Oberman, A: Exercise and the primary prevention of cardiovascular disease. Am J Cardiol (Suppl) 55:10D, 1985.
23. Paffenberger, RS Jr, Wing, AL and Hyde, RT: Physical activity as an index of heart attack risk in college alumni. Am J Epidemiol 108:161, 1978.
24. Peters, RK, Cady, LD, Jr, Bischoff, DP, et al: Physical fitness and subsequent myocardial infarction in healthy workers. JAMA 249:3052, 1983.
25. Shaw, LW, for the National Exercise and Health Disease Project: Effects of a prescribed supervised exercise program on mortality and cardiovascular morbidity in patients after a myocardial infarction. Am J Cardiol 48:39, 1981.
26. Wood, PD, Stefanick, ML, Dreon, DM, et al: Changes in plasma lipids and lipoproteins in over-weight men during weight loss through dieting as compared with exercise. N Engl J Med 319:1173, 1988.
27. Schwartz, RS: The independent effects of dietary weight loss and aerobic training on high density lipoproteins and apolipoprotein A-1 concentrations in obese men. Metabolism 36:165, 1987.
28. Thompson, PD, Lazarus, B, Cullinane, E, et al: Exercise, diet or physical characteristics as determinants of HDL-levels in endurance athletes. Atherosclerosis 46:333, 1983.
29. Williams, PT, Wood, PD, Haskell, WL, et al: The effects of running mileage and duration on plasma lipoprotein levels. JAMA 247:2674, 1982.
30. Peltonen, P, Marniemi, J, Hietanen, E, et al: Changes in serum lipids, lipoproteins and heparin releasable lipolytic enzymes during moderate physical training in man: A longitudinal study. Metabolism 30:518, 1981.
31. Wood, PD, Haskell, WL, Blair, SN, et al: Increased exercise level and plasma lipoprotein concentrations: A one-year randomized, controlled study in sedentary, middle-aged men. Metabolism 32:31, 1983.
32. Warwick, PM and Garrow, JS: The effect of addition of exercise to a regimen of dietary restriction on weight loss, nitrogen balance, resting metabolic rate and spontaneous activity in three obese women in a metabolic ward. Int J Obes 5:25, 1981.
33. Hadjiolova, I, Mintcheva, L, Dunev, S, et al: Physical working capacity in obese women after an exercise programme for body weight reduction. Int J Obes 6:405, 1982.
34. Woo, R, Garrow, JS, and Pi-Sunyer, FX: Voluntary food intake during prolonged exercise in obese women. Am J Clin Nutr 36:478, 1982.
35. Garrow, JS: Effects of exercise on obesity. Acta Med Scand (Suppl) 711:67, 1986.
36. Wilmore, JH: Body composition in sport and exercise: Directions for future research. Med Sci Sports Exerc 15:21, 1983.
37. Richter EA, Ruderman, NB, and Schneider, SH: Diabetes and exercise. Am J Med 70:201, 1981.
38. Berger, M, Berchtold, P, Cuppers, HJ, et al: Metabolic and hormonal effects of muscular exercise in juvenile type diabetics. Diabetologica 13:355, 1977.
39. Koivisto, VA and Felig, P: Effects of leg exercise on insulin absorption in diabetic patients. N Engl J Med 298:79, 1978.
40. Dandona, P, Hooke, D, and Bell, J: Exercise and insulin absorption from subcutaneous tissue. Br Med J 1:479, 1978.
41. Holloszy, JO, Schultz, J, Kusnierkiewicz, J, et al: Effects of exercise on glucose tolerance and insulin resistance. Acta Med Scand (Suppl.) 711:55, 1986.
42. Morgan, WP: Anxiety reduction following acute physical activity. Psychiatr Ann 9:141, 1979.
43. Folkins, CH and Sime, WE: Physical fitness training and mental health. Am Psychol 36:373, 1981.
44. Brown, BJ: The effect of an isometric strength program on the intellectual and social development of trainable retarded males. Am Correct Ther J 31:44, 1977.
45. Greist, JH, Klein, MH, Eischens, RR, et al: Running as treatment for depression. Comp Psychiatr 20:41, 1979.
46. Orava, S, Puranen, J, and Ala-Ketola, L: Stress fractures caused by physical exercise. Acta Orthop Scand 49:19, 1978.
47. Herring, SA and Nilson, KL: Introduction to overuse injuries. Clin Sports Med 6:225, 1987.
48. Koplan, JP, Siscovick, DS, and Goldbaum, GM: The risks of exercise: A public health view of injuries and hazards. Pub Health Rep 100:189, 1985.
49. Siscovick, DS, Weiss, NS, Fletcher, RH, et al: The incidence of primary cardiac arrest during vigorous exercise. N Engl J Med 311:874, 1984.
50. Thompson, PD, Funk, EJ, Carlton, RA, et al: Incidence of death during jogging in Rhode Island from 1975 through 1980. JAMA 247:2535, 1982.

51. Haskell, WL: Cardiovascular complications during exercise training of cardiac patients. Circulation 57:920, 1978.
52. Thompson, PD, Stern, MP, Williams, P, et al: Death during jogging or running: A study of 18 cases. JAMA 242:1265, 1979.
53. Diamond, GA and Forrester, JS: Analysis of probability as an aid in the clinical diagnosis of coronary artery disease. N Engl J Med 300:1350, 1979.
54. McNeer, JF, Margolis, JR, Lee, KL, et al: The role of the exercise test in the evaluation of patients for ischemic heart disease. Circulation 57:64, 1979.
55. Kaul, S, Finkelstein, DM, Homma, S, et al: Superiority of quantitative exercise thallium-201 variables in determining long-term prognosis in ambulatory patients with chest pain: A comparison with cardiac catheterization. J Am Coll Cardiol 12:25, 1988.
56. Gibbons, RJ, Fyke, FE, Clements, IP, et al: Noninvasive identification of severe coronary artery disease using exercise radionuclide angiography. J Am Coll Cardiol 11:28, 1988.
57. Ward, A, Malloy, P, and Rippe, J: Exercise prescription guidelines for normal and cardiac populations. Cardiol Clin 5:197, 1987.
58. American College of Sports Physicians: Guidelines for Exercise Testing and Prescription, ed 3. Lea & Febiger, Philadelphia, 1986.
59. Terjung, RL: Peripheral adaptations in skeletal muscle induced by exercise training. Heart Failure 3:93, 1988.
60. Ewart, CK, Stewart, KJ, Gillian, RE, et al: Usefulness of self-efficacy in predicting overexertion during programmed exercise in coronary artery disease. Am J Cardiol 57:557, 1986.
61. DeBacker, G, Jacobs, R, Prineas, R, et al: Ventricular premature contractions: A randomized non-drug intervention trial in man. Circulation 59:762, 1979.
62. Barnard, RJ, MacAlpin, R, Kattus, AA, et al: Ischemic response to sudden strenuous exercise in healthy men. Circulation 48:936, 1973.
63. American College of Sports Physicians: Guidelines for Exercise Testing and Prescription, ed 3. Lea & Febiger, Philadelphia, 1986.
64. American Heart Association: Exercise Program Coordinator's Guide. American Heart Association, Dallas, 1984.
65. Grimby, G and Saltin, B: Physiological effects of physical conditioning. Scand J Rehab Med 3:6, 1971.
66. Graham, TE: Lactate metabolism during submaximal and maximal exercise. Heart Failure 3:77, 1988.
67. Moss, AJ, DeCamilla, J, Davis, H, et al: The early posthospital phase of myocardial infarction: Prognostic stratification. Circulation 54:58, 1976.

CHAPTER 14

Effects of Smoking
on the Cardiovascular System

Jack P. Strong, M.D.
Margaret C. Oalmann, Dr. P.H.

"Cigarette smoking should be considered the most important of known modifiable risk factors for coronary heart disease in the United States." This dramatic statement was the conclusion of the overall findings of the 1983 Public Health Service Report on the Health Consequences of Smoking.[1] Thus, the concept of the causal role of smoking on coronary heart disease (CHD) has evolved from a suspicion in the 1960s to a certainty in this decade.

The first Surgeon General's Report on The Health Consequences of Smoking in 1964 pointed out that "the causative role of these risk factors, including cigarette smoking in coronary heart disease, though not proven, is suspected strongly enough to be a major reason for taking countermeasures against them. It is also more prudent to assume that the established association between cigarette smoking and coronary heart disease has causative meaning than to suspend judgment until no uncertainty remains."[2] In 1979, the magnitude of the epidemiologic, pathologic, clinical, and experimental evidence had grown to the point that the Surgeon General's report concluded: "Smoking is causally related to coronary heart disease in the common sense of that idea and for the purpose of preventive medicine."[3]

Yet, according to data from the National Health Survey, 30 percent of persons 18 years of age and over smoked cigarettes in 1985, some 21 years after the first report. Among these smokers, 88 percent were conscious of the association between smoking and heart disease.[4] This observation is one important reason for emphasizing further the relationship of smoking and cardiovascular diseases, particularly CHD. Another reason is that modification of tobacco usage seems more feasible and straightforward in the prevention of some cardiovascular diseases, particularly CHD, than the more complex measures necessary to change other risk factors, such as habitual dietary pattern, serum lipid levels, and levels of blood pressure. Promoting the avoidance of tobacco usage to reduce the risk of cardiovascular disease seems a rather straightforward measure, posing no hidden risks for individuals nor for the American population.

In this chapter, the magnitude of the problem is defined, and current evidence for the relationship of smoking and various forms of cardiovascular disease is reviewed under the headings of CHD, cerebrovascular disease, atherosclerotic peripheral vascular disease, and atherosclerosis, condensing the massive amount of information summarized and reviewed in the 1983 Report of the Surgeon General as well as reports published afterwards. Special emphasis is placed on the effect of smoking on the extent and severity of atherosclerotic arterial lesions. Tobacco smoking may have its effect at different stages in the long sequence of events from the initiation and progression of lesions, to stenosis and occlusion with clinically significant ischemic damage to the heart, brain, or lower extremities.

DEFINING THE PROBLEM

Cardiovascular disease, especially CHD, is currently the most important health problem for the American public. Mortality statistics indicate that in 1987 all cardiovascular diseases accounted for over 46 percent of all deaths (968,240 out of 2,105,361 total deaths) and that approximately 25 percent of deaths from all causes are the result of CHD.[5,6] Even though mortality from all cardiovascular disease and particularly for CHD and cerebrovascular disease has decreased in the last two decades, cardiovascular disease accounts for more than twice as many deaths as all cancers combined.

A comprehensive review of the world literature for more than 40 years, including the results of epidemiologic observations covering many millions of person-years on the relationship between cigarette smoking and CHD, is found in the 1983 Public Health Service Report on the Health Consequences of Smoking. The consensus of previous reports from the Public Health Service and from other scientific bodies throughout the world was succinctly stated in this sentence: "Cigarette smoking is causally related to coronary heart disease; it and elevated levels of serum cholesterol and hypertension constitute the major risk factors for contracting and dying from this disease."[1]

The economic impact of smoking for all diseases is of huge proportion. The Office of Technology Assessment estimates that for employers, the yearly direct health-care cost and indirect productivity cost of smoking is $65 billion, equivalent to an estimated productivity loss and health care cost of $2.17 per pack of cigarettes sold.[7-9] Smokers have a 50 percent higher absenteeism rate than non-smokers, are 50 percent more likely to be hospitalized, and have a job-related accident rate that is twice as high.[10]

The overall economic cost of cardiovascular disease per year in the United States is estimated at $102 billion, corresponding to $48 billion direct health expenditures, $13 billion indirect cost of morbidity, and $41 billion indirect cost of mortality.[11] Heart disease accounts for more total days of annual hospital care (30,781,000 in 1983) than any other disease.[12] Average length of hospital stay for those with cerebrovascular disease is 10.4 days, heart attacks 10.0 days, and congestive heart failure 8.6 days.[13] About two thirds of myocardial infarction patients do not recover completely, and 88 percent under the age of 65 are unable to return to their usual occupations.[14] Forty percent of stroke patients require special services and 10 percent require total care.[15] Thus, the contribution of smoking to cardiovascular disease is large and has an enormous impact on health care cost in the United States.

CORONARY HEART DISEASE

Although the relationship of smoking to peripheral vascular disease has been suspected since the turn of the nineteenth century, Howard was the first to observe in 1934 that the increasing incidence of coronary heart disease might be associated with the progressive increase in cigarette smoking noticed after World War I.[1] In 1958, Hammond and Horn published the first major prospective study disclosing a link between cigarette usage and CHD.[16,17] These investigators, who had set out primarily to study the effect of cigarette smoking on cancer, found that smokers had a 70 percent greater risk of dying from CHD than nonsmokers, and that heavy smokers had CHD mortality rates approximately two and one half times greater than nonsmokers. They also reported a consistent dose-response relationship between the number of cigarettes consumed per day and the risk of developing CHD.

Numerous additional epidemiologic studies on the relationship between cigarette usage and CHD were reported before 1964, when the first major U.S. Public Health Service review was published. The findings in these studies, carried out in United Kingdom, Canada, Sweden, Japan, Switzerland, and the United States, were remarkably uniform in that smokers had much higher death rates from CHD than nonsmokers despite the diversity of the populations studied and the different methodologies used. However, the Surgeon General's advisory committee on smoking and health in 1964 was unwilling to conclude that the association had causal significance.

One of the most conclusive studies was the investigation by Doll and Hill on British doctors from whom information concerning smoking habits was obtained. Death certificates of those who died were used to assay the cause of death.[18,19] This study involved 34,400 men who responded to the questionnaire about their smoking habits. Follow-up questionnaires were sent 6, 15, and 20 years after the initiation of the study. The 20-year mortality from that study was reported in 1976, at which time 10,072 deaths had been identified[20] (Table 14–1). The death rate for smokers of all forms of tobacco was 37 percent higher than the death rate for nonsmokers. Furthermore, a definite dose-response relationship was observed; the mortality was less in those who stopped smoking than in those who continued to smoke; and the relative effect on mortality from CHD in smokers as compared with nonsmokers was greatest in the younger age group of male physicians.

Results of the Framingham Study conducted by the U.S. Public Health Service basically confirmed the observations made by Hammond and Horn in regard to cigarette smoking (see Fig. 1–3) and provided basic information on the relationship of other risk factors, such as serum cholesterol levels and blood pressure levels, to CHD.[21] An important additional finding in the Framingham Study was the synergistic effect of cigarette smoking with other CHD risk factors, resulting in a risk greater than the sum of the individual risks.[1]

The 1983 Surgeon General's report listed the following succinct conclusions in regard to CHD:

1. Cigarette smoking is a major cause of CHD in the United States for both men and women. Because of the number of persons in the population who smoke and the increased risk that cigarette smoking represents, it should be considered the most important of the known modifiable risk factors for CHD.

Table 14–1. Mortality by Age in Nonsmokers and Current Cigarette Smokers: Selected Causes; Numbers of Deaths in Parentheses.

| Age (in years) | Annual Death Rate per 100,000 Men* | | | |
| | Nonsmokers | Current Smokers, Smoking Only Cigarettes: #/day | | |
		1–14	15–24	>25
	Ischemic heart disease			
<45	7 (3)	46 (12)	61 (22)	104 (18)
45–54	118 (32)	220 (38)	368 (90)	393 (69)
55–64	531 (79)	742 (91)	819 (123)	1025 (125)
<65	166 (114)	278 (141)	358 (235)	427 (212)
65–74	1190 (83)	1866 (134)	1511 (101)	1731 (81)
75	2432 (92)	2719 (113)	2466 (50)	3247 (27)
	Myocardial degeneration			
<65	6 (4)	6 (3)	9 (6)	23 (11)
65–74	44 (3)	124 (9)	186 (12)	204 (9)
75	945 (40)	1932 (79)	1307 (21)	2114 (11)
	Cerebral thrombosis			
<65	10 (6)	18 (9)	14 (9)	22 (11)
65–74	131 (9)	166 (12)	353 (23)	290 (13)
>75	1039 (41)	985 (41)	1397 (26)	1448 (10)

*Indirectly standardized for age to make the four entries in any one line comparable.
From Doll and Peto,[20] p. 1529, with permission.

2. Overall, cigarette smokers experience a 70 percent greater CHD death rate than do nonsmokers. Heavy smokers, those who consume two or more packs per day, have CHD death rates between two and three times greater than nonsmokers.

3. The risk of developing CHD increases with increasing exposure to cigarette smoke, as measured by the number of cigarettes smoked daily, the total number of years one has smoked, and the degree of inhalation, and with an early age of initiation.

4. Cigarette smokers have a twofold greater incidence of CHD than do nonsmokers, and heavy smokers have an almost fourfold greater incidence.

5. Cigarette smoking is a major independent risk factor for CHD, and it acts synergistically with other risk factors (most notably, elevated serum cholesterol and hypertension) to greatly increase the risk of CHD.

6. Women have lower rates for CHD than do men. In particular, CHD rates for women are lower prior to the menopause. A part of this difference is due to the lower prevalence of smoking in women, and for those women who do smoke, to the tendency to smoke fewer cigarettes per day and to inhale less deeply. Among those women who have smoking patterns comparable with male smoking patterns, the increments in CHD death rates are similar for the two sexes.

7. Women who use oral contraceptives and who smoke increase their risk of a myocardial infarction by a factor of approximately tenfold compared with women who neither use oral contraceptives nor smoke.

8. Cigarette smoking has been found to significantly elevate the risk of sudden death. Overall, smokers experience a two to four times greater risk of sudden death than nonsmokers. The risk appears to increase with increasing dosage as measured by the number of cigarettes smoked per day and diminishes with cessation of smoking.

9. The CHD mortality ratio for smokers compared with nonsmokers is greater for the younger age groups than for the older age groups. Although the smoker-to-nonsmoker mortality ratio narrows with increasing age, smokers continue to experience greater CHD death rates at all ages.

10. Cigarette smoking has been estimated to be responsible for up to 30 percent of all CHD deaths in the United States each year. During the period 1965 to 1980, there were over 3 million premature deaths from heart disease among Americans attributed to cigarette smoking. Unless smoking habits of the American population change, perhaps 10 percent of all persons now alive may die prematurely of heart disease attributable to their smoking behavior. The total number of such premature deaths may exceed 24 million.

11. Cessation of smoking results in a substantial reduction in CHD death rates compared with those of persons who continue to smoke. Mortality from CHD declines rapidly after cessation. Approximately 10 years following cessation the CHD death rate for those ex-smokers who consumed less than a pack of cigarettes daily is virtually identical to that of lifelong nonsmokers. For ex-smokers who had smoked more than one pack per day, the residual risk of CHD mortality is proportional to the total lifetime exposure to cigarette smoke.

12. Epidemiologic evidence concerning reduced tar and nicotine or filter cigarettes and their effect on CHD rates is conflicting (see Fig. 1–4). No scientific evidence is available concerning the impact on CHD death rates of cigarettes with very low levels of tar and nicotine.

13. Smokers who have used only pipes or cigars do not appear to experience substantially greater CHD risks than nonsmokers.

Studies published after the 1983 report are in general agreement with the major findings just summarized. The age-adjusted rate of sudden deaths is significantly greater in male smokers (41/1000) than in nonsmokers (18/1000) in the Framingham CHD study 26-year follow-up data.[22] A 13-year follow-up of men who survived a first episode of unstable angina or myocardial infarction for 2 years suggests that continued smoking increases the rate of sudden death in those with less severe initial attacks and that the effect of smoking on fatal reinfarctions is more apparent in those with a complicated clinical presentation. Overall, mortality in those who continued to smoke was significantly higher (82.1 percent) than in those who stopped smoking (36.9 percent).[23] Cigarette smoking was second only to systolic blood pressure as a risk factor for total CHD, fatal CHD, and acute coronary insufficiency among 14 biologic and life-style factors measured in Japanese men living in Hawaii and even exceeded the association of blood pressure with nonfatal myocardial infarction.[24] A high prevalence of cigarette smoking was found to be the major contributing risk factor to high mortality rates found in a retrospective study in young British Army soldiers with CHD.[25]

CEREBROVASCULAR DISEASE

Vascular diseases of the central nervous system represent a public health problem of major proportions because together they constitute the third leading cause of death, after CHD and cancer, in the United States. Elevated blood pressure has been the most important risk factor consistently found in all epidemiologic studies for all major varieties of stroke, including intracerebral hemorrhage, occlusive atherosclerotic cerebrovascular disease, and some forms of subarachnoid hemorrhage. The relationship of serum lipids and lipoproteins to cerebrovascular disease is not as clear as for CHD, probably because the various subtypes of cerebrovascular disease are not readily distinguishable in epidemiologic studies.

There is a growing body of evidence for a positive association between smoking and cerebrovascular disease. Data from numerous recent prospective mortality studies have shown an association between cigarette smoking and cerebrovascular disease, with the risk being most evident in the younger age groups. The increased risk in smokers diminishes with increasing age, and little or no effect is noted after age 65. Inasmuch as there are several distinct forms of cerebrovascular diseases, each with a different pathogenesis, the relationship of smoking to cerebrovascular disease is more complex and unclear than is the case for tobacco usage and CHD. No consistent dose-effect relationship between level of cigarette smoking and incidence or mortality from all cerebrovascular disease not further subclassified was observed in studies summarized in the 1983 Surgeon General's report. Nevertheless, some studies that differentiated among the various forms of cerebrovascular disease (for example, the study of British physicians by Doll and Hill) have indeed found not only a 1.5 relative risk for cerebral thrombosis for heavy smokers in men but also a strong dose-response relationship in this same category of cerebrovascular disease.[20]

Additional evidence on the relationship of smoking and cerebrovascular disease has been derived from studies published after the 1983 summary in the Surgeon General's report. In 1986, the Honolulu Heart Program reported a 12-year follow-up study on smoking and stroke (Table 14–2). Subjects who smoked at study entry and 6 years later had a two to three times higher relative risk for thromboembolic stroke than nonsmokers, and the risk for hemorrhagic stroke was increased four to six times. No clear dose-response trends were observed for thromboembolic strokes. There was a definite dose-response effect in the risk of hemorrhagic stroke among heavy smokers, being three to four times higher than in nonsmokers and two times higher than in more moderate smokers.[26–28]

Data from a New Zealand study[29,30] indicate that the relative risk of stroke for persons smoking 1 to 20 cigarettes a day is 3.3 times that of nonsmokers, whereas for heavy smokers (more than 20 cigarettes a day), it is 5.6.

In the Framingham Study, 69 percent of subarachnoid and intracerebral hemorrhage cases and 29 percent of controls had a history of prior heavy smoking.[31] The 1988 Framingham report on cigarette smoking as a risk factor for stroke concludes that "the risk of stroke increased with the increasing number of cigarettes smoked consistent with a quantitative relationship between smoking and stroke incidence." It concluded that "the risk of stroke among smokers had decreased

Table 14–2. Age-Adjusted Incidence of Stroke Over 12-Year-Period
According to Number of Cigarettes Smoked per Day.

Number of Cigarettes Smoked	Subjects at Risk	Incidence of Stroke* (Number of First Events)		
		Thromboembolic Strokes	*Hemorrhagic Strokes*	*All Strokes*
0	4437	17.1 (78)	6.0 (27)	25.6 (117)
1–9	195	30.6 (6)	10.2 (2)	46.0 (9)
10–19	590	27.3 (17)	9.8 (6)	40.2 (25)
20–29	1464	40.0 (58)	11.7 (17)	55.1 (80)
30–39	635	28.8 (16)	24.5 (14)	59.5 (33)
>39	551	28.8 (14)	18.0 (9)	49.5 (24)

*Expressed as number of subjects per 1000.
From Abbott, Yin, Reed, et al,[26] p. 718, with permission.

significantly by two years after quitting and reverted to the lower level seen in non-smokers within five years after stopping."[32]

It is clear that adequate control of hypertension and of cardiac disease that might give rise to embolic stroke are important approaches in the prevention of cerebrovascular disease. Nevertheless, cigarette smoking cessation also has an important role in stroke prevention. The Carter Center report concludes that about 11 percent of stroke cases could be prevented if smoking is stopped.[33]

ATHEROSCLEROTIC PERIPHERAL VASCULAR DISEASE

The relationship between cigarette smoking and peripheral vascular disease has been well recognized since 1904, when Erb concluded that smokers showed a higher percentage of intermittent claudication than nonsmokers.[1] U.S. Public Health Service reviews of the evidence associating cigarette smoking with peripheral arterial occlusive disease have confirmed the clinically recognized strong association. Furthermore, data from the Framingham study indicate that cigarette smoking is one of the major risk factors in the development of intermittent claudication.[34,35] The Lipid Research Clinics Prevalence Study reported in 1986 that 48 percent of men with intermittent claudication were current smokers, whereas only 30 percent of men without the disease were current smokers[36] (Table 14–3). Men with peripheral vascular disease are at increased risk of abdominal aortic aneurysm, 20 percent, compared with a control group, 2 percent.[37] The 1983 Surgeon General's report concludes that "cigarette smoking is the most powerful risk factor predisposing to atherosclerotic peripheral arterial disease" and that "smoking cessation plays an important role in the medical and surgical management of atherosclerotic peripheral vascular disease."

ATHEROSCLEROSIS

Atherosclerosis is that specific form of arteriosclerosis characterized by accumulation of lipid in the intima of large elastic arteries and the medium-sized muscular arteries. In addition to lipid, smooth muscle cells and macrophages (with and without intracellular lipid inclusions), connective tissue, and various blood com-

Table 14–3. Adjusted[A] Means and Proportions of Selected Cardiovascular Risk Factors for Men with and Men without Intermittent Claudication.

	Claudication History	
Study Variable	*Yes[B]*	*No*
Number of participants	21	4671
Lipid levels (mg/dl)		
Triglyceride	176.4	148.6
Cholesterol	207.7	216.4
HDL-cholesterol	35.6	46.4
LDL-cholesterol	142.7	145.8
VLDL-cholesterol	29.3	24.3
Quetelet Index	2.66	2.66
Systolic blood pressure (mm Hg)	128.5	129.5
Diastolic blood pressure (mm Hg)	77.9	82.6
Hypertension (%)[C]	12	20
Smoking (% current)	48	30
Cigarettes/day (smokers only)	29.7	23.9
Drinking (% yes)	50	71
Alcohol (g/day)	16.4	19.4
Regular exercise (% yes)[D]	11	28

[A]Adjusted for age, estimating adjusted means with age set at 55 years of age.

[B]Significance testing was not done because there were so few participants with claudication.

[C]Blood pressure $\geq$ 160 systolic or $\geq$ 95 diastolic or on medication for hypertension.

[D]Answer to question, "Do you regularly engage in strenuous exercise or hard physical labor?"

From Pomrehn, Duncan, Weissfeld, et al,[36] p. 102, with permission.

ponents accumulate in the lesions. Complications, including necrosis and ulceration of plaques, hemorrhage into plaques and thrombosis over atherosclerotic plaques, occur and result in arterial narrowing and occlusion. In the case of the aorta, atherosclerosis may be complicated by destruction of the media, dilatation, and aneurysm formation.

Atherosclerosis is clinically significant because it is the underlying cause of CHD (coronary occlusion, coronary thrombosis, myocardial infarction, and angina pectoris) and of one major type of cerebral vascular disease (cerebral thrombosis with infarction). It also causes aortic aneurysms and sets the stage for arteriosclerotic peripheral vascular disease.

Inasmuch as cigarette smoking is a major risk factor for CHD, cerebral infarction, peripheral vascular disease, and other clinically significant sequelae of atherosclerosis, a key question is whether cigarette smoking has an effect on the early development of arterial lesions, the progression of arterial lesions, the terminal occlusive events, or a combination of these. Studies in the past two decades specifically designed to answer questions dealing with the association between cigarette smoking habits and the development of atherosclerotic lesions in various arterial beds have done much to clarify the relationship. A large body of evidence from autopsy studies with retrospective smoking data as well as prospective studies with autopsy follow-up indicates that cigarette smoking has a significant positive association with the basic atherosclerotic lesions in the artery.

SMOKING AND AORTIC ATHEROSCLEROSIS

The effects of smoking are most striking on aortic atherosclerosis. A strong and significant positive association has been found in almost every study evaluating this relationship. The evidence for the relationship between cigarette smoking and aortic atherosclerosis was summarized in the 1983 Surgeon General's report[1] and in a review article by Solberg and Strong.[38] Five retrospective autopsy studies and three prospective epidemiologic studies of cardiovascular disease with autopsy follow-up showed positive and significant associations between cigarette smoking habits and quantitative measures of atherosclerotic lesions in the aorta. A positive relationship between cigarette smoking and calcification of the thoracic aorta as seen on chest x-rays was observed in one additional study.

The relationship of smoking and atherosclerosis in deceased men in New Orleans has been the subject of five reports describing the general findings and providing detailed information.[39-43] Atherosclerotic raised lesions in the abdominal aorta are more extensive in the heavy smokers than in the nonsmokers, with a definite gradient trend of increased lesions with increased smoking. Differences between heavy smokers and nonsmokers in extent of raised atherosclerotic lesions were statistically significant. Furthermore, multivariate analysis indicated that there were statistically significant differences among three categories of smokers (heavy, light to moderate, and nonsmokers) for lesions in the abdominal aorta. Two of the studies were specifically focused on the effect of cigarette smoking on fatty streaks (the earliest gross visible lesions of atherosclerosis) and raised atherosclerotic lesions (the more advanced stage of the atherosclerotic process).[42,43] Results strongly suggest that smoking has a role in the progression of fatty streaks to the more advanced stage of atherosclerosis.

In 1981, Auerbach and Garfinkel concluded that the extent of atherosclerotic lesions increased with number of cigarettes smoked but also that aortic aneurysms were eight times more frequent among those who smoked one to two packs of cigarettes per day than in nonsmokers[44,45] (Table 14-4).

Subsequent to these retrospective autopsy studies, three prospective epidemiologic studies with autopsy follow-up confirmed the positive relationship between smoking and atherosclerotic lesions in the aorta[46-48] (Table 14-5). Both the Surgeon General's report and the review by Strong and Solberg[38] concluded that the effect of smoking on atherosclerosis is more pronounced in the aorta than in the coronary arteries.

SMOKING AND CORONARY ATHEROSCLEROSIS

A significant positive relationship between cigarette smoking and atherosclerotic lesions in the coronary arteries is observed in the highest-risk populations for CHD. The relationship between cigarette smoking and gross atherosclerotic lesions in the coronary arteries has been particularly studied by Auerbach and colleagues and by Strong and Richards. Auerbach and coworkers[49] found more coronary atherosclerosis in smokers than in nonsmokers and a progressive increase in the extent of atherosclerosis with increased amounts of cigarette smoking. The detailed study

Table 14–4. Percentage of Cases (Adjusted for Age) with Advanced Thickening of Blood Vessels in the Left Ventricular Wall by Cigarette-Smoking Habits: Group **A** (1955–60) and Group **B** (1970–77).

Smoking Habits	Subepicardial Arteries		Myocardial Arteries		Myocardial Arterioles	
	A	**B**	**A**	**B**	**A**	**B**
All cases						
Never regularly	29.6	19.6	2.8	4.7	1.8	5.1
1 pack/day	60.1	41.9*	30.4	21.5*	34.7	28.6
1–2 packs/day	83.6	55.6	65.5	32.8*	77.0	45.4*
2 or more packs/day	91.9	64.4	85.4	40.4*	89.5	53.6*
Excluding cases with coronary heart disease, diabetes, or hypertension						
Never regularly	18.5	8.9	0	2.5	1.3	2.5
1 pack/day	56.7	36.4*	31.5	19.4*	36.2	25.5*
1–2 packs/day	81.3	54.0*	64.2*	30.4*	76.1	43.6*
2 or more packs/day	90.6	61.3*	84.8	38.8*	87.9	51.5*

*Difference in percentages between **A** and **B** groups statistically significant p <0.05

From Auerbach and Garfinkel,[45] p. 767, with permission.

of smoking and atherosclerosis in deceased men in New Orleans, conducted with many precautions and special concerns about evaluation of lesions, collection of smoking information, and problems of autopsy selection, indicated that atherosclerotic involvement of the coronary arteries is more extensive in heavy smokers than in nonsmokers for both black and white men in both the total autopsy sample and in the basal group (accidents, cancer, infections, and miscellaneous causes of death unrelated to atherosclerotic disease).[39-43] The 1983 report from the U.S. Public Health Service tabulates all the autopsy studies on smoking and coronary atherosclerosis with details of the methodology used. Most, but not all, of these studies show a significant positive relationship between smoking and lesions in the coronary arteries.

One prospective epidemiologic study of cardiovascular disease with autopsy follow-up showed a significant relationship of cigarette smoking to atherosclerotic lesions in the coronary arteries. The Honolulu Heart Study, characterized by careful documentation of selected major risk factors, including cigarette smoking habits during life, and by standardized evaluation of atherosclerotic lesions at autopsies, revealed significant positive associations between cigarette smoking and measures of atherosclerotic lesions in both the coronary arteries and aorta.[47] No significant relationship between cigarette smoking habits and lesions in the coronary arteries was observed in the Oslo Heart Study; aortic lesions were not evaluated in that study.[50] The Puerto Rico Heart Study showed a positive significant relationship

Table 14–5. Association of Atherosclerosis in Aorta
with Antemortem Characteristics: Simple Correlation
Coefficients (Puerto Rico Heart Health Program).

	Correlation Coefficients		
Characteristics Measured at Exam 1	Total (120)	Rural (31)	Urban (89)
Systolic blood pressure	0.25	0.27	0.24
Diastolic blood pressure	0.19	0.29	0.16
Serum cholesterol	0.29	0.36	0.28
Age, exam 1	0.31	0.39	0.29
Relative weight	−0.08	−0.22	−0.06
Physical activity	−0.18	−0.21	−0.14
Blood glucose	0.14	0.05	0.17
Hematocrit	0.23	0.33	0.21
Education	−0.08	−0.23	−0.03
Income	0.01	−0.01	−0.01
Cigarettes smoked	0.32	0.37	0.31
Calories (24-hour recall)	−0.24	−0.55	−0.12
Starch (24-hour recall)	−0.19	−0.45	−0.07
Alcohol (24-hour recall)	−0.18	−0.39	−0.18
Total fats (24-hour recall)	−0.19	−0.49	−0.11
Triglycerides (fasting)	0.11	0.53	0.04
Ventricular rate	0.07	0.11	0.05
Vital capacity	−0.29	−0.28	−0.29

From Sorlie, Garcia-Palmiere, Castillo-Staab, et al,[46] p. 349, with permission of
the publisher.

between the extent of atherosclerotic lesions in the aorta and cigarette smoking habits but not with the extent of coronary atherosclerosis.[46]

SMOKING AND AORTIC AND CORONARY ATHEROSCLEROSIS

A more recent report from the Honolulu Heart Project compares two different
methods of evaluating gross atherosclerotic lesions and relates them to risk factors
for CHD.[51] Cigarette smoking in cigarette pack years is positively and significantly
correlated with aortic atherosclerotic lesions as measured by both methods in the
total autopsy sample and also in the basal noncardiovascular disease group. In the
basal group, cigarette pack years is positively and significantly correlated with coronary lesions by one method of grading and positively but not significantly correlated by the other method by multivariate analyses. This report concludes that
"blood pressure, serum cholesterol, and cigarette smoking appeared to be independent antecedent predictors for atherosclerosis in both the coronary arteries and the
aorta."

Current available evidence concerning the relationship of cigarette smoking
and atherosclerotic lesions in the aorta and coronary arteries suggests that cigarette
smoking has an aggravating and accelerating effect on the development of atherosclerotic lesions in the artery wall and that such effect is not limited to events leading to the occlusive episode. These findings do not rule out the possibility that cig-

arette smoking could also be associated with other events precipitating thrombosis, hemorrhage, or vasoconstriction leading to occlusion and ischemia.

SMOKING AND CEREBRAL ATHEROSCLEROSIS

The relationship between cigarette smoking and atherosclerosis in the cerebral vasculature has not been fully investigated. Sternby[48] found that cigarette smokers had more extensive raised lesions in the basilar artery than nonsmokers. This study was based on a subsample of 60 autopsy subjects from a prospective study of cardiovascular disease in Malmo, Sweden. Holme and associates[52] found a positive but not statistically significant correlation between raised lesions in the cerebral vessels and the number of cigarettes smoked in the Oslo Heart Study. The limited amount of information available on cigarette smoking and atherosclerosis in the cerebral vasculature does not lead to a clear conclusion.

POSSIBLE MECHANISMS RELATING TOBACCO USAGE AND ATHEROSCLEROSIS

Although the aggravating effect of cigarette smoking on the atherosclerotic lesions seems established beyond doubt, the specific mechanisms of such effect have not yet been elucidated. Of the 4000 or more different compounds identified in tobacco smoke, nicotine and carbon monoxide are the constituents most often singled out as having both supporting data and a rational role in the pathogenesis of atherosclerotic lesions. Other cigarette smoke constituents such as hydrogen cyanide, oxide of nitrogen, and carbon disulfide have been studied for possible pathogenic cardiovascular effects, but they are less suspect than carbon monoxide and nicotine.[53,54]

Studies of the effect of whole tobacco smoke[55] have suggested that cigarette smoking often causes slight to moderate elevation of total serum cholesterol concentration and that smoking may decrease HDL concentrations and elevate LDL concentrations—changes in lipoproteins that have been associated with increased amounts of atherosclerosis as well as with increased risk of CHD. McGill's review indicated that, in regard to smoking and the hemostatic system, smoking seemed to have little or no effect on clotting action but marked effects on platelets.[55] Platelet interaction with the arterial wall conceivably could lead to progression of established atherosclerotic lesions or possibly play some role in the occlusive mechanism in persons who already have extensive arterial disease.

THE EFFECT OF CESSATION OF CIGARETTE SMOKING

Switching to lower-yield tar and nicotine brands of cigarettes may have some value in decreasing cancer risk but may not reduce the risk for CHD. Compensatory behaviors (smoking more cigarettes, inhaling more deeply and for a longer period of time) could lead to increased atherogenesis via the greater intake of carbon monoxide, hydrogen cyanide, and nitrous oxide.[10]

Numerous studies have consistently shown that persons quitting cigarette smoking experience a substantial decrease in CHD mortality, with improved life expectancy as compared with those who continued smoking. Ex-smokers experience overall mortality ratios that decline as the number of years of cessation increases. The overall mortality ratios of ex-smokers after 15 years of cessation are similar to those of persons who have never smoked.[7] The CHD death rate for ex-smokers declines rapidly after cessation. After 3 years of not smoking, the CHD death rate for ex-smokers who smoked less than one pack a day is almost identical to that of lifelong nonsmokers.[56] These reports indicate a more favorable outcome from smoking cessation than was estimated in the 1983 Surgeon General's report. Smoking cessation improves the prognosis of arteriosclerotic peripheral vascular disease and has a favorable impact on vascular patency following reconstructive coronary arterial surgery.[1,10]

The 1983 Surgeon General's report cites four intervention trials conducted involving mortality follow-up of individual men for 5 to 10 years. The relative reductions in CHD mortality in each of the four intervention studies involving individual follow-up are reasonably consistent with the reduction in CHD risk factors, and for the combination of all four studies the reduction in CHD mortality is statistically significant.

Data published after the 1983 report strengthen earlier findings. After 10 years of follow-up in the Whitehall study, CHD mortality was 18 percent lower in the intervention group than in the controls.[57] The MRFIT project showed that those who quit smoking, in both the control and the intervention groups, had significantly lower CHD mortality rates than those who continued to smoke. The authors estimate that elimination of major risk factors reduces CHD mortality rates by two thirds in 35- to 45-year-old men and by half in 46- to 57-year-old men.[58,59] It is important to recognize that although the excess relative risk in CHD associated with smoking diminishes with increasing age, the absolute excess risk is large at all ages for both sexes. Indeed, a recent report from the Coronary Artery Surgery study concludes that, even in persons with clinical evidence of coronary artery disease, smoking cessation lessens the risk of death or of myocardial infarction in older (65 years of age or over) as well as younger (30 to 50 years of age) persons.[60]

Since 1968, CHD mortality in the United States has decreased 27 percent. Available data suggest that prevention of controllable risk factors might be responsible for such decline in CHD mortality rates. Trends in smoking, cholesterol, and blood pressure, translated into mathematical equations and related to CHD mortality rate, give the following predictions: A 5 mg per dl drop in mean cholesterol level would produce a 4.3 percent drop in mortality rate; a 2 mmHg drop in diastolic blood pressure would produce an 8.7 percent decline; a 20 percent decline in the amount of cigarette smoking would produce a 10 percent decline. If all three occurred—and there is some evidence they did—a 22 percent decline would be expected, which is very near the observed 27 percent decline in CHD mortality rate during this past two decades in the United States.[61]

INTERVENTION ISSUES

Among the health promotion goals set for 1990 in the United States is the reduction below 25 percent of the proportion of adult smokers.[62,63] This set of major objectives for improving health and quality of life for the American people was proclaimed in 1979,[64] based on the observation that the majority of deaths in the United States are due to fewer than a dozen conditions, with heart disease ranked first and stroke third.[65] Other studies concur to indicate that the same conditions are responsible for the majority of morbidity, disability, and health care costs in this country.[66–69]

The predominant causes of morbidity, mortality, and disability are for the most part preventable, but they are only partially responsive to medical care. Available morbidity and mortality data suggest that focusing on about 10 risk factors could potentially prevent between 40 and 70 percent of all deaths, one third of acute disability, and two thirds of chronic disability.[70] It is important to note there is no risk factor that raises the risk of one disease while simultaneously lowering the risk of another.

Smoking, obviously one of these 10 important causes of disability, has been designated as the single most important preventable cause of death.[1] It is prevalent throughout society, and there is no reason to believe that any population can smoke cigarettes or use tobacco in other forms without increasing the risk of death from several diseases, particularly cardiovascular disease. Of particular importance to the physician are the following observations: Tobacco has been determined to be addicting, and nicotine is the addicting substance in tobacco;[71] data from intervention studies show that people at high risk seem no more motivated to change their behavior than people at lower risk;[72-75] and populations seem to respond as well to multiple risk factor intervention as to single risk factor intervention.[70]

Physicians should encourage their patients, young or old, with cardiovascular disease or without, to quit smoking if this "most important of known modifiable risk factors" is to be conquered in the near future (see Chapter 15). Furthermore, in any risk factor intervention effort (for example, lowering serum lipid levels, controlling blood pressure, or controlling diabetes), adding emphasis on cessation of smoking seems not only feasible but effective.

REFERENCES

1. U.S. Department of Health and Human Services: The Health Consequences of Smoking: Cardiovascular Disease, A Report of the Surgeon General. Office on Smoking and Health. Rockville, MD: DHHS (PHS) 84-50204, 1983.
2. U.S. Public Health Service: Smoking and Health: Report of the Advisory Committee to the Surgeon General of the Public Health Service. Centers for Disease Control, PHS No. 1103, 1964.
3. U.S. Department of Health, Education, and Welfare: Smoking and Health: A Report of the Surgeon General. Office on Smoking and Health, DHEW (PHS) 79-50066, 1979.
4. National Center for Health Statistics: Health Promotion and Disease Prevention, United States, 1985. Data from the National Health Survey. DHHS Publication No. (PHS) 88-1591, Series 10, No. 163, 1988.
5. National Center for Health Statistics: Advance report of final mortality statistics, 1986. DHHS Publication No. (PHS) 88-1120, (Suppl) 37(6):16, 1988.
6. National Center for Health Statistics: Annual Summary of Births, Marriages, Divorces, and Deaths: United States, 1987. DHHS Publication No. (PHS) 88-1120, 36(13):18, 1988.
7. U.S. Department of Health and Human Services: Disease Prevention/Health Promotion: The Facts. Office of Disease Prevention and Health Promotion. Rockville, MD. DHHS (PHS), Bull Publishing Co., Palo Alto, CA, 1988.
8. American Heart Association: 1986 Heart Facts. American Heart Association, Dallas, TX, 1985.
9. National Center for Health Statistics: Health, United States, 1985. Public Health Service, Washington, D.C. DHHS Publication No. (PHS) 86-1232, 1985.
10. American Heart Assocation: Why Risk Heart Attack: Seven Ways to Guard Your Heart. Dallas, TX: American Heart Association, 1981.
11. National Heart Lung and Blood Institute: Fact Book, Fiscal Year 1985. National Institutes of Health, Bethesda, MD, 1985.
12. Graves, EJ: Utilization of short-stay hospitals: United States 1983 annual summary. Vital and Health Statistics. Series 13 (83). DHHS (PHS) 85-1744, 1985.
13. Dennison, CF: 1984 Summary: National Hospital Discharge Survey: Advance data from vital and health statistics. (112). DHHS (PHS) 85-1250, 1985.

14. Kannel, WB, Thom, TJ, and Hurst, FW: Incidence, prevalence, and mortality of cardiovascular diseases. The Heart, 6th ed., Mc-Graw-Hill, New York, 1986, p 560.

15. Positioning for Prevention: An Analytical Framework and Background Document for Chronic Disease Activities. Report of the Chronic Disease Planning Groups. Centers for Disease Control. U.S. Department of Health and Human Services, 1986.

16. Hammond, EC and Horn, D: Smoking and death rates—Report on forty-four months of follow-up of 187,783 men. I. Total mortality. JAMA 166:1159, 1958.

17. Hammond, EC and Horn, D: Smoking and death rates—Report on forty-four months of follow-up of 187,783 men. II. Death rates by cause. JAMA 116:1294, 1958.

18. Doll, R and Hill, AB: Mortality in relation to smoking: Ten years' observations of British doctors. Br Med J 1(5395):1399, 1964.

19. Doll, R and Hill, AB: Mortality in relation to smoking: Ten years' observations of British doctors. Br Med J 1(5396):1460, 1964.

20. Doll, R and Peto, R: Mortality in relation to smoking: 20 years' observations on male British doctors. Br Med J 2(6051):1525, 1976.

21. Dawber, TR: The Framingham Study. The Epidemiology of Atherosclerotic Disease. Harvard University Press, Cambridge, 1980.

22. Kannel, WB and McGee, DL: Epidemiology of sudden death: Insights from the Framingham Study. In Josephson, ME (ed): Sudden Cardiac Death. Cardiovascular Clinics, Volume 15. FA Davis, Philadelphia, 1985, p 93.

23. Daly, LE, Mulcahy, R, Graham, IM, et al: Long-term effect on mortality of stopping smoking after unstable angina and myocardial infarction. Br Med J 287(6388):324, 1983.

24. Yano, K, Reed, DM, and McGee, DL: Ten-year incidence of coronary heart disease in the Honolulu Heart Program. Relationship to biologic and lifestyle characteristics. Am J Epidemiol 119:653, 1984.

25. Lynch, P: Coronary risk profile of young soldiers with coronary heart disease. J Royal Army Medical Corps 131:38, 1985.

26. Abbott, RD, Yin, Y, Reed, DM, et al: Risk of stroke in male cigarette smokers. N Engl J Med 315:717, 1986.

27. Abbott, RD, Donahue, RP, MacMahon, SW, et al: Diabetes and the risk of stroke: The Honolulu Heart Program. JAMA 257:949, 1987.

28. Stemmerman, GN, Hayashi, T, Resch, JA, et al: Risk factors related to ischemic and hemorrhagic cerebrovascular disease at autopsy: The Honolulu Heart Study. Stroke 15:23, 1984.

29. Bonita, R: Cigarette smoking, hypertension and the risk of subarachnoid hemorrhage: A population-based case-control study. Stroke 17:831, 1986.

30. Bonita, R, Scragg, R, Stewart, A, et al: Cigarette smoking and risk of premature stroke in men and women. Br J Surg 293:6, 1986.

31. Sacco, RL, Wolf, PA, Bharucha, NE, et al: Subarachnoid and intracerebral hemorrhage: Natural history, prognosis, and precursive factors in the Framingham Study. Neurology 34:847, 1984.

32. Wolf, PA, D'Agostino, RB, Kannel, WB, et al: Cigarette smoking as a risk factor for stroke: The Framingham Study. JAMA 259:1025, 1988.

33. Haynes, SG, et al: Closing the Gap for Cardiovascular Disease: The Carter Center Health Policy Project Interim Summary. The Carter Center of Emory University, Atlanta, GA, 1984.

34. Kannel, WB: Epidemiology studies of smoking in cerebral and peripheral vascular disease, In Wynder, EL, Hoffman, D, and Gori, GB (eds): Modifying the Risk for the Smoker. Volume 1. Proceedings of the Third World Conference on Smoking and Health, New York, June 1975. DHEW (NIH) 76-1221:257, 1976.

35. Kannel, WB and Shurtleff, D: The Framingham study: Cigarettes and the development of intermittent claudication. Geriatrics 28:61, 1973.

36. Pomrehn, P, Duncan, B, Weissfeld, L, et al: The association of dyslipoproteinemia with symptoms and signs of peripheral arterial disease: The Lipid Research Clinics program prevalence study. Circulation (Suppl I) 73:I-100, 1986.

37. Allardice, JT, Allwright, GJ, Wafula, JMC, et al: High prevalence of abdominal aortic aneurysm in men with peripheral vascular disease: Screening by ultrasonography. Br J Surg 75:240, 1988.

38. Solberg, LA, and Strong, JP: Risk factors and atherosclerotic lesions. A review of autopsy studies. Arteriosclerosis 3:187, 1983.

39. Strong, JP, Richards, ML, McGill, HC, Jr, et al: On the association of cigarette smoking with coronary and aortic atherosclerosis. J Atheroscler Res 10:303, 1969.

40. Strong, JP, and Richards, ML: Cigarette smoking and atherosclerosis in autopsied men. Atherosclerosis 23:451, 1976.

41. Patel, YC, Eggen, DA, and Strong, JP: Obesity, smoking and atherosclerosis: A study of interassociations. Atherosclerosis 36:481, 1980.

42. Patel, YC, Kodlin, D, and Strong, JP: On the interpretation of smoking risks in atherosclerosis. J Chron Dis 33:147, 1980.

43. Tracy, RE, Toca, VT, Strong, JP, et al: Relationship of raised atherosclerotic lesions to fatty streaks in cigarette smokers. Atherosclerosis 38:347, 1981.

44. Auerback, O and Garfinkel, L: Atherosclerosis and aneurysm of the aorta in relation to smoking habits and age. Chest 78:805, 1980.

45. Auerbach, O and Garfinkel, L: Myocardial mural arterial fibrosis and cigarette smoking: A comparative study 1955–1960 versus 1970–1977. Bull NY Acad Med 57:759, 1981.

46. Sorlie, PD, Garcia-Palmiere, MR, Castillo-Stado, MI, et al: The relation of antemortem factors to atherosclerosis at autopsy. Am J Pathol 103:345, 1981.

47. Rhoads, GG, Blackwelder, WC, Stemmerman, GN, et al: Coronary risk factors and autopsy findings in Japanese-American men. Lab Invest 38:304, 1978.

48. Sternby, NH: Atherosclerosis, smoking and other risk factors. In Gotto, AM Jr, Smith, LC, and Allen, B (eds): Atherosclerosis V. Proceedings of the Fifth International Symposium on Atherosclerosis, 1969, Houston, TX. Springer-Verlag, New York, 1980.

49. Auerbach, O, Hammond, EC, and Garfinkel, L: Smoking in relation to atherosclerosis of the coronary arteries. N Engl J Med 273:775, 1965.

50. Holme, I, Solberg, LA, Weissfeld, L, et al: Coronary risk factors and their pathway of action through coronary raised lesions, coronary stenoses and coronary death: Multivariate statistical analysis of an autopsy series: The Oslo Study. Am J Cardiol 55:40, 1985.

51. Reed, DW, Strong, JP, Hayashi, T, et al: Comparison of two measures of atherosclerosis in a prospective epidemiology study. Arteriosclerosis 8(6):782, 1988.

52. Holme, I, Enger, SC, Helgeland, A, et al: Risk factors and raised atherosclerotic lesions in coronary and cerebral arteries: Statistical analysis from The Oslo Study. Arteriosclerosis 1:250, 1981.

53. U.S. Public Health Service: The Health Consequences of Smoking. A Report of the Surgeon General: 1971. U.S. Department of Health, Education, and Welfare, Public Health Service, Health Services and Mental Health Administration, DHEW Publication No. (HSM) 71-71-7513:3, 1971.

54. McMillan, GC: Evidence for components other than carbon monoxide and nicotine as etiological factors in cardiovascular disease. In Wynder, EL, Hoffmann, D, and Gori, GB (ed): Modifying the Risk for the Smoker. Vol. 1. Proceedings of the Third World Conference on Smoking and Health, New York, June 2–5, 1975. U.S. Department of Health, Education, and Welfare, Public Health Service, National Institutes of Health, National Cancer Institute, DHEW Publication No. (NIH)76-1221, pp 363–367, 1976.

55. McGill, HC Jr: Potential mechanisms for the augmentation of atherosclerosis and atherosclerotic disease by cigarette smoking. Preventive Medicine 8:390, 1979.

56. Rosenberg, L, Kaufmann, DW, Helmrich, SB, et al: The risk of myocardial infarction after quitting smoking in men under 55 years of age. N Engl J Med 313:1511, 1985.

57. Kuller, L: Risk factor reduction in coronary heart disease. Mod Concepts Cardiovasc Dis 53:7, 1984.

58. Kannel, WB, Neaton, JD, Wentworth, D, et al: Overall and coronary heart disease mortality rates in relation to major risk factors in 325,348 men screened for the MRFIT. Am Heart J 112:825, 1986.

59. Prevention of Coronary Heart Disease, Report of a WHO Expert Committee. WHO Tech. Rep. Ser. 678, Geneva 1982.

60. Hermanson, B, Omenn, GS, Kronmal, RA, et al: Beneficial six-year outcome of smoking cessation in older men and women with coronary artery disease. Results from the CASS registry. N Engl J Med 319:1365, 1988.

61. Feinleib, M: Changes in cardiovascular epidemiology since 1950. Bull NY Acad Med 60:449, 1984.

62. Department of Health and Human Services. Promoting health/preventing disease—Objectives for nation. DHEW (PHS) 80-55071. U.S. Government Printing Office, Washington, D.C., 1980.

63. Health promotion data for the 1990 objectives. Estimates from the National Health Interview Survey of Health Promotion and Disease Prevention: United States, 1985. National Center for Health Statistics, Hyattsville, MD. DHHS (PHS) 86-1250 (VHS no. 126), 1986.

64. Office of the Assistant Secretary for Health and the Surgeon General: Healthy People: The Surgeon General's Report on Health Promotion and Disease Prevention. DHEW (PHS) 79-55071, 1979.

65. White, CC, Tolsma, PD, Haynes, SG, et al: Cardiovascular disease. In Amler, RW and Dull, HB (eds): Closing the Gap—The Burden of Unnecessary Illness. Oxford University Press, NY, 1987.

66. Colvez, A and Blanchet, M: Disability trends in the United States population 1966–76: Analysis of reported cases. Am J Public Health 71:464, 1981.

67. Dean, AG, West, DJ, and Weir, WM: Measuring loss of life, health, and income due to disease and injury. Public Health Rep 97:38, 1982.

68. National Center for Health Statistics: Prevalence of Selected Chronic Conditions, United States, 1983–85. DHHS Publication No. (PHS) 88-1250, No. 155, 1988.

69. National Center for Health Statistics: 1987 Summary: National Hospital Discharge Survey. DHHS Publication No. (PHS) 88-1250, 1988.

70. Kottke, TE: Disease and risk factor clustering in the United States: The complications for Public Health Policy. In Integration of Risk Factor Interventions. U.S. Department of Health and Human Services, 1986.

71. U.S. Department of Health and Human Services: The Health Consequences of Smoking: Nicotine Addiction. DHHS Pub No (PHS) 88-8406. U.S. Department of Health and Human Services, Public Health Service, Office of Smoking and Health, 1988.

72. Maccoby, N, Farquhar, JW, Wood, PD, et al: Reducing the risk of cardiovascular disease: Effects of a community-based campaign on knowledge and behavior. J Commun Health 3:100, 1977.

73. Salonen, J, Heinonen, O, Kottke, T, et al: Change in health behavior in relation to estimated coronary heart disease risk during a community-based CVD prevention program. Int J Epidemiol 10:343, 1981.

74. Salonen, JT, Puska, P, Kottke, T, et al: Coronary risk factor clustering patterns in eastern Finland. Int J Epidemiol 10:203, 1981.

75. Multiple Risk Factor Intervention Trial Research Group: Multiple risk factor intervention trial: Risk factor changes and mortality results. JAMA 248:1465, 1982.

CHAPTER 15

Modification of the Smoking Habit

Leonard G. Hudzinski, Ph.D.

Who among you believes the now-echoed emphasis of Surgeon General C. Everett Koop, who repeats with every opportunity, "The public cannot be told too often that smoking is the major preventable cause of death and disease in our nation."? From the pioneering work of Alton Ochsner in the 1930s[1] to the present, evidence continues to mount supporting the accuracy of this position.

Numerous studies show that: (1) 85 percent of smokers want to quit, (2) physicians hold the most influence in helping patients quit, and (3) 38 million of 54 million smokers see a physician at least once a year.[2] However, most smokers who are interested in stopping do not want to attend a formal treatment program.[3] Despite the fact that most physicians believe it is their responsibility to encourage their patients to stop smoking, many fail to advise smokers to abstain from tobacco use.[4] *Surveys indicate that most adult smokers have never been told by their physician to stop smoking.*[5,6]

The good news, the important news of this chapter, is that although many treatment methods have been tried over the past 20 years to help patients stop smoking, several studies emphasize the power of brief intervention in the physician's office. Russell reports that nothing has yielded better results than some degree of "simple attention and support, which produces abstinence rates of 10 to 25 percent at the end of one year."[7] Russell has shown that 1 to 2 minutes of physician advice and provision of an educational leaflet can result in a one-year "cure rate of 5.1 percent." This rate was 17 times greater than the 0.3 percent cure rate for individuals in a control group who did not receive physician advice to quit smoking.

In 1983, Russell's studies went one step further.[11] With a sample of 1354 people, he replicated his earlier study using different physicians, different patients, and another comparison group; he also added to the physician's advice to patients the option of treatment with nicotine gum. At the level of significance of 0.001, the one-year "cure-rate" doubled. In summary, *the 1- to 2- minute physician message has been shown to substantially influence the number of patients who quit smoking.*

The less dependent and the more motivated persons are to stop smoking, and the better their family supports cessation of smoking, the more likely they are to benefit from brief intervention.

Mortality among smokers with coronary heart disease (CHD) is 70 percent greater than among nonsmokers. In addition to being the single largest cure of cancer mortality, smoking is considered to be the major cause of chronic lung disease, causing approximately 80 percent of bronchitis and 90 percent of emphysema. It is little wonder that some employers, especially those in health-related activities, have concluded that smoking on their premises is inconsistent with their corporate goals and public image. Increasingly, businesses are banning smoking in the workplace. A recent report from the Public Health Service indicates that smoking costs United States employers $26 billion in lost productivity per year.[8] Not only do smokers retire or die earlier than nonsmokers, they are estimated to take a minimum of 33 percent more days off, representing 81 million working days lost each year. In addition, data reveal that employers have been paying extremely high health insurance costs because smokers use health care benefits up to 50 percent more than nonsmokers. Smokers tend to have approximately twice as many industrial accidents as nonsmokers, resulting in additional treatment and compensation costs to employers. Management is becoming increasingly aware of the financial advantage an organization realizes with a policy of smoking cessation. One analysis estimates that the cost per year to a corporation for each smoker on the payroll is approximately $5,600.[9] The study states that this amount was arrived at by including the costs of excess medical care; premature mortality and disability; increased absenteeism; excess fire and industrial accident risks; lost time due to smoking breaks; costs resulting from property damage; physical depreciation on equipment, furniture, and fixtures; excess maintenance requirements; and involuntary smoking by workers who must breathe the smoke of their co-workers. A much more conservative estimate is that company savings approach $624 per year for each smoker who quits.

Researchers have found that nonsmokers who breathe cigarette smoke may inhale the equivalent of one to two cigarettes per day. Evidence suggests that there is no safe level of exposure to some of the harmful contents of tobacco. Research indicates that tobacco smoke may expose nonsmokers to more toxic and active concentrations of harmful substances than smokers inhale directly. Worksite contaminants from tobacco often reach levels exceeded by environmental and occupational regulations. Tobacco smoke is irritating to many and can exacerbate symptoms of asthma, bronchitis, and allergy.[10] There is increasing evidence that exposure to tobacco smoke may cause disease, including lung cancer, in otherwise healthy adults. One estimate indicates that as many as 5000 lung cancer deaths in the United States may result from passive smoking.

Smoking is so pervasive in our society that many physicians fail to consider the important effect of tobacco on medications they prescribe for their patients. If your patient smokes, it is essential that you weigh this information carefully. There are more than 3000 components in cigarette smoke, of which only a small number have been investigated regarding their pharmacologic effects on the body. Dawson and associates note that "with about one-third of the population smoking tobacco, there is a potential for a high incidence of altered drug disposition and drug response."[12] They indicate that smoking increases, decreases, accelerates, and decelerates the metabolism of various drugs. The authors conclude that "the knowledge that is presently available regarding the effect of smoking on the disposition of selected drugs requires that smoking and its effects be considered as a covariant in drug actions and interactions."

The difference we find in patients' reactions to drugs may be due in part to smoking. Clearly, smoking influences metabolism, the kinetics of drugs, and their resulting pharmacologic activity. The physician should address the patient's present level of smoking and may have to modify drug dosage accordingly. Interactions of tobacco with medications are numerous and may be significant; medical therapy can be seriously undermined by smoking. For example, cigarette smoking tends to accelerate the metabolism of many drugs. Propranolol, commonly used to treat selected heart problems, high blood pressure, and migraine, is now considered less effective when used in the "average" dose by a smoker. The high degree of first-pass metabolism of propranolol keeps its bioavailability low, and cigarette smoking can reduce its bioavailability even further. In a recent trial examining the effects of beta-blockers on heart attacks, levels of propranolol were significantly lower in cigarette smokers than in nonsmokers. For this reason, the response to propranolol and its resulting therapeutic benefits may be lessened in cigarette smokers.

The chemical properties in tobacco activate the sympathetic nervous system, provoking the release of catecholamines. This activation is an important mechanism that affects the way in which the body uses drugs. Cigarette smoking can decrease blood flow to the skin and fat tissue, which can impede the absorption of insulin. The disappearance rate of insulin from subcutaneous tissue in smokers is only one half that in nonsmokers, presumably because of constriction of blood vessels.[13]

Beta-blockers are less effective than normal in relieving angina in cigarette smokers. Not only may smoking induce coronary spasm, but calcium-channel blockers may be less effective in smokers; in fact, cigarette smoking may antagonize the effect of calcium-channel blockers on coronary spasm.

Pain killers, such as propoxyphene, are also less effective in cigarette smokers than in nonsmokers. These drugs have excessive first-pass metabolism that is probably increased by smoking. Reduced therapeutic efficacy may be due at least partially to reduced bioavailability.

Smoking also affects the actions of psychotropic drugs. Sedation from benzodiazepines and the neuroleptic effect of chlorpromazine seem to be lessened in cigarette smokers, apparently as the result of a stimulant effect of nicotine on the brain. Nicotine is a complex drug that can provide an individual with powerful, immediate satisfaction, including alleviation of fatigue and stress. This drug can stimulate beta endorphins and vasopressin, which can increase stress tolerance, reduce pain, and at times improve concentration.

What benefits could outweigh the undoubtedly serious risks of smoking? It goes without saying that it is difficult to understand why a physician would justify a patient's smoking. In summary, the physician needs to know the patient's current smoking level and, in some cases, may have to adjust doses of medication accordingly, if prescribing medications. In some instances, patients may benefit by taking medication at bedtime and refraining from smoking thereafter.

Emphasize smoking cessation to your patients who smoke. Ask all patients who smoke if they have thought about quitting. If they indicate an interest in cessation, you can play one of three roles in helping the patient quit: (1) You can work with the patient in a 1- to 2-minute session, supplemented by low-cost, self-help materials and possibly a prescription for nicotine gum, (2) You can initiate brief interventions in your office, using a nurse or psychology/social work counselor to consult with patients, (3) The patient can be referred to a commercial or comprehensive smoking cessation program that may be associated with a hospital, psychology department, or medical school. Remember, most smokers who are interested in cessation of smoking do not want to attend a formal treatment program. Unlike smoking clinics, which solicit interested people, many smokers seen in a physician's office have mixed feelings about the prospect of stopping use of tobacco. At minimum, your goal should be to plant the seed that encourages patients to consider changing their smoking behavior. Smoking cessation is a process that evolves over time rather than a single event. The smoker moves through stages from a lack of interest in stopping smoking to contemplating the idea, to a concerted effort to stop, and finally to maintaining abstinence. On a cost/benefit scale, whether you intervene at one of these points and work with the patient, refer the patient to your nurse or associate for more intensive work, or suggest enrollment in a comprehensive smoking cessation program may depend on the patient's expressed motivation to change.

By understanding the patient's reasons for smoking, you can help establish the level of your intervention. It is advisable to use the least intrusive, least expensive intervention methods first. If they fail, then use progressively more intensive treatment methods. It is important to assess the patient's commitment and readiness to stop smoking. Toward this end, you may find that information from patients concerning their prior attempts to quit smoking, brands of cigarettes they have smoked, their awareness of the risks of smoking, and the reasons why they smoke are useful in planning a treatment strategy. Empirical evidence suggests that the stronger the brand of cigarette smoked and the longer the patient has been smoking that brand, the more difficulty the patient will experience in attempting to stop smoking. On the other hand, the more frequently the patient has attempted to quit smoking in the past, the greater the likelihood that he or she will eventually abstain from cigarette use. Each smoker can be identified by one of approximately six reasons for use of tobacco, documented in the Horns test,[14] which shows how smokers use cigarettes. Keep in mind that smoking may be characterized by one or a combination of the following factors. Knowing these factors may help you decide the level of your involvement with a particular patient. National trends suggest that the following percentages constitute the prime motives for smoking:

STIMULATION—10 PERCENT. This type of smoker is stimulated by cigarettes. They help him to wake up in the morning, to organize his energies, and to keep him going. Many smokers report that while smoking they experience a sharpening of intellectual capacity and increased impulse control.

HANDLING: SENSORY MOTOR MANIPULATION—10 PERCENT. This type of smoker enjoys manipulating a cigarette with his hands and watching the smoke while exhaling, and he generally makes a production of lighting the cigarette, holding it, and flicking its ashes.

PLEASURABLE RELAXATION—15 PERCENT. This smoker gets real, honest pleasure from smoking, especially after dinner or a cocktail. He or she tends to smoke to accentuate or enhance pleasurable feelings accompanying a state of well-being.

CRUTCH: TENSION REDUCTION—30 PERCENT. This negative-affect type of smoker uses cigarettes for their sedative effect in moments of stress, tension, or discomfort. He uses cigarettes to help cope with problems. Substitutions generally do not help this type of smoker.

CRAVING: PSYCHOLOGIC ADDICTION—25 PERCENT. This type of smoker feels dependent on tobacco use and alternates between positive and negative feelings regarding smoking. The person is constantly aware when he or she is not smoking and begins craving the next cigarette when he or she puts out the present one.

HABIT—10 PERCENT. The habitual smoker gets little satisfaction from the habit and performs it automatically. This type of smoker may not even be aware he or she has a lighted cigarette. When smoking, there is little awareness of the act of smoking. It is important for this type of person to develop awareness and to understand the pattern of his or her smoking.

For patients who are ready to stop, as well as for those who are not, it is important to provide a firm, clear message about the risks of smoking and the benefits of stopping. Smokers are generally aware of the risks of smoking; however, they are more likely to respond to information that applies directly to them. If a patient has not thought about stopping before, he or she may not be influenced by a single message. A clear, brief suggestion to stop smoking can play a critical role in the patient's attitude toward smoking cessation in the future. On subsequent patient visits, the physician should continue to provide a 1- to 2-minute concise message about smoking and offer assistance in quitting.

A short, specific, firm message can be highly effective. Make your message clear-cut on the benefit of cessation. You might target a patient's specific symptoms, for example, shortness of breath. You can tell patients that this symptom almost always improves within a few weeks after they stop smoking. Point out life expectancy gains resulting from cessation; estimates suggest that smokers in their 30s who stop smoking increase life expectancy by 8 to 9 years. Persons 65 years of age who stop smoking increase their longevity by 3 to 4 years.

When patients you are counseling experience symptoms caused by smoking, such as pronounced cough or shortness of breath, expect the effectiveness of your advice to be multiplied. Your message should not be ambiguous because smokers often try to rationalize that the advice they are hearing does not apply to them. Do not emphasize adverse health consequences of smoking; rather, accentuate the positive medical benefits patients will realize with cessation. Make the message simple and brief. Most smokers respect the authority and advice of their physicians.

Do not advise switching to low-tar/nicotine cigarettes or switching to a pipe or cigar. Do not advise a tapering method. The most effective method of stopping is to quit "cold turkey," by stopping abruptly.

Nicotine chewing gum, Nicorette, is a major breakthrough in the treatment of patients who want to stop smoking. The rationale for this form of nicotine substitute is that it helps to wean smokers from cigarettes by providing an alternative source of nicotine while at the same time avoiding the other damaging components in cigarette smoke, namely carbon monoxide and tar. By successively decreasing the amount of nicotine gum chewed, the patient becomes comfortably tolerant to lower blood levels of nicotine and is eventually able to discontinue use of nicotine altogether.

Nicotine resin chewing gum, Nicorette, is a sugar-free gum that contains nicotine, the addictive substance in tobacco. In the United States, nicotine gum is available by prescription in a 2-mg dose. A blood nicotine level comparable to one half of one cigarette is achieved by 2 mg of this prescription. The patient who will benefit most from this form of therapy is a heavy smoker (about 25 cigarettes per day) who is dependent on nicotine. The gum should not be used by pregnant or nursing women, patients who have had a recent myocardial infarction, or those with life-threatening arrhythmias. In summary, the gum is safer than smoking because it does not contain the tars, irritants, and carbon monoxide found in cigarette smoke. The highly dependent smoker who begins using nicotine gum should be counseled on its correct use and contraindications. Nicotine gum, however, should not be used without counseling by a physician.

One study examined the cost effectiveness of using nicotine gum as an adjunct to physician counseling against smoking during routine office visits. The findings of the study indicate that the cost per year in lives saved with this intervention ranged from $4113 to $9473 for both men and women, depending on their age. The study concluded that nicotine gum was a cost-effective adjunct to physician advice.

Unfortunately, many abstaining smokers, free from tobacco for months or even years, resume its use, generally as a result of anxiety, stress, or depression, or if they are drinking alcohol. Evidence indicates that smokers are more likely to relapse under stress if they are ill-prepared with new coping skills to handle stress. Physicians should beware of becoming frustrated with patients' failures to quit smoking or their rationalizations for smoking. Keep in mind that any attempt to quit smoking should be considered a learning experience for the patient rather than a failure and should be encouraged. Most smokers report two to four unsuccessful attempts before they succeed at quitting.

A careful review of issues concerning smoking relapse can be found in the proceedings of the National Conference on Smoking Relapse.[15] Indeed, much of the recent work in this area originates with the 1974 observation of Hunt and associates[16] that smoking relapse rates are remarkably similar to those of other addictions involving alcohol and heroin. Because it is likely that a patient who quits smoking will relapse (60 percent of smokers relapse within the first 3 months of quitting), continue to encourage smoking cessation and guard against the abstinence violation effect. This effect is a common rationalization that some smokers use in order to give up abstinence or control over smoking. The effect is an immediate reaction to smoking one cigarette; the smoker rationalizes that as a result of one episode of smoking he or she is no longer able to abstain and therefore may as well continue to smoke. These patients may feel dejected and may express a sense of personal failure. Remember to encourage these patients and emphasize that the more often they seriously attempt to quit, the more likely it is that they will succeed in achieving abstinence.

Techniques involved in relapse prevention generally include analysis of the smoker's high-risk situations. The physician should review with the patient the emotional states he or she experiences and the situations in which the patient feels most likely to resume smoking. If a patient breaks abstinence, the physician should repeat the cycle of the 1- to 2-minute clear, cogent message on the benefits of stopping smoking. The messages given should be consistent. The likelihood of abstinence from smoking increases after the patient has experienced one or two failed attempts to quit.

A six-, nine-, or 12-month follow-up is crucial to evaluate the patient's progress, and is perhaps as important as initial counseling promoting cessation. Keep in mind that 85 percent of patients who want to stop smoking look to their physician for support and encouragement.

REFERENCES

1. Ochsner, AD and DeBakey, M: Primary pulmonary malignancy. Surg Gynecol Obstet 68:435, 1939.
2. American Society of Internal Medicine: Stop Smoking Campaign for Physicians, 1101 Vermont Avenue NW, Washington, DC 20005, 1987.

3. Schwartz, JL and Dubitzky, M: Expressed willingness of smokers to try ten smoking withdrawal methods. Pub Health Rep 82:855, 1967.

4. Rimer, EK, Strecher, VJ, Keintz, MK, et al: A survey of physicians' views and practices about patient education for smoking cessation. Prev Med 15:92, 1986.

5. Cummings, KM, Giovino, G, Sciandra, R, et al: Physician advice to quit smoking: Who gets it and who doesn't. Am J Prev Med 3:69, 1987.

6. Anda, RF, Remington, PL, Sienko, EG, et al: Are physicians advising smokers to quit? The patient's perspective. JAMA 257:1916, 1987.

7. Russell, MH, Wilson, C, and Taylor, C: Effect of general practitioners' advice against smoking. Behav Med J 2:231, 1979.

8. Dartnell Institute of Business Research: Smoking in the office—is it a problem? Targ Sur 9:1, 1977.

9. Kristein, M: The Economics of Health Promotion at the Work Site (pamphlet). American Health Foundation, New York, 1982.

10. US Department of Health and Human Services: The Health Consequences of Involuntary Smoking, a Report of the Surgeon General. Public Health Service, Office of Smoking and Health, Rockville, MD, 5, 1986.

11. Russell, MH, Merriman, R, Stapleton, JN, et al: Effect of nicotine chewing gum as an adjunct to general practitioner advice against smoking. Br Med J 287:1782, 1983.

12. Dawson, GW, Vestal, RE, and Jusko, WJ: Smoking and Drug Metabolism in Nicotine and the Tobacco Smoking Habit, Balfourd DJK Edition, Pergamon Press, New York, 1984.

13. Benowitz, NL: The role of the pharmacist in smoking cessation, a continuing education program. Journal of New Developments in Clinical Medicine, Communications Media for Education, Inc., Princeton Junction, NJ, 1988.

14. Horn, D: An approach to office management of the cigarette smoker. Dis Chest 54:203, 1968.

15. Shumaker, SA and Grunberg, NE: Smoking Relapse. In National Working Conference on Smoking Relapse, Lawrence Erlbaum Associates, London, 1985.

16. Hunt, WA, Barnett, LW, and Branch, LG: Relapse rates in addiction programs. J Clin Psychol, 27:455, 1971.

Index

A page number in *italics* indicates a figure. A "t" following a page number indicates a table.

231